Manual of Rheumatology and Outpatient Orthopedic Disorders

Manual of Rheumatology and Outpatient Orthopedic Disorders

Diagnosis and Therapy

Department of Orthopedic Surgery
Division of Rheumatic Diseases
Hospital for Special Surgery
Cornell University Medical College
New York City

Editors

John F. Beary III, M.D.
Assistant Professor of Medicine, Georgetown University School of Medicine; Attending Physician, Georgetown University Hospital, Washington, D.C.; Formerly Fellow, Division of Rheumatic Diseases, Cornell University Medical College, New York City

Charles L. Christian, M.D.
Professor of Medicine, Cornell University Medical College; Physician-in-Chief, Hospital for Special Surgery, New York City

Thomas P. Sculco, M.D.
Assistant Professor of Clinical Surgery (Orthopedic), Cornell University Medical College; Assistant Attending Orthopedic Surgeon, Hospital for Special Surgery, New York City

Associate Editor

Allan Gibofsky, M.D.
Assistant Professor of Medicine, Cornell University Medical College; Assistant Attending Physician, Hospital for Special Surgery, New York City

Foreword by

John L. Decker, M.D.
Chief, Arthritis and Rheumatism Branch, National Institute of Health, Bethesda, Maryland

Little, Brown and Company
Boston

To the memory of John L. Marshall, D.V.M., M.D., Associate Professor of Surgery (Orthopedic) and Director of the Sports Medicine Service at the Hospital for Special Surgery. His contributions to sports medicine have been many, and his loss is deeply felt by his family, colleagues, and the amateur and professional athletes he served.

Foreword

Making and acting upon a decision are the critical events in any patient-physician encounter, although it is uncommon for either the patient or the physician to recognize the significance of this sequence. As the physician's experience with the problem at hand increases, the decisions and consequent actions often become more and more instinctual. In the early days of aviation, pilots, distrusting their primitive and frequently failing instruments, were said to have flown "by the seat of the pants"; so, too, the physician may go with the "feel" of the situation. This handbook is built on facts. It describes the acquisition of needed facts from the physician-patient encounter in rheumatic disease, the integration of that data into a decision, and the actions that logically result from those decisions. It constitutes not only a reasonable substitute for experience for the younger physician but also an excellent yardstick against which the older can measure performance.

There was a time not long ago when the patient with rheumatoid arthritis was viewed as a collection of inflamed joints. The very concept of the disease as a systemic affliction, developed by clinicians of yesteryear such as Bauer, Ragan, Copeman, and Hench, was critical to the development of rheumatology as a discipline of internal medicine, while placing perhaps undue emphasis on systemic features. These pages help to restore the concepts that all that hurts is not systemic disease, that articular symptoms are the major feature of rheumatoid arthritis, and that those who would deal with diseases manifesting musculoskeletal pain must also be aware of local afflictions such as march fracture, tennis elbow, and slipped capital femoral epiphysis. They represent the happy juxtaposition of the medical and orthopedic surgical expertise of the Hospital for Special Surgery, a hospital with an enviable tradition of cooperation and of excellence in both disciplines.

The pearls are numerous and genuine, and yet no one will consider the manual all-encompassing. It would not be easy to compress a more practical and useful clinical introduction into fewer pages. The reader will use it as such: a personal introduction to the complex and fascinating pathophysiology of human locomotor disease.

John L. Decker

Preface

The busy practitioner often has a perception that medical information is unlimited while the time to absorb it is not. The success of the Little, Brown Manual Series is related to this medical "information explosion." The manuals present important diagnostic and therapeutic information in a succinct, easily retrievable, and clinically useful format.

Musculoskeletal and rheumatic complaints account for about 15% of the patients seen by primary care physicians. We hope this book will meet the need of internists, family physicians, rheumatology trainees, house officers, and students for current, useful information on rheumatologic disorders and office orthopedic problems.

All authors are present and past members of the Division of Rheumatic Diseases or the Department of Orthopedic Surgery at the Hospital for Special Surgery. Of course, some clinical problems have more than one potential solution; in such instances, for the sake of clarity and brevity, we detail the approach used at our hospital. Areas of controversy are identified, but again the authors state specifically the therapeutic regimen currently used at the Hospital for Special Surgery.

Features of the book include coverage of joint aspiration and injection techniques, differential diagnosis of common patient presentations, and treatment of office orthopedic disorders (fracture therapy is covered in the *Manual of Acute Orthopedic Therapeutics*). The rheumatic disease chapters are arranged alphabetically to assist reader access, and appendixes containing frequently needed, clinically important material that is difficult to commit to memory, such as neurologic dermatomes and optimal patient weights, are included.

We are grateful to senior faculty members who reviewed the manuscript. They include Drs. Philip D. Wilson, Jr., Chairman of the Department of Orthopedic Surgery, Carl Berntsen, Lawrence Kagen, William Kammerer, Michael Lockshin, and Paul Phillips.

Our artist Lynn Thompson ably illustrated the book. Susan Cunningham typed the final manuscript and performed numerous tasks to keep the book on schedule. Vivian Sanchez and Kathy Fallon also assisted with draft typing. Finally, we express special appreciation to Kathleen O'Brien, Medical Series Development Editor at Little, Brown, who skillfully assisted us to prepare a book which we hope you will agree is concise and practical.

J. F. B.
C. L. C.
T. P. S.
A. G.

Contents

III
Diagnosis and Therapy

IV
Appendixes

Manual of Rheumatology and Outpatient Orthopedic Disorders

I. Musculoskeletal Data Base

1. Musculoskeletal History and Physical Examination

Emmanuel Rudd

The musculoskeletal or locomotor system, like other body systems, can be defined anatomically and assessed functionally. Lower extremities support the weight of the body and allow ambulation. They require proper alignment and stability. Upper extremities reach, grasp, and hold, thus allowing self-care, feeding, and work. They require mobility and strength. Diseases and disorders of the musculoskeletal system disturb the anatomy and interfere with function.

Musculoskeletal History

The history of patients with rheumatic complaints should include: (1) reason for consultation and nature of complaints, (2) chronologic review of present illness with emphasis on the locomotor system, (3) consequences of time and disease and present functional assessment, (4) past medical, surgical, and trauma history, (5) review of systems, social history, and present medical care, and (6) family history.

These queries cover the spectrum of rheumatic complaints: pain, stiffness, joint swelling, lack of mobility, physical handicap, and fear of future disability and handicap.

The interviewer should be flexible and tactful. Interrupting the patient with too many questions should be avoided; the interviewer should merely guide the flow of information. The objective is to define the patient's complaints and goals and to identify areas of musculoskeletal involvement that can be scrutinized on physical examination.

I. History of rheumatic disease

A. Note why the patient came to the physician and what **symptoms** bother him most.

B. Determine duration, mode of onset, and pattern of progression of musculoskeletal complaints.

    1. Chronicity.

    2. Intermittency with remissions and exacerbations.

C. Record **severity of disease** as revealed by a chronologic review of:

    1. Ability to work through the months or years.

    2. Need for hospitalization or home confinement.

    3. When applicable, ability to do household chores.

    4. Activities of daily living and personal care.

    5. Landmarks of significant functional change, such as retirement from work; need for household help; assistance for personal care; and use of cane, crutches, or wheelchair.

D. Assessment of **current functional ability:**

    1. At home. Independence or reliance on help from family members and others.

    2. At work. Transportation and job requirements.

    3. At recreational and social activities.

    4. Review of typical 24-hour period, focusing on abilities to transfer, ambulate, and perform personal care.

E. Obtain an **overview of management** for rheumatic disease.

1. List the **medications** used in the past with emphasis on duration of treatments, favorable or unfavorable effects, and possible adverse reactions. Present drug regimen and patient's compliance.

2. Instruction in and compliance with a therapeutic exercise program.

3. Surgical procedures on joints, benefits and liabilities.

F. Determine **patient's understanding** of disease or disorder, goals, and expectations.

G. Record **psychosocial consequences** of disease:

1. Anxiety, depression, insomnia.

2. Economic impact of handicap and present means of support.

3. Family interrelationships.

4. Use of community resources.

II. **Past history and review of systems.** Follow traditional lines of questioning with special emphasis on diseases and system disorders related to rheumatic complaints and diseases of connective tissue. Especially inquire about iritis, sicca symptoms of mouth or eyes, Raynaud symptoms, diarrhea, urethral discharge, or skin rash.

III. **Family history.** Inquiry about arthritis and rheumatic disease in parents and siblings often elicits vague and unreliable statements about arthritis and rheumatism; rarely are such diagnoses reliable. The presence of severely handicapped relatives with rheumatoid arthritis or other severe rheumatic disease might cause significant psychologic impact on the patient and should be brought out in the interview.

Physical Examination with Emphasis on Rheumatic Disease

Five subjects of physical examination that should be recorded are (1) gait, (2) neck and back, (3) muscles, (4) upper extremities, and (5) lower extremities.

The patient should be properly attired in a short gown, open at the back to allow examination of the entire spine. Examination should be methodical and start with observation of patient's attitude, comfort, apparent state of nutrition, and method of rising from a chair and sitting down. The gait is described, and note is made of a limp or use of cane or crutches. The patient is examined while standing, sitting, and supine. The examiner should rely mainly on inspection. When using palpation and manipulation, the examiner should be gentle and forewarn the patient of potentially painful maneuvers.

I. **Standing position**

A. Examining front and back, **note posture** (cervical lordosis, scoliosis, dorsal kyphosis, lumbar lordosis). Check if pelvis is level by putting one finger on each iliac crest and noting asymmetry. Note also if a tilt of the trunk to one side exists.

B. **Examine alignment of lower extremities** for flexion deformity of knees, genu varum (bowlegs), or genu valgum (knock-knees).

C. **Observe position of ankles and feet** (varus or valgus heels, flat feet, inversion or eversion of the feet).

D. **Check for trunk motion** on forward bending (with rounding of the normal thoracolumbar spine), lateral flexion to each side with motion normally starting at the lumbosacral level, and hyperextension.
The extent of spinal flexion can be assessed with a metal tape measure. One end of the tape is placed at the C7 spinous process, and the other end is placed at S1 with the patient standing erect. The patient is then asked to bend forward, flexing the spine maximally. The measuring tape will reveal an increase of 4 in. with normal spine flexion; 3 in. of the total increase result from lumbar spine (mea-

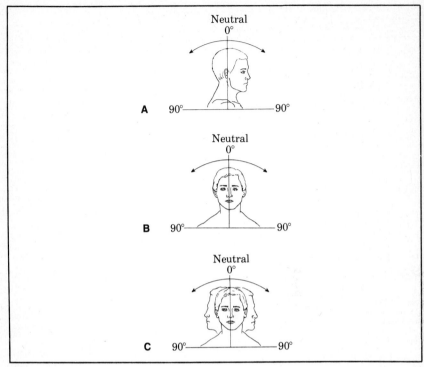

Figure 1-1. Neck motion. A. Flexion and extension. B. Lateral bending. C. Rotation.

sured from spinous processes T12 to S1) mobility in normal adults. These measurements are useful for serial evaluation of patients with spondyloarthropathy.

II. Seated position

A. Observe head and neck motion in all planes (Fig. 1-1).

B. Examine thoracolumbar spine motion with pelvis fixed: observe rounding and straightening of back, lateral flexion to each side, and rotation to right and left.

C. Check temporomandibular joints: palpate, examine lower jaw motion, and measure aperture between upper and lower teeth with mouth fully open.

D. Proceed with the rest of the routine examination of the head and neck; describe eye, ear, nose, and throat findings.

E. Upper extremities

1. Shoulders

a. Note normal **contour** or "squaring" caused by deltoid atrophy. Palpate anteriorly for soft tissue swelling and laterally under the acromion for tendon insertion tenderness.

b. Functional evaluation of the entire shoulder complex is assessed by elevating both arms from 0 degrees along sides of body to 180 degrees straight above the head. Quantitate internal rotation by having patient reach with dorsum of hands the highest possible level of the back (Fig. 1-2); quantitate external rotation by noting the position behind neck or head that hands can reach.

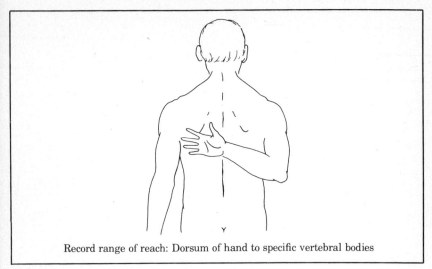

Record range of reach: Dorsum of hand to specific vertebral bodies

Figure 1-2. Internal rotation of shoulder, posterior view.

    c. Isolate **glenohumeral joint motion** from the scapulothoracic motion by fixing the scapula. Holding both hands, assist the patient in abducting arms to the normal maximum of 90 degrees and note restriction of motion on either side. To determine internal and external rotation of glenohumeral joint on each side, the examiner places one hand on the shoulder *to prevent scapular motion* and, with the other hand, assists each arm to full external rotation of 90 degrees and full internal rotation of 70 degrees (Fig. 1-3).

2. Elbows

    a. Inspect each elbow for **maximum extension** to 0 degrees and full flexion to 140 degrees. Less than full extension is reported in degrees as flexion deformity or lack of extension.

    b. Inspection and palpation may reveal presence of **olecranon bursitis** or soft tissue swelling of **synovitis,** which is felt in the fossae between the olecranon and lateral epicondyle or between the olecranon and medial epicondyle.

    c. **Subcutaneous nodules and tophi** should be sought in the olecranon bursa and over the extensor surface of the elbow and forearm.

3. Wrist and hands

    a. Inspect and palpate wrists; metacarpophalangeal (MP), proximal interphalangeal (PIP), and distal interphalangeal (DIP) joints of fingers; and carpometacarpal (CM), MP, and interphalangeal (IP) joints of thumbs (Fig. 1-4). Note shape and deformity.

    b. **Soft tissue swelling** has a spongy consistency and should be sought on the dorsum of the wrist distal to the ulna and over the radiocarpal joint. On the volar surface, the normal step-down from hand to forearm may be obliterated by soft tissue swelling. Volar synovitis may be associated with carpal tunnel syndrome.

    c. All **finger joints** should be examined by inspection and palpation for soft tissue swelling, capsular thickening, and bony enlargement.

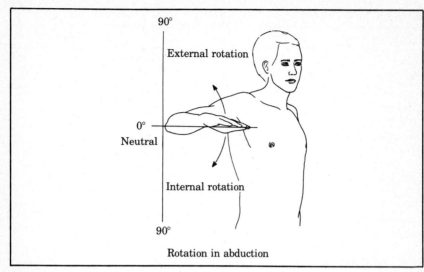

Figure 1-3. Shoulder rotation (with arm in abduction).

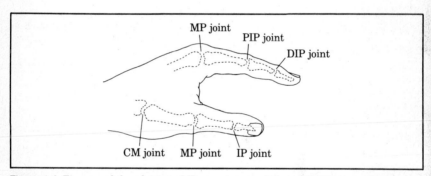

Figure 1-4. Finger and thumb joints. MP = metacarpophalangeal; PIP = proximal interphalangeal; DIP = distal interphalangeal; CM = carpometacarpal; and IP = interphalangeal.

d. **Average wrist motion** is dorsiflexion to 75 degrees, palmar flexion to 70 degrees, ulnar deviation of 30 degrees, and radial deviation of 20 degrees (Table 1-1).

e. **Fist** is described as 100% when all fingers reach palm of the hand and the thumb closes over fingers. Halfway fist closing is recorded as 50%; less than 50% and 75% are other possible intermediate measurements. The distance from fingertips to palm can also be recorded.

f. **Grip** is quantitated by noting patient's maximum strength in grasping two fingers of the examiner. Pinch is assessed by the force necessary to break patient's pinch between index finger and thumb.

g. **Pronation and supination** are combined functions of elbow and wrist and are determined by having patient hold forearm horizontal and thumb up.

Table 1-1. Average Joint Motion

Joint Motion	Normal Value
Spine	
Cervical	
Forward flexion	40°
Lateral bending	30°
Extension	30°
Rotation	60°
Thoracic	
Rotation with pelvis fixed	45°
Chest expansion	>6 cm
Lumbar	
Forward flexion	90°
Lateral bending	30°
Extension	30°
Upper Extremities	
Shoulder	
Abduction (arm at side and elevation above head)	180°
Rotation (arm in abduction to 90°)	
Internal	70°
External	90°
Elbow	
Flexion	140°
Extension	0°
Forearm	
Pronation	75°
Supination	85°
Wrist	
Extension	75°
Flexion	70°
Unlar deviation	30°
Radial deviation	20°
Fist (in percentage)	
Full fist	100%
Lower Extremities	
Hip	
Flexion	120°
Extension	0°
In flexion	
Internal rotation	25°
External rotation	35°
Abduction	45°
Adduction	25°
In extension	
Abduction	60°
Adduction	30°

Table 1-1 (Continued)

Joint Motion	Normal Value
Knee	
Flexion	130°
Extension	0°
Ankle	
Flexion	15°
Extension	35°
Hindfoot	
Inversion-eversion (subtalar); in percentage	
Full motion	100%

Pronation and supination are measured in degrees from the neutral position with the hand turning palm up and palm down (Fig. 1-5).

F. While the patient is sitting, customary physical examination of the **neck and chest** should be performed; it should include examination of sternoclavicular joints and measurement of chest expansion.

III. Supine patient

A. Start with the standard physical examination of **abdomen** and then proceed to the examination of **lower extremities.**

B. Alignment of the **knees** is compared to alignment noted on weight bearing (sec. **I.B.**). Palpate pedal pulses. Record degrees of active straight leg-raising on each side.

C. Hips

1. Hip function is screened by gently rolling each lower extremity and noting the freedom of motion of the **"ball and socket" joint.** Rolling also allows the measurement of **internal and external rotation** of the hip joint in extension.

2. With one hand fixing the pelvis, the other hand is used to move each hip to the normal 60 degrees of full **abduction** and to the normal 25 degrees of **adduction** while the hip is held in extension.

3. Each hip joint is then examined in **flexion.** Both lower extremities are flexed at knees and hips and carried toward the chest, thus giving the maximum angle (120 degrees) of flexion of each hip.

4. **Normal hip extension** is to 0 degrees. In order to avoid overlooking a hip flexion deformity for which accentuation of lumbar lordosis may compensate, the examiner keeps one lower extremity flexed over the chest, thus flattening the lumbar spine, while instructing the patient to extend fully the opposite leg (Fig. 1-6).

5. With the hip in 90 degrees of flexion, the joint is evaluated for internal rotation (25 degrees), external rotation (35 degrees), abduction (45 degrees), and adduction (25 degrees) (Fig. 1-6).

D. Knees

1. By inspection and palpation, note position and mobility of **patellae.** Knee extension-flexion range is 0 to 130 degrees.

2. **Soft tissue swelling** is elicited by bimanual examination. Demonstrate intraarticular fluid by the **patellar click sign:** while compressing the suprapatel-

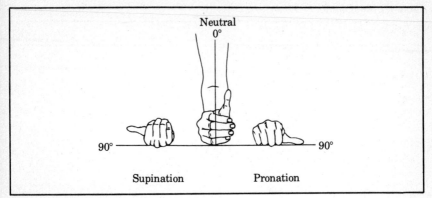

Figure 1-5. Forearm pronation and supination.

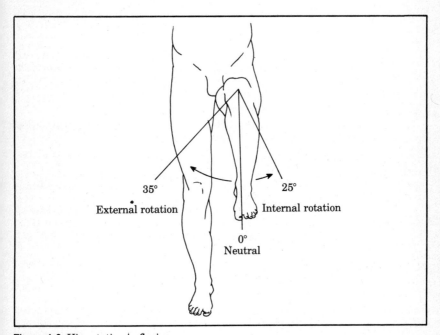

Figure 1-6. Hip rotation in flexion.

lar pouch with one hand, push the patella against underlying fluid and femoral condyle with the index finger of the other hand to elicit a click.

For the detection of a small amount of effusion, use the **bulge sign.** This maneuver is best executed by placing both hands on the knee in order that the index fingers meet on the medial joint margin and the thumbs meet on the lateral aspect of the joint. Through a firm stroking motion of the fingers above and below the patella, fluid is "milked" into the interior of the joint, and the medial aspect of joint becomes flat. The thumbs are then pushed suddenly and firmly into the lateral joint margin, thus producing a bulge of fluid on the medial side of the joint. A delayed fluid wave or bulge will appear on the medial aspect between the patella and the femur.

Table 1-2. Graduations of Muscle Weakness

Grade	Muscle Involvement
0	No muscle contraction
1	Flicker or trace of contraction
2	Active movement possible with gravity eliminated
3	Active movement possible against gravity
4	Active movement possible against gravity and resistance*
5	Normal muscle power

*In judging myopathic weakness, grade 4/5 encompasses a very wide range from slight to severe involvement. Accordingly, some observers subdivide this grade into 4−, 4, and 4+; however, such divisions are difficult to define in objective terms.
Source: Gardner-Medwin, D., and Walton, J. N.   A classification of the neuromuscular disorders and a note on the clinical examination of the voluntary muscles. In J. N. Walton (Ed.), *Disorders of the Voluntary Muscle.* Boston: Little, Brown, 1969. P. 432.

> **3. Popliteal area** is examined for presence of a synovial cyst. (This observation should also be made when the patient is standing because standing makes the cyst more prominent.)
>
> **4. Knee stability** is evaluated by stressing medial and lateral collateral ligaments. Anteroposterior stability is assessed by holding the knee flexed with the foot firmly anchored on the bed and using both hands to pull and push the leg (drawer sign).

E. Ankles and feet

> **1. Synovial soft tissue swelling** of ankles at both malleoli should be distinguished from periarticular edema and fat pads.
>
> **2. Normal ankle motion** is 15 degrees flexion and 25 degrees extension.
>
> **3. Subtalar motion,** which allows inversion and eversion of the foot, is best reported as a percentage of normal with 100% meaning full mediolateral motion.

F. Toes. By inspection and palpation, note:

> **1. Alignment** and cock-up deformity with dorsal subluxation of metatarsal joints, and hammertoes with flexion at PIP and DIP joints. Also observe corns and calluses.
>
> **2. Soft tissue swelling** and presence of inflammation, which are best documented by mediolateral squeezing across the metatarsal joints; pain may be elicited.

G. Muscle examination. Proximal and distal, note:

> **1.** On inspection, muscle **wasting** and muscle **atrophy.**
>
> **2.** On palpation, muscle **tenderness.**
>
> **3.** On testing motion, muscle **strength** (Table 1-2).

H. Neurologic examination

> **1.** Standard evaluation of **tendon reflexes.**
>
> **2. Impairment of nerve root function** must be sought with care, and motor and sensory deficits recorded.
>
> **3.** Look for **nerve entrapment** secondary to joint pathology (e.g., carpal tunnel syndrome).

IV. Systematic examination and joint chart

> **A.** Inspection, palpation, and movement of joints reveal swelling, tenderness, temperature and color changes over the joint, crepitation, and deformity.

1. **Tenderness** on direct pressure over the joint, and **stress pain** produced when the joint, at the limit of its range of motion, is nudged a little farther, are important findings of inflammation.

2. **Crepitation** is a palpable or audible sensation with joint motion caused by roughened articular or extraarticular surfaces rubbing each other.

3. **Deformity** is caused by bony enlargement, subluxation, and ankylosis in abnormal positions.

B. Quantitation of findings

1. **Range of motion** is reported in degrees and, when practical, in percentage of normal (i.e., the fist and the subtalar motions). See Table 1-1 for average values.

2. **Swelling and tenderness** are arbitrarily reported in grades 1, 2, and 3, which indicate size and severity ranging from minimal to severe.

3. Other physical signs of joint abnormality include **warmth and erythema over the joint** and should be expressed as grades 1, 2, or 3 (mild, moderate, or severe).

Assessment of Joint Structure and Function

Rheumatic disease history and systematic method of examination allow assessment of:

I. **Degree of joint inflammation.** Number of acute joints and their location and degree of involvement.

II. **Structural damage and deformity.** Malalignment, subluxation, and instability. Findings are reported by a count of joints deformed or limited in their motion.

III. **Function.** Assessment is based on:

A. Joint range of motion.

B. Muscle strength (grip strength, abduction of shoulders, straight leg raising, rising from squatting and sitting positions, and walking on toes). See Table 1-2.

C. Activities of daily living: mobility, personal care, special hand functions, and work and play activities.

D. Function can be reported in four classes based on the American Rheumatism Association classification:

Class 1 Normal function without or despite symptoms
Class 2 Some disability but adequate for normal activity without special devices or assistance
Class 3 Activities restricted; special devices or assistance required
Class 4 Totally dependent

IV. **Extraarticular features.** Examination is completed by recording specific findings important in rheumatic diseases, such as subcutaneous nodules, nail changes, rash, abnormal eye findings, sicca signs, lymphodenopathy, leg ulcers, and visceral involvement such as splenomegaly, pleural or pericardial signs, and neurologic abnormalities.

In conclusion, a comprehensive history focused on the musculoskeletal system and psychosocial consequences of disease, followed by a complete physical examination with a detailed musculoskeletal and joint evaluation, is the clinical basis for diagnosis and individualized management of rheumatic disease.

2. Rheumatologic Laboratory Tests

H. Hallett Whitman III

Laboratory studies outlined in this chapter are helpful in the diagnosis and treatment of rheumatic diseases. They should always be interpreted in the context of a careful history and physical examination. Serologic or biochemical values that either contradict the clinical diagnosis or will substantially change the intended therapy should always be viewed with caution. This chapter discusses erythrocyte sedimentation rate (ESR), C-reactive protein, autoantibodies, complement, and other tests helpful in the serologic evaluation of rheumatic diseases. Uric acid metabolism will be discussed in Chapter 23 and synovial fluid analysis in Chapter 4.

I. Acute phase reactants

A. Erythrocyte sedimentation rate (ESR). The rate of fall in millimeters per hour of red blood cells (RBCs) in a standard glass tube (Westergren method) is a time-honored measurement of inflammation. Methods other than Westergren have been found to be less reliable. RBCs in inflammatory disorders tend to form stacks (rouleaux) that presumably result from increased levels of fibrinogen and thus sediment more rapidly. Falsely low ESRs are found in sickle cell disease, anisocytosis, spherocytosis, polycythemia, or heart failure. Prolonged storage of blood to be tested or tilting of the calibrated tube will increase the ESR.
Normal Westergren ESR values are 0 to 15 mm/hr for males and 0 to 20 mm/hr for females. The ESR is largely of value if it is normal, thus tending to exclude *active* inflammatory disorders such as acute rheumatic fever, systemic lupus erythematosus (SLE), rheumatoid arthritis (RA), or temporal arteritis-polymyalgia rheumatica (TA-PMR). It is useful in following the course (including therapeutic responses) of chronic inflammatory disorders.

B. C-reactive protein (CRP). CRP is an acute phase reactant serum protein that is not present in normal serum and was originally identified by its ability to give a precipitin reaction with pneumococcal C-polysaccharide. It is now commonly measured by a latex agglutination test and is performed with particles coated with serum that is hyperimmune to CRP.
CRP levels rise rapidly under any inflammatory stimulus, and then fall if inflammation subsides. CRP testing may be performed on freeze-stored serum, which is its major advantage compared to ESR testing.

II. Rheumatoid factor.
Rheumatoid factors (RF) are primarily associated with RA but are also found in other disorders (see Table 2-1). They are immunoglobulins with specificity for the Fc portion of IgG. Multiple Ig classes have RF activity but conventional serologic systems detect only IgM components.

A. Method. Agglutination of IgG-coated latex particles is the method used in most laboratories for measuring IgM RF. The test can be qualitative, that is, concerned with the positivity or negativity of agglutination, or quantitative, using serial dilutions of the test sera. There are many other serologic systems for detection of RF, including bentonite flocculation and a variety of hemagglutination procedures.

B. The molecular characteristics of RF and complexes formed with IgG are shown in Table 2-2.

C. Interpretation. About 75% of RA patients have IgM RF, and patients with extraarticular disease are usually RF positive. Since IgM RFs are not specific for RA and only 75% of patients with RA have IgM RFs, the test is helpful only when combined with clinical information (Table 2-1).

Table 2-1. Frequency of Rheumatoid Factor as Measured by Latex
Agglutination in Rheumatic and Nonrheumatic Diseases

Disease	Approximate Frequency (%)
Sicca syndrome	90
Cryoglobulinemia and purpura	90
Rheumatoid arthritis	75
Mixed connective tissue disease	25
Polymyositis	20
Systemic lupus erythematosus	20
Systemic sclerosis (scleroderma)	20
Juvenile rheumatoid arthritis	10
Subacute bacterial endocarditis	40
Chronic interstitial pulmonary fibrosis	35–60
Pulmonary silicosis	30–50
Aging (>60 years)	15–50
Waldenström disease (macroglobulinemia)	28
Cirrhosis	25
Infectious hepatitis	25
Leprosy	25
Tuberculosis	15
Trypanosomiasis	15
Sarcoidosis	10
Syphilis	10

III. **Antinuclear antibodies.** A wide array of antibodies to nuclear and cytoplasmic cellular antigens is found in lupus and other rheumatic diseases through immunofluorescence, radioimmunoassay, and immunodiffusion. Different profiles of antinuclear antibodies in rheumatic diseases have been described and correlated with clinical features. The LE-cell test is obsolete as a result of its poor sensitivity compared to ANA assay. (Some aspects of the clinical application of ANA data are discussed in Chap. 26.)

A. **Indirect immunofluorescent ANA.** Immunofluorescence (IF) technique employs a cellular substrate, usually a thin section of frozen rat liver or kidney, placed on a glass slide. A cytocentrifuge preparation of white blood cells or cells in tissue culture can also be used. Test sera diluted 1 : 10 or greater are added to the tissue, incubated, and then washed off. Fluorescein-labeled antibodies reactive with all immunoglobulins or specific for human IgG, IgM, or IgA are then layered over the sections, incubated, and washed off. Immunofluorescent microscopy detects the presence of antibodies in the test sera bound to nuclear components.

Through indirect immunofluorescence, a variety of patterns representing antibodies to different cellular antigens can be detected. Percent ANA positivity and patterns of immunofluorescence observed are shown in Table 2-3.

ANA studies are usually reported by pattern, intensity of fluorescence (1+ to 4+), and titer. Values of 3+ or 4+ (bright, brightest) are considered significant. Once positive ANA activity has been documented in a patient's serum, there is seldom need to repeat the test unless dramatic changes in the patient's therapy or condition have taken place. Steroids or immunosuppressive therapy may change the ANA positivity, titer, or pattern, but most laboratories do not rely on serial changes in ANA to monitor disease activity. The usefulness of ANA is not its specificity but rather its sensitivity and technical simplicity. A positive ANA (diffuse or peripheral pattern) is strongly suggestive, although not diagnostic, of

Table 2-2. Molecular Characteristics of Rheumatoid Factor
and Complexes Formed with IgG

Rheumatoid Factor	Sedimentation Constant (S)	Sedimentation Constant (S) of Complexes Formed with IgG	Comment
IgM (penta-meric)	19S	22S	Only Ig class of RF detected by conventional serologic tests
IgG	7S	10–15S (intermediate complexes)	Concentration of intermediate complexes higher in synovial fluid than in serum; in high concentration, intermediate complexes may produce serum hyperviscosity; intermediate complexes may form insoluble complexes with IgM RF
IgM (low molecular weight)	8S	?	Detectable level of 8S IgM correlates with severe systemic diseases, including vasculitis

SLE. Greater diagnostic specificity derives from determining reactivity of positive ANA sera with nuclear constituents such as DNA, Sm antigen, or nRNP (see below).

B. Anti-DNA antibodies. Antibodies to DNA are measured at the Hospital for Special Surgery (Cornell University Medical College) by the Farr method (% DNA binding). An equal volume of test serum diluted 1:10 and radiolabeled C_{14} *Eschericia coli* double-stranded DNA are incubated at 37°C for one hour and refrigerated overnight. Saturated ammonium sulfate is then added to the mixture; this step precipitates out *all antibodies and any bound DNA*. The mixture is then centrifuged and the top half is counted as supernatant (S). The remaining precipitate is redissolved in saline and counted as precipitate (P). Percent DNA binding is calculated by the following formula:

% DNA binding = P − S/P + S × 100

Other methods for measuring double-stranded DNA antibodies are outlined and reviewed by Chubick (*Ann. Intern. Med.* 89:186, 1978).

Similar methods may be used for measuring antibodies to single-stranded DNA. Since even highly purified DS-DNA may have single-stranded regions or nicks exposing single-stranded antigenic determinants, the conventional Farr assay probably measures a small amount of binding to SS-DNA as well as antibodies to DS-DNA. Significant binding by sera in a DS-DNA Farr assay (greater than 30%) is generally found only in lupus or mixed connective tissue disease (MCTD). Antibodies to single-stranded DNA are found in SLE and a variety of other conditions, including drug-induced SLE and liver disease.

C. Antibodies to other nuclear constituents. The heterogeneity of antinuclear antibodies, evident from varied patterns of ANA, has been verified in immunochemical studies employing soluble components derived from nuclei. In addition to DNA, several other antigens have been partially characterized. The procedures for this detection of such specificities are largely confined to research laboratories; the nomenclature and conclusions regarding disease association are in evolution. Table 2-4 summarizes the current state of study regarding the cellular location of the antigens, immunofluorescence patterns, methods of detection, and primary disease associations.

Several of the antinuclear specificities are associated with "speckled" ANA pattern (Sm, nRNP, SS-A, SS-B, RANA). Most of them can be expressed with multiple nuclear substrates, but at least one antigen (RANA) is present only in

Table 2-3. Patterns of Antinuclear Immunofluorescence*

Disease	Diffuse (Homogeneous)	Peripheral (RIM)	Speckled	Nucleolar	% ANA Positivity
Lupus	++	++	+	ϕ	90 or greater
MCTD	ϕ	ϕ	+	ϕ	90 or greater
RA	+	ϕ	+ϕ	ϕ	30–50
Sicca syndrome	ϕ	ϕ	+	+	50–70
Scleroderma	ϕ	ϕ	+	+	70 or greater
Drug-induced SLE	+	+	ϕ	ϕ	90 or greater
Polymyositis	+ϕ	+ϕ	+ϕ	+ϕ	20
Aging (>60 years)	+ϕ	+ϕ	+ϕ	+ϕ	20
Chronic liver disease	+ϕ	+ϕ	+ϕ	+ϕ	20
Idiopathic pulmonary fibrosis	+ϕ	+ϕ	+ϕ	+ϕ	10
Pneumoconiosis	+ϕ	+ϕ	+ϕ	+ϕ	10

*ANA patterns may vary considerably, and different tissue or cellular substrates may give different patterns and degrees of staining
+ = common; ++ = most common; ϕ = less common; +ϕ = variable pattern; MCTD = mixed connective tissue disease.

human B lymphocyte lines. The two antinuclear specificities most characteristic of SLE are anti-DS DNA and anti-Sm. High titers of anti-nRNP are usually associated with a mixed or undifferentiated pattern of MCTD; however, none of these reactivities can be considered diagnostic of anything.

IV. **Complement.** The complement system, composed of 18 different plasma proteins, is a major effector of the humoral immune system. Activation of the system by immune complexes or polysaccharides can occur through two pathways, the classical or the alternative. Both pathways eventually cleave C_3 with subsequent activation of the terminal components (C_5 to C_9), leading to lysis of target cells and the generation of multiple mediators of inflammation and anaphylaxis (Fig. 2-1). Serial measurements of complement levels may be helpful in guiding the therapy of SLE patients (see Chap. 26).

A. **Quantification** of complement or its components can be performed by hemolytic assays or by immunodiffusion using antisera specific for individual components.

1. **Total hemolytic complement** (CH_{50}), measured in hemolytic units, assays the ability of the test serum to lyse 50% of a standardized suspension of sheep red blood cells coated with rabbit antibody.

2. By using stable intermediate complexes of complement components or sera known to be deficient in various components, **functional assays of individual components** have been developed.

3. C_3, C_4, **properdin, and factor B** quantitative determinations by radial immunodiffusion are widely used clinical measurements.

B. **Complement deficiency states.** Deficiencies of early classical pathway components C_1 through C_4 (of which C_2 and C_4 are the most common) are associated with SLE-like syndromes and an increased incidence of infection. Terminal component deficiencies C_5 through C_9 have also been associated with rheumatic syndromes and an increased incidence of infection, particularly *Neisseria*. Deficiency of the inhibitor of C_1 esterase is associated with hereditary angioedema, and deficiency of C_3b inactivator is associated with increased incidence of infection.

C. **Associations and interpretation.** CH_{50} measurements are often low in SLE, cryoglobulinemia, and systemic vasculitis as a result of consumption by circulating or fixed immune complexes. Since numerous complement components are heat labile, all test sera must be kept frozen at $-20°C$ and assayed within two weeks or frozen at $-70°C$ and assayed within two years. Table 2-5 summarizes the serum and synovial fluid CH_{50} determinations in various rheumatic diseases.

V. **Other serologic tests**

A. **Lupus anticoagulant.** The lupus anticoagulant that inhibits the activation of thrombin can be identified by a **prolonged partial thromboplastin time** and a normal or slightly prolonged thromboplastin time in the absence of anticoagulant therapy. Specific factors in SLE sera that inactivate factors VII, XI, and XII have also been identified. Clinically significant bleeding is rare.

B. **False positive serologic tests for syphilis.** False positive serologic tests for syphilis are present in as many as 25% of lupus patients. The test is frequently positive in patients with the lupus anticoagulant; antibodies against phospholipid antigens contained in coagulation factors and STS reagents *may* be responsible for both phenomena.

C. **Hepatitis B (HB) serologic tests** (see Chap. 42). Syndromes associated with chronic HB surface antigen (HBs) include polyarteritis (approximately 30% of cases), essential mixed cryoglobulinemia (variable reported associations, up to 30%), and membranoproliferative glomerulonephritis. Patients with HBs positive polyarteritis usually express HBe antigen, have antibodies to HB core antigen, and have immune complexes containing HBs reactants.

Table 2-4. Antibodies to Nuclear and Cytoplasmic Antigens

Antigen	Cellular Location	Immuno-fluorescence Pattern	Method of Detection	Disease Association	% Positivity	Comments
Native (ds)DNA	N	P, D	RIA, IP, HA, CIE	SLE	65	Relatively specific for SLE
Denatured (SS)DNA	N	P, D	RIA, IP, HA, CIE	SLE	10	Much lower specificity for SLE than anti-ds DNA
				Drug-induced SLE	60	
				RA	10	
				Hepatitis	10	
				SS	<10	
				Biliary cirrhosis	<10	
Extractable nuclear antigen						
RNase sensitive (nRNP)	N	SP	IP, HA, CIE	MCTD or overlap	100	ENA is a crude preparation that contains many nuclear antigens
RNase insensitive (Sm)	N	SP	IP, HA, CIE	SLE	50	High specificity for SLE but less sensitive than (ds)DNA
SS-B (Ha, La)	N	SP	IP, CIE	SS	40–60 (much lower in SS with RA)	Primary SS
SS-A (Ro)	N, B-lymphocyte lines	SP	IP	SS	40–60 (much lower in SS with RA)	SS; also seen in SLE

RANA	N, B-lymphocyte lines	SP	IP	RA	65	EB virus–induced antigen similar to EBNA
DNA-Histone (sNP)	N	P, D	LE test IP	SLE	50	Antigen responsible for LE phenomenon
Cytoplasmic ribosomes	C	Cytoplasmic, granular	IP RIA	SLE	70	Test not uniformly available
PM-1	N	SP	IP	Polymyositis Dermatomyositis	50 20	Antigen poorly characterized
Histone	N	D	IF	SLE Drug-induced SLE	30–50	Test not uniformly available

Abbreviations
N = nucleus
C = cytoplasm
P = peripheral
D = diffuse
SP = speckled
sNP = soluble nucleoprotein
nRNP = nuclear ribonucleoprotein
Sm = Smith antigen
PM-1 = polymyositis 1
RANA = rheumatoid arthritis nuclear antigen
SS = sicca syndrome
SLE = systemic lupus erythematosis
MCTD = mixed connective tissue disease
RIA = radioimmunoassay
IP = immunoprecipitation
LE = LE-cell test
HA = hemagglutination
CIE = counterimmunoelectrophoresis

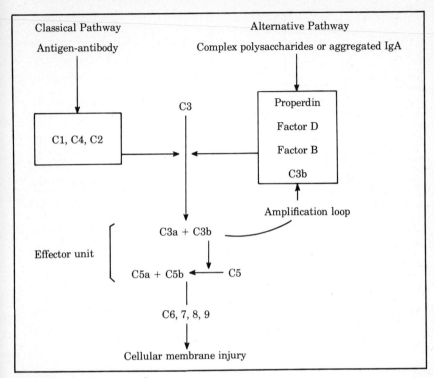

Figure 2-1. Complement pathways.

Table 2-5. Complement Levels in Serum and Synovial Fluid

Diagnosis	Serum	Synovial Fluid
Normal	→	50% of serum level
Rheumatoid arthritis	↑ →	↓ →
RA vasculitis	↓ →	↓ →
SLE	↓ →	↓ →
Drug-induced SLE	→	→
Polymyositis	→	→
Scleroderma	↓ →	→
Sicca syndrome	↓ →	→
Vasculitis	←→	←→
Rheumatic fever	↑ →	→
Gout	↑ →	←→
Pseudogout	↑ →	←→
Septic arthritis	←→	←→
HLA-B27 associated arthropathies	↑ →	↑ →
Cryoglobulinemia	↓ →	↓ →

↑ = elevated; ↓ = down; → = normal; ←→ = variable.

2. Rheumatologic Laboratory Tests   **21**

D. Immune complex assays. Several procedures have been developed for the detection and quantification of immune complexes in sera and other biologic fluids. Principles employed include size and solubility variables of complexes (versus monomeric immunoglobulins), reactivity of complexes with complement (or its components), and affinity of complexes for receptors on cell membranes.

Among these procedures, the two that have been most extensively applied are (1) the **Raji cell assay,** which is based on the attachment of complexes to human lymphoblastoid cells through surface Fc and complement receptors, and (2) the **C1q-binding assay** (as well as other techniques that depend on the affinity of purified **C1q** for immune complexes).

Although immune complex assays are promising research tools, a variety of problems such as standardization and avoidance of artefacts make them inappropriate for routine clinical application.

E. Cryoglobulins. The simplest test for immune complexes, which is based on their diminished solubility in the cold, is to observe for cryoprecipitation of sera at 0°C to 5°C. Although it lacks sensitivity and is not readily quantified, cryoprotein screening is the basis for identification of a relatively common immune complex syndrome called mixed, or essential, cryoglobulinemia. Cryoproteinemia is also a common feature of SLE and other pathologic states associated with immune complex phenomena. Blood to be studied for cryoproteins should not be processed by routine laboratory procedures: after clotting in a 37°C bath, serum should be separated by a brief centrifugation at room temperature and an aliquot examined for precipitation after two days at 0°C to 5°C. Turbidity caused by protein versus lipid can be differentiated by centrifugation in the cold. Small amounts of cryoprotein (less than 30 μg/ml when quantified) may be seen in a wide variety of pathologic sera and have questionable significance. Sera with very large quantities of cryoprotein almost invariably contain monoclonal immunoglobulins; the sera can be subjected to "cryocrit" measurements in calibrated hematocrit tubes.

Bibliography

Alspaugh, M., and Maddison, P.   Resolution of the identity of certain antigen-antibody systems in systemic lupus erythematosus and Sjögren's syndrome. *Arthritis Rheum.* 22:796, 1979.

Chubick, A.   An appraisal of tests for native DNA antibodies in connective tissue diseases. *Ann. Intern. Med.* 89:186, 1978.

Cohen, A. S.   *Laboratory Diagnostic Procedures in the Rheumatic Diseases* (2nd ed.). Boston: Little, Brown, 1975.

Cooper, N. R.   The Complement System. In H. H. Fundenberg (Ed.), *Basic and Clinical Immunology* (2nd ed.). Los Angeles: Lange, 1978.

LeRoy, E. C., Maricq, H. R., and Kaheleh, M. B.   Undifferentiated connective tissue syndromes. *Arthritis Rheum.* 23:341, 1980.

Notman, D. D., Kurata, T., and Tan, E. M.   Profiles of antinuclear antibodies in systemic rheumatic diseases. *Ann. Intern. Med.* 83:464, 1975.

3. Arthrocentesis and Intraarticular Injection

Richard Stern

I. **Arthrocentesis.** Arthrocentesis is a safe and relatively easy procedure that plays both diagnostic and therapeutic roles in the management of arthritis patients. It should be included in the initial evaluation of every patient with a joint effusion, especially those with monarthritis. Subsequent synovial fluid analysis can lead to a specific diagnosis in infectious and crystal-induced arthritis and can be of help in differentiating an inflammatory process such as rheumatoid arthritis from a non-inflammatory state.

A. Diagnostic indications

   1. As part of an initial evaluation.

   2. To rule out superimposed infection in an already diseased joint.

B. Therapeutic indications

   1. Relief of pain by drainage of an effusion.

   2. Installation of medication.

   3. Drainage of a septic joint.

   4. Drainage of hemarthrosis (correct any coagulation disorder first).

C. Contraindications

   1. Infection in overlying skin or soft tissue.

   2. Severe coagulation disorder.

II. **Intraarticular injection.** Joint injection is primarily used to deliver intraarticular corticosteroids to treat inflammed joints, bursae, or tendons. Contraindications are the same as for arthrocentesis. Cortisone should not be injected into a joint until infection (including that caused by mycobacteria or fungi) has been excluded. There is some evidence that repeated injection of cortisone into the small joints of the hand may lead to deformity. Similarly, cortisone injections into tendon insertions may result in rupture. Large joints should not be injected more than 3 or 4 times per year, or 10 times cumulatively. Small joints should be injected less often, not more than 2 or 3 times per year, or 4 times cumulatively.

III. **Supplies**

A. Aseptic skin preparation materials

   1. Sterile gloves.

   2. Iodine solution.

   3. Alcohol solution.

   4. Sterile gauze pads.

B. Local anesthesia materials

   1. 1% lidocaine for skin, subcutaneous tissues, and joint structure.

   2. Ethyl chloride spray for skin.

C. Sterile needles from size 18- to 25-gauge, depending on the size of the joint. Inflamed joint fluids may be thick and require a large needle for removal.

D. Syringes from size 3 cc to 50 cc, depending on the joint and amount of effusion.

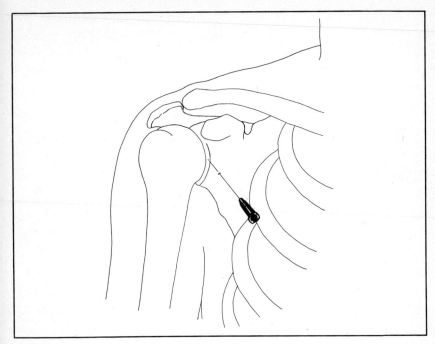

Figure 3-1. Arthrocentesis of the shoulder, anterior approach.

E. Tubes for synovial fluid analysis

1. Chemistry tube for glucose.

2. Hematology tube (with EDTA) for cell count and differential.

3. Sterile tube for cultures and smears.

4. Heparinized tube for crystal analysis. Ascertain that a powdered anticoagulant, which may interfere with crystal identification, is not used.

5. Cytology bottle (if neoplasm suspected).

IV. **Technique.** The most important maneuver before aspirating a joint is to locate the appropriate landmark and mark it with an indelible felt pen.
Generous **local anesthesia** of the overlying skin and subcutaneous tissues is recommended. Long-acting intraarticular steroid preparations may induce a crystal synovitis 24 hours after the injection, which soon abates spontaneously. Further, the needle itself may traumatize the joint, especially if the joint is small; for this reason, the patient should be warned of possible short-term aggravation of symptoms in the injected joint and receive appropriate analgesia instructions.

A. **Shoulder.** The shoulder may be entered either anteriorly or posteriorly.

1. **Anterior approach** (Fig. 3-1). With the patient's hand in the lap and the shoulder muscles relaxed, the glenohumeral joint can be palpated by placing one's fingers between the **coracoid process** and the humeral head. As the shoulder is internally rotated, the humeral head can be felt turning inward and the joint space can be felt as a groove just lateral to the coracoid. When the skin over this area is anesthetized, a 20- or 22-gauge needle can be inserted lateral to the coracoid (avoid the thoracoacromial artery which runs on the medial aspect of

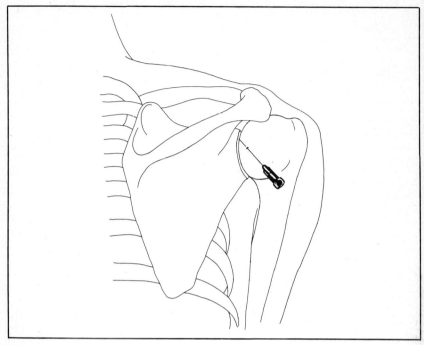

Figure 3-2. Arthrocentesis of the shoulder, posterior approach.

the coracoid). The needle is directed dorsally and medially into the joint space. The needle should be directed slightly superiorly to avoid the neurovascular bundle.

   2. **Posterior approach** (Fig. 3-2). The posterior aspect of the shoulder joint is identified with the patient's arm maximally internally rotated. This position is achieved by placing the patient's ipsilateral hand on the opposite shoulder. The humeral head can then be palpated by placing a finger posteriorly along the **acromion** while the shoulder is rotated. The needle is inserted about 1 cm inferior to the **posterior tip of the acromion** and directed anteriorly and medially.

B. **Elbow** (Fig. 3-3). The **elbow joint** can be identified by placing the patient's relaxed arm in the lap. With the palm facing the patient, flex the elbow to a 45-degree angle. Place your finger on the **lateral epicondyle** and note the shallow depression distal to it, which represents the elbow joint. A 22-gauge needle is introduced perpendicular to the joint.

C. **Wrist** (Fig. 3-4). Wrist aspiration is performed on the dorsal aspect just distal to the radius or ulna as indicated by clinical examination.

   1. **Radial entry.** The hand and the wrist are relaxed in a slightly flexed position. The joint space can be located by palpating the edge of the distal radius just medial to the **thumb extensor tendon.** A 22-gauge needle should be directed into the joint from the dorsal aspect.

   2. **Ulnar entry.** Keep the wrist in the same relaxed position. The joint space can be identified by palpating just distal to the **distal ulna.** The 22-gauge needle is directed in a volar and radial direction.

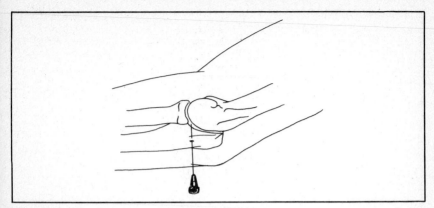

Figure 3-3. Arthrocentesis of the elbow.

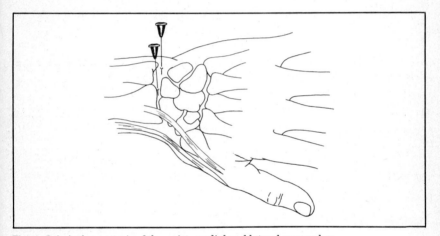

Figure 3-4. Arthrocentesis of the wrist, medial and lateral approaches.

D. Ankle (Fig. 3-5)

The ankle may be difficult to enter. For both approaches, the foot is first placed at about a 45-degree angle of plantar flexion.

1. **Medial approach.** A 22-gauge needle is placed about one-half in. proximal and lateral to the distal end of the **medial malleolus.** The flexor hallucis longus tendon is just lateral to this point. The needle is directed 45 degrees posterior, slightly upward, and lateral.

2. **Lateral approach.** A 22-gauge needle is placed about one-half in. proximal and medial to the distal end of the **lateral malleolus.** The needle should be directed 45 degrees posterior, slightly upward, and medial.

E. Knee (Fig. 3-6)

The knee is the largest and easiest joint to enter. It may be entered either medially or laterally. The patient should be supine with the knee comfortably extended to relax the quadriceps muscle. If one can gently rock the patella medially and laterally, relaxation is adequate. Grasping the medial and lateral margins of the patella, a skin mark can be made that corresponds to the inferior plane of the

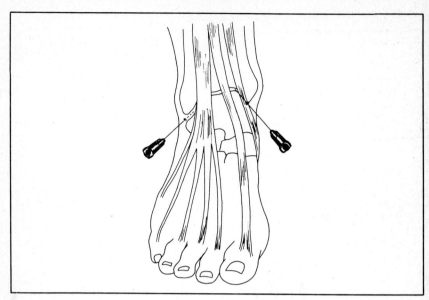

Figure 3-5. Arthrocentesis of the ankle, medial and lateral approaches.

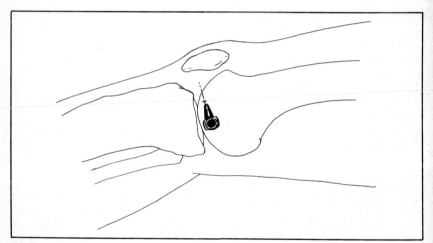

Figure 3-6. Arthrocentesis of the knee, medial approach.

Table 3-1. Intraarticular Therapy Regimens

Joint	Needle Gauge	Dosage of Methylprednisolone Acetate (mg)
Knee; shoulder	16–24	40–80
Wrist; ankle; elbow	20–22	10–40
Interphalangeal	25	5–10

patella. It is generally easier to aspirate at the medial aspect of the joint. After anesthetizing the skin and subcutaneous tissue, an 18-gauge needle is introduced in a direction parallel to the plane of the posterior surface of the patella. With thick exudative effusions, a larger bore needle may be required. Drainage of the knee bursa can be facilitated by compressing the suprapatellar pouch during aspiration. With large knee effusions, the distended suprapatellar pouch can be aspirated directly from either the medial or lateral aspect of the quadriceps muscle mass.

F. **Small joints of the hands and feet.** These joints may be difficult to enter. Occasionally the effusion bulges and facilitates aspiration. Often a corticosteroid injection can be made just adjacent to the joint rather than within it; and one obtains an equivalent clinical response.

   1. **The metacarpophalangeal (MCP) joint** can be easily palpated on its dorsal, lateral aspect with the finger slightly flexed and relaxed. The joint is entered on the dorsal-lateral aspect using a 22-gauge needle. Because it is a ball (distal metacarpal) and cup (first phalanx) joint, the needle should not be directed at a 90-degree angle but rather distally at about a 60-degree angle.

   2. **The metatarsophalangeal (MTP) joint** is aspirated in a fashion similar to that for a MCP joint.

   3. **The proximal interphalangeal (PIP) joint** margin is barely palpable but may be felt on its dorsal aspect just distal to the skin crease. The joint is entered from the dorsal aspect with a 25-gauge needle that is directed slightly distally.

   4. **The distal interphalangeal (DIP) joint** is extremely small and difficult to enter. The technique is the same as for aspirating the PIP joint.

G. **Other joints.** There are external landmarks that can direct aspiration and injection of the hip joint, but success in this venture requires some experience. When the goal of aspiration is to secure synovial fluid for diagnostic studies, arthrocentesis should be performed under fluoroscopic control, employing a small injection of radiopaque dye to verify that the needle is in the hip joint bursa. The spinal and sacroiliac joints cannot be entered safely in an outpatient setting. If diagnostic material is needed from these joints, an open surgical procedure is required.

V. **Intraarticular medications.** At our institution, we use the long-acting insoluble corticosteroid preparation, methylprednisolone acetate. The dose varies with the size of the joint. Dosages and appropriate needle sizes are summarized in Table 3-1.

4. Synovial Fluid Analysis

Richard Stern

Synovial fluid analysis is an extremely useful diagnostic tool in the evaluation of rheumatic diseases. It should be included in the initial evaluation of most arthritic conditions. It can yield a specific diagnosis in infectious and crystal-induced arthritis and can be helpful in the diagnosis of other arthritic diseases.

I. Synovial fluid studies

A. Gross examination alone can be quite helpful in establishing the nature of a joint fluid. After allowing air bubbles to clear, a heparinized specimen is examined for:

1. Color. Normal synovial fluid is straw colored. Inflammatory fluids range from yellow to greenish yellow. Hemarthrosis occurs in patients with coagulation disorders, trauma, neoplasms, and tuberculosis arthritis, and in patients receiving anticoagulant therapy.

2. Clarity. Normal synovial fluids are clear enough to read print through. As inflammation increases from mild to marked, the fluid becomes first translucent and then opalescent.

3. Viscosity. Synovial fluid viscosity is tested by allowing a drop of fluid to fall from the needle tip. Normal synovial fluids are quite viscous, and a "string" of fluid will form. Because viscosity is decreased in inflammatory synovial fluids, no string sign is seen.

4. Mucin clot. If 1 ml of synovial fluid is added to 3 ml of 2% acetic acid, a firm mucin clot will form. When acetic acid is added to an inflammatory fluid, a poor clot results.

B. Cell count is performed on a counting chamber. However, because there are often few cells present, the initial count can be taken undiluted. If there are too many cells to count, appropriate dilution can be made with normal saline. (Diluents for white blood cells, WBCs, precipitate mucin.) Often both red blood cells (RBCs) and WBCs can be counted on the same chamber.

C. Crystal examination is performed using polarizing microscopy of a specimen of heparinized fluid (see Chap. 23). A useful mnemonic for differentiating urate crystals from calcium pyrophosphate is "U-Pay-Peb": *U*rate crystals *pa*rallel to the polarizer's axis appear *y*ellow; urate crystals *pe*rpendicular to the polarizer's axis appear *b*lue. The opposite is true for the calcium pyrophosphate crystals of pseudogout.

D. Microbiologic studies

1. Stains should include both Gram and acid-fast methods.

2. Cultures should include routine bacterial studies. Fungal and mycobacterial cultures are ordered as necessary. Fluids suspected of harboring gonococci should be plated on Thayer-Martin material at the bedside as gonococci are fastidious and difficult to grow.

E. Biochemical studies

1. Glucose. Synovial fluid glucose determination, when interpreted with a simultaneous serum value, is helpful in diagnosing infectious arthritis. In bacterial infection or tuberculosis, the synovial fluid glucose will be less than half the serum value. Occasionally, low values may be seen in rheumatoid arthritis.

2. Protein does not provide additional useful information and should not be routinely ordered.

Table 4-1. Synovial Fluid Analysis

Classification	Condition	Gross Examination			Microscopic Examination			Biochemical Examination		Microbiologic Examination
		Color	Clarity	Viscosity	WBC/mm^3	%NTP	Crystals	Glucose (%serum)	Complement	Culture/Smear
Normal	Normal	Yellow	Translucent	High	<200	<25	0	Same	Normal	0
Group 1 (noninflammatory)	Osteoarthritis	Yellow	Transparent	High	<2,000	<25	0	Same	Normal	0
	Trauma	Pink or red	Transparent	High	<2,000	<25	0	Same	Normal	0
	SLE	Yellow	Translucent	Slightly decreased	0–9,000	<25	0	Same	Normal	0
Group 2 (inflammatory)	Acute rheumatic fever	Yellow	Translucent	Slightly decreased	0–60,000	25–50	0	Same	Normal	0
	Pseudogout	Yellow or white	Translucent or opaque	Low	50–75,000	90	+	Same	Normal	0
	Gout	Yellow or white	Translucent or opaque	Low	100–160,000	90	+	Same	Normal	0
	Rheumatoid arthritis	Yellow or purulent	Translucent or opaque	Low	3,000–50,000	50–75	0	75–100	Normal or low	0
Group 3 (purulent)	Tuberculosis	Purulent	Opaque	Low	2,500–100,000	50	0	50–75	Normal or low	+
	Bacterial arthritis	Purulent	Opaque	Low	50,000–300,000	>90	0	<50	Normal or low	+*

*Often negative in gonococcal arthritis.
WBC = white blood cells; SLE = systemic lupus erythematosus; NTP = neutrophils.

3. **Complement** may be decreased in rheumatoid arthritis, but the test is rarely helpful for diagnosis because synovial fluid complement is usually normal in early rheumatoid arthritis.

II. **Diagnosis by fluid group** (Table 4-1). Synovial fluid can be divided into three groups based on the degree of inflammation.

A. **Group 1 fluids** are clear, transparent, and have few white cells on cell count. They include normal, osteoarthritic, and SLE joint fluids.

B. **Group 2 fluids** generally have a higher white count and are not as clear as group 1 fluids; they appear translucent. This group includes fluids from most noninfectious, inflammatory arthritic conditions such as gout, pseudogout, and rheumatoid arthritis. Leukemia or lymphoma occasionally present in this category, but the differential count reveals greater than 90% mononuclear cells.

C. **Group 3 fluids** are opalescent or purulent. Group 3 fluids include those from bacterial infections and tuberculosis (although joint fluid from gonococcal arthritis can be either group 2 or group 3). Group 3 fluids typically have 50,000 to 300,000 white cells per mm^3 which are mostly neutrophils. Occasionally the synovial fluid from an inflammatory arthritic condition such as rheumatoid arthritis may have as many as 50,000 to 75,000 white cells per mm^3 and appear opalescent or even purulent. As Table 4-1 shows, there is considerable overlap between the various arthritic diseases; this table is meant to serve as a guideline rather than a rigid set of criteria.

5. Immunogenetic Aspects of Rheumatic Diseases

Allan Gibofsky

The efforts of numerous investigators over the past three decades have resulted in the recognition of a major histocompatibility complex in humans consisting of the alleles of at least five closely linked loci on the short arm of autosomal chromosome 6. The antigens that the genes of this region coded were first detected on white blood cells and, therefore, were originally referred to as human leukocyte antigens (HLAs). Initially these antigens primarily interested transplantation physicians since similarity between donor and recipient seemed to influence allograft survival; soon, however, the hypothesis was advanced that certain clinical conditions might be associated with one or more antigens of this system. A large number of diseases have been studied, and individual or combinations of antigens have appeared with greater frequency than would be expected in the normal population. This increase is particularly true for rheumatic disease and related syndromes with features of altered immunoreactivity, where, as will be discussed, the strongest and most significant associations were demonstrated. This chapter will review the basic concepts of immunogenetics, emphasizing the potential significance of the HLA system antigens in clinical rheumatology.

I. Immunogenetic nomenclature

A. **Gene.** Segment of DNA that directs the synthesis of a polypeptide chain or protein.

B. **Allele.** Alternative form of the same gene, resulting from mutation or duplication.

C. **Locus.** The position of a gene on any given chromosome.

D. **Genotype.** The genetic composition of the individual.

E. **Phenotype.** The observed expression of the genotype.

F. **Haplotype.** Closely linked loci, transmitted as a unit from each parent; two haplotypes constitute the genotype.

G. **Alloantigen.** Product of the A, B, C, or DR loci; recognized on the cell surface by specific antibody.

H. **Determinant.** Product of the HLA-D locus; recognized by cell-cell interaction in the mixed lymphocyte culture technique.

II. Major histocompatibility system

A. **Loci definition.** The relationship among the various loci that comprise the HLA system is shown in Figure 5-1. Five closely linked loci, A, B, C, D, and DR, were defined at the Eighth International Histocompatibility Workshop in 1980; the alleles of each are shown in Table 5-1. The products of the A, B, and C series are defined using serologic reagents, most often with a lymphocytotoxicity assay. The determinants of the D locus are defined by cell-cell interaction in the mixed lymphocyte culture.

Initial studies directed towards the development of serologic methods for the detection of HLA-D antigens have resulted in the recognition of yet another antigenic system, preferentially expressed on the surface of B-lymphocytes. This B-cell system has extensive biologic and chemical homologies with the I region antigens of the murine histocompatibility system and has also been termed Ia. These Ia alloantigens were primarily recognized with alloantibodies that developed as a result of immunization with paternal antigens during pregnancy, or in the sera of renal transplant recipients who become immunized against nonmatching antigens present on the homograft. These human Ia determinations are

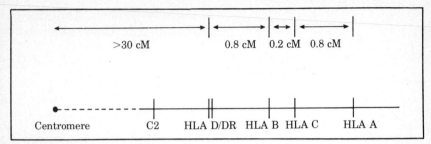

Figure 5-1. Map of major histocompatibility (MHC) region of human chromosome 6. Distances are in centimorgans (cM).

highly polymorphic and have certain alloantigenic specificities related closely to HLA-D alleles; for this reason, these particular Ia phenotypes were designated HLA-DR to indicate their close relationship with the determinants of the HLA-D locus.

B. Genetics of inheritance. The antigens of this system are inherited in classical Mendelian fashion. Unlike those phenotypic characteristics that exhibit dominant and recessive forms (e.g., eye color and ABO type), the HLA antigens are *codominant:* if a gene has been inherited from either parent, the corresponding HLA antigen will be expressed on the cell surface. Given the number of alleles at each locus, the number of possible phenotypic combinations is very large, indicating the enormous immunogenetic heterogeneity of an outbred population. Thus the finding that a particular antigen's frequency in a patient group is different from that seen in normals is likely to prompt intense interest in the biologic role of this system in the regulation of the immune response and disease susceptibility.

III. Disease associations. Of the many conditions thus far investigated and shown to be associated with particular alleles of the HLA system, the rheumatic diseases have been the most important. While the associations are high, they are neither absolute nor diagnostic; the presence of an antigen is not the sole determinant in disease pathogenesis for it occurs with low frequency in disease-free individuals as well. Nevertheless, knowledge of the association may prove useful in permitting subdivisions of clinical groups within the larger population (e.g., pauciarticular juvenile rheumatoid arthritis). This knowledge could facilitate the search for possible etiologic agents, and confirm or refute the following suggested mechanisms for HLA and disease associations:

1. The HLA antigen might be structurally similar to the antigenic component of an infectious agent.
2. The HLA antigen may be a part of a neoantigen, formed in combination with an infectious agent.
3. The HLA antigen may be a receptor for an infectious or environmental toxin.
4. There may be a deficiency of one or more complement system components.
5. There may be linkage disequilibrium with one or more immune response genes.

A. Ankylosing spondylitis. The most significant association of any HLA antigen occurs in this disease. Between 85% and 90% of Caucasian patients have HLA-B27, which seems to be a marker for seronegative axial arthropathy in this group. Ethnic differences may be important as well since the antigen occurs with different frequency in both patient and control non-Caucasian groups. The lower association in Pima Indians and American blacks, groups in which the disease itself is less frequent, would suggest that B27 is not involved directly in the disease pathogenesis but rather may be linked to the predisposing gene. Thus far, no HLA-D or DR association has been recognized, which suggests that susceptibility to ankylosing spondylitis involves mechanisms different from those involved in the other rheumatic diseases.

Table 5-1. Alleles of the Human HLA System

HLA-A	HLA-B			HLA-C	HLA-D	HLA-DR
1	5	w41		w1	w1	1
2	7	w42		w2	w2	2
3	8	w44		w3	w3	3
9	12	w45		w4	w4	4
10	13	w46		w5	w5	5
11	14	w47		w6	w6	w6
25	15	w48		(new)	w7	7
26	17	w49		w7 (CVE)	w8	
28	18	w50		w8 (T8, T9)	w9	w8 (IA8)(DuB15)
29	27	w51			w10	w9 (4w7)
w19	37	w52			w11 (included in Dw7)	w10 (ST-1)
w23	40	w53			(new)	
w24	w4	w54			w12 (DH0, DB4)	
w30	w6 (new)					
w31	w16	w55(22.1)(8w55)				
w32	w21	w56(22.2)(8w56)				
w33	w22	w57(17.1—long)	(8w67)			
w34	w35	w58(17.2—short)	(8w68)			
w36	w38	w59(8.2)	(8w69)			
w43	w39	w60(40.1)	(8w60)			
	w43	w61(40.2)	(8w61)			
		w62(15.1)	(8w64)			
		w63(15.2)	(8w65)			

w = provisional workshop assignment.

35

B. Reiter syndrome. Nearly 80% of Caucasian patients with the classical triad of symptoms have the antigen B27. This antigen is also seen in slightly lower frequency in incomplete forms of the syndrome. It has been suggested that the reactive arthritis seen following infection with *Yersinia* or *Salmonella* infection is comparable to the form of Reiter syndrome following bacterial dysentery. In these conditions as well, HLA-B27 is increased.

C. Rheumatoid arthritis. The B-lymphocyte alloantigen HLA-DR4 has been reported in 60% to 80% of Caucasian patients with classical adult seropositive RA, as compared to 24% to 28% of controls. A slightly lower association has also been reported for the corresponding mixed lymphocyte culture determinant HLA-DW4. In contrast, no HLA association was detected in adult patients with clinically similar, seronegative disease, which suggests that seronegative and seropositive RA have different immunogenetic bases.

D. Systemic lupus erythematosus (SLE). Both HLA-DR antigens DR2 and DR3 were found to be increased in Caucasian patients with SLE. This immunogenetic diversity would support the clinical diversity seen in this disease. There have been some data suggesting that clinical subgroups of patients with SLE show an association with one or the other HLA-DR antigen—for example, with DR3 in skin disease or DR2 in vasculitis—but not necessarily with both.

E. Sicca syndrome. Caucasian patients with primary sicca syndrome show a strong association with HLA-DW3 and the related B-cell antigen HLA-DR3. Of interest was the recent report that HLA-DR4 is increased in frequency in patients with secondary sicca syndrome, which no doubt reflects the high incidence of RA seen in this population.

F. Psoriatic arthritis. The HLA antigens A26, B38, Cw6, DR4, and DR7 have been reported increased in patients with psoriatic arthritis. In addition, B27 has been reported increased in patients with axial skeletal disease. Different antigens have been reported associated with skin disease alone.

G. Inflammatory bowel disease (IBD). Patients with IBD and ankylosing spondylitis show an increased frequency of HLA-B27. No increase in the frequency of this antigen is seen in patients with enteropathic peripheral arthritis as a manifestation of IBD.

H. Behcet disease. The HLA antigen B5 is increased in Caucasian patients with this condition. The association is even more significant in Oriental patients.

I. Lyme arthritis. HLA-DR2 is increased in Caucasian patients with this disorder, which is presumed to result from an infection transmitted by a tick bite.

J. C2 deficiency. The gene coding for the second component of complement is located on chromosome 6 and is part of the major histocompatibility complex. Fu and associates have reported several family studies of patients with C2 deficiency and a SLE-like illness in whom the deficient C2 gene segregated with the same haplotype (A10-B18).

K. Rheumatic fever. In two groups of patients with this disease, a non-HLA-D related B-cell alloantigen Ia883 has been reported, respectively, in 71% and 75% of patients. The relationship of this alloantigen to other genes located within the major histocompatibility complex remains to be determined.

L. Juvenile rheumatoid arthritis. HLA-B27 has been reported in 40% of patients with combined pauciarticular and axial disease. Associations with the B-cell alloantigens HLA-DR5 and HLA-DRw8 have also been reported.

Bibliography

Gibofsky, A., et al. Disease associations of the Ia-like human alloantigens. Contrasting patterns in rheumatoid arthritis and systemic lupus erythematosus. *J. Exp. Med.* 148:1728, 1979.

Suciu-Foca, N.   The HLA system in human pathology. *Pathobiol. Annu.* 9:81, 1979.

Terasaki, P. I. (Ed.). *Hiscompatibility Testing 1980.* Copenhagen: Munksgaard, 1980.

Winchester, R. J., and Kunkel, H. G.   The human Ia system. In *Advances in Immunology,* Vol. 29. New York: Academic, 1980.

II. Clinical Presentations

6. Monarthritis

John F. Beary III

I. Acute monarthritis

A. Infectious arthritis is the most important condition to diagnose because permanent joint injury can be prevented by prompt, specific antibiotic therapy. Bacteria are the most frequent cause of acute infectious arthritis. Viral arthritis is difficult to document with currently available technology and is usually polyarticular.

The diagnosis of bacterial arthritis is suggested by a focus of infection contiguous to the joint, traumatic penetration of the joint, a focus of infection in another area of the body that can reach the joint by hematogenous spread, or a history of fever, rigor, or extramarital sexual contact.

The diagnosis is confirmed by joint aspiration, which is mandatory in initial evaluation of monarthritis. The white blood cell count in the joint fluid is frequently, but not always, greater than 50,000/mm^3. The infectious agent may be identified with a gram-stained smear, but the highest priority is *prompt* innoculation of the specimen on appropriate bacteriologic media. A complete discussion of infectious arthritis is found in Chapter 24.

B. Crystal-induced disease

1. **Gout** classically presents as a severe monarthritis of the first metatarsophalangeal joint (podagra), but any joint or bursa may be affected. Other features suggesting the diagnosis include male sex, monarthritis or oligoarthritis of lower extremity joints, complete recovery between episodes, and hyperuricemia. The diagnosis is confirmed by examination of synovial fluid under compensated, polarized light (see Chap. 23). Urate crystals are needle shaped and have strong negative birefringence.

2. **Pseudogout** is suggested by occurrence in an elderly patient, large joint involvement (especially of the knee), and radiographic evidence of chondrocalcinosis. The diagnosis is confirmed by demonstration of calcium pyrophosphate dihydrate crystals in synovial fluid. The crystals are rhomboid shaped and exhibit weak positive birefringence.

C. Trauma. A history of relevant injury is present. Diagnostic evaluation may demonstrate hemarthrosis or juxtaarticular fracture.

D. Internal derangement of the knee is suggested by a history of trauma, episodes of joint locking or "giving way," and tenderness at the joint margin. Diagnosis is confirmed by arthrography or arthroscopy, which may demonstrate meniscal or ligamentous tears, or cartilage bodies free in the joint.

E. Nontraumatic hemarthrosis is suggested by a history of a bleeding disorder such as hemophilia, or of the use of anticoagulant drugs. Joint neoplasms such as synovial hemangioma and pigmented villonodular synovitis must also be considered in the differential diagnosis and can be identified with synovial biopsy.

F. Atypical presentation of a polyarticular disease, particularly rheumatoid arthritis, should be considered. However, any syndrome that is ordinarily characterized by polyarthritis may present as monarticular disease.

A prolonged observation period of many months may be required before more typical features of rheumatoid arthritis, such as symmetric polyarthritis, rheumatoid nodules, or rheumatoid factor, appear. It is better to classify such patients as having monarthritis of undetermined etiology rather than label them with a premature diagnosis. The diagnosis of monarticular rheumatoid arthritis requires rigorous elimination of other causes of monarthritis, especially infection and crystal-induced synovitis.

II. Chronic monarthritis. Arthritis that persists for more than two months is defined as chronic monarthritis. The following disorders should be considered in the differential diagnosis.

A. Infectious arthritis should have highest priority in differential diagnostic consideration. Mycobacteria and fungi must be considered as well as bacteria in evaluation of chronic monarthritis. An immunosuppressed host, history of tuberculosis exposure, evidence of pulmonary disease, and positive purified protein derivative (PPD) skin test are features that suggest the diagnosis of tuberculous arthritis. Diagnosis may be confirmed by synovial fluid examination and culture. If synovial fluid studies are nondiagnostic, synovial biopsy is recommended to obtain tissue for pathologic and microbial studies.

B. Rheumatoid arthritis may present as chronic monarthritis. The oligoarticular form of juvenile rheumatoid arthritis is an important consideration (see Chap. 25). Months of observation may be required before more typical features (polyarticular pattern, rheumatoid nodules, or rheumatoid factor) appear.

C. Osteoarthritis usually has an insidious onset. Initially pain occurs with activity. Features that support the diagnosis of osteoarthritis include occurrence in an elderly patient; presence of physical stresses related to occupation, athletics, or obesity; and involvement of distal interphalangeal or first carpometacarpal joints of the hand. Hips, knees, and lumbar spine are frequently involved. Radiographic findings of joint space narrowing, subchondral bony sclerosis, and osteophyte formation are typical. Laboratory studies are normal.

D. Internal derangement of the knee (see sec. **I.D.**) may, if untreated, cause secondary degenerative joint disease.

E. Osteonecrosis is suggested by monarticular pain in a shoulder, hip, or knee; presence of a risk factor such as alcoholism or corticosteroid therapy; and the radiographic finding of a periarticular bone lucency with a sclerotic margin. However, radiographic studies may be negative for weeks after onset of symptoms, and diagnosis of early osteonecrosis is best made by radionuclide bone scan (see Chap. 29).

F. Articular neoplasms are among the least common causes of monarthritis. Benign conditions include pigmented villonodular synovitis, synovial chondromatosis, and hemangioma. Malignant joint neoplasms include synovial sarcoma and metastatic bone tumors. The diagnosis is established by synovial biopsy.

G. Sarcoidosis arthropathy is a rare cause of monarthritis and is usually nondestructive. Hilar adenopathy and uveitis are extraarticular features that suggest the diagnosis of sarcoidosis. Synovial biopsy demonstrates noncaseating granulomas in most patients with arthropathy.

7. Polyarthritis

Stephen Paget

I. Acute polyarthritis. Individual chapters discuss in greater detail most of the conditions considered in the differential diagnosis of polyarthritis (two or more inflamed joints).

A. Infectious arthritis

1. **Bacterial.** Because three-quarters of patients with gonococcal (GC) arthritis present with a migratory polyarthritis, the gonococcus is the most common bacteria associated with such a clinical picture. Meningococci may present in a similar manner, but joint infections with staphylococci, pneumococci, and streptococci tend to be monoarticular. Clues to the presence of gonococci include associated gonococcal infection in other areas (e.g., urethra, cervix, rectum, and pharynx), vesiculopustular skin lesions, tenosynovitis, history of venereal disease, and history of sexual promiscuity. As always, the diagnosis of infectious arthritis is confirmed by joint aspiration and appropriate synovial fluid and other cultures. A complete discussion of bacterial infectious arthritis is found in Chapter 24.

    Acute migratory polyarthritis in children and young adults that begins shortly after a streptococcal infection suggests acute rheumatic fever (ARF). According to the modified Jones criteria, the presence of two major, or one major and two minor, criteria is considered diagnostic of ARF in the setting of a recent streptococcal infection (see Chap. 38).

2. **Viral.** The most common viral-related polyarthritis is associated with hepatitis B infection. In the prodromal (preicteric) phase of the disease, some patients develop a rheumatoid arthritis–like polyarthritis associated with an urticarial or purpuric rash. This disorder usually clears with the appearance of jaundice; can be diagnosed by the presence of hepatitis B surface antigen and elevated transaminase levels in the serum; and is related to the presence of immune complex deposition in joints and skin. Rubella viral (German measles) infection or rubella vaccine can be associated with a self-limited form of polyarthritis. Lyme disease, probably caused by an arthropod-borne agent, can lead to monoarticular or polyarticular arthritis and can be associated with the rash of erythema chronicum migrans (see Chap. 10).

    Infections caused by *Rickettsia,* fungi, and parasites can, at times, lead to polyarticular disease, although clearly not as often as the disorders mentioned above.

B. Rheumatoid arthritis (RA) and juvenile rheumatoid arthritis (JRA). Although RA in the majority of patients has an insidious onset, it may be acute and fulminating. Clues to the presence of this disorder in both its adult and juvenile forms include the symmetrical involvement of the small joints of hands, wrists, and feet (or joints other than the distal interphalangeals), the prominence of morning stiffness, and systemic features such as fever, fatigue, malaise, and anemia. The presence in serum of rheumatoid factor and the elevation of the ESR are helpful laboratory findings which are often present.

C. Systemic lupus erythematosus (SLE) and other connective tissue diseases. SLE can present as an acute RA-like polyarthritis. The associated systemic features that suggest the diagnosis of SLE are fever, skin rash (e.g., discoid lupus or facial erythema in a butterfly distribution), serositis, and renal, hematologic, or central nervous system disorders. Antinuclear antibody tests (ANA) are positive in more than 90% of patients with active SLE. Polymyositis, dermatomyositis, scleroderma, undifferentiated connective tissue syndromes, and polyarteritis

43

nodosa can also present, either initially or during their course, as acute polyarthritis. In general, other characteristic clinical manifestations of these disorders help in differential diagnosis. At times, however, long periods of observation are necessary before the exact diagnosis becomes clear.

D. Seronegative spondyloarthropathies. This term comprises a group of diseases that share the following clinical features: spondylitis, sacroiliitis, and uveitis. The HLA-B27 antigen is positive in most patients and, by definition, the serum of most patients with these disorders is negative for rheumatoid factor.

1. In **ankylosing spondylitis,** a disease that has its major effect upon the spine, peripheral joint involvement indistinguishable from RA may be seen in as many as 35% of patients at some stage; peripheral joint involvement may be the initial manifestation of the disease in 20% of cases.

2. **Reiter syndrome** is diagnosed by the clinical triad of polyarthritis, conjunctivitis, and urethritis or diarrhea. Other distinguishing features include sausage-shaped, inflamed digits, circinate balanitis, and a pustulokeratotic palm and sole skin rash called keratodermia blennorrhagica.

3. **Psoriatic arthritis** can be a highly inflammatory process most characteristically presenting as an asymmetrical polyarthritis of the interphalangeal joints of the fingers and toes. Psoriatic lesions may be found in the adjacent nails, and a history of chronic psoriasis can be elicited.

4. **Enteropathic arthritis** is that form of polyarthritis associated with underlying inflammatory bowel disease (ulcerative colitis or regional enteritis). Although such an arthritis may occur before clinically apparent bowel disease, some parallel pattern in the course of the bowel and joint disease activity commonly exists. Small distal joints of the hands and feet are much less commonly affected in enteropathic arthritis than in RA, while an asymmetrical involvement of knees and ankles is typical of this disorder.

E. Crystal-induced disease

1. **Gout.** As many as one-third of patients with gout can present with polyarticular arthritis. Clinical features in favor of gout are male sex, acute onset, history of podagra (arthritis of the big toe joints) or renal stones, family history of gout or stones, the presence of tophi, and hyperuricemia. The definitive diagnosis is based on the demonstration of negatively birefringent, needle-shaped crystals in synovial fluid polymorphonuclear leukocytes.

2. **Pseudogout.** When acute, this type of arthritis commonly involves three or fewer large, lower extremity joints, especially the knee. Inflammatory changes secondary to calcium pyrophosphate dihydrate crystals can be marked and of intensity similar to gout. Helpful clinical hints include: normal uric acid, presence on x-ray of chondrocalcinosis and, most importantly, the identification of weakly positively birefringent, rhomboid-shaped crystals in the synovial fluid.

F. Serum sickness. Approximately 10 to 14 days after contact with an allergen (e.g., heterologous serum or penicillin), an allergic patient will develop a febrile reaction associated with an acute, at times migratory, polyarthritis. This immune complex–related illness can be diagnosed by the history of drug intake, the appropriate latent period, the presence of a systemic illness (urticaria, adenopathy, nephritis, and neuritis), and abnormal laboratory tests (increased erythrocyte sedimentation rate, increased white blood cell count, eosinophilia, and decreased complement).

G. Sarcoidosis. This granulomatous disease can present as an acute polyarthritis in a pattern known as Löfgren syndrome; that is, association with hilar adenopathy, erythema nodosum, and fever. Ankles and knees are by far the joints most commonly involved. Involvement is symmetrical; often inflammation is periarticular and joint motion may be normal.

H. Henoch-Schönlein purpura. In its fully developed state, this vasculitic syndrome consists of nonthrombocytopenic purpura, arthralgia or mild arthritis, abdominal pain, gastrointestinal hemorrhage, and renal disease. Two-thirds of patients develop a nondeforming polyarthritis, usually after the onset of purpura.

I. Hematologic disorders. Polyarthritis may be the presenting or early manifestation of hematologic diseases such as leukemia, lymphoma, and sickle cell disease. These disorders can be diagnosed by their associated clinical findings, bone marrow examination, or tests for the presence of abnormal hemoglobins. Synovial fluid cytology studies may assist in diagnosis of the neoplastic disorders.

II. Chronic polyarthritis. Arthritis that persists for more than two months is defined as chronic polyarthritis. The following entities can cause this problem.

A. Rheumatoid arthritis usually begins as a slowly progressive polyarthritis with a strong tendency toward symmetrical joint involvement. Other clinical features include female predominance (female-male ratio of 3 : 1), prolonged early morning stiffness, development of typical hand deformities such as ulnar deviation, subcutaneous nodules (20% patients), and positive tests for rheumatoid factor (80% patients).

B. Connective tissue diseases

    1. Systemic lupus erythematosus (SLE). A symmetric, generally nondeforming, nonerosive polyarthritis is a common manifestation of SLE. Although the arthritis can be RA-like, other clinical findings that suggest SLE are fever, skin rash, serositis, nephritis, and central nervous system disease. Although SLE remains a clinical diagnosis, positive tests for the serum antinuclear antibody, found in more than 90% of patients with active disease, are confirmatory of this disorder. Anti-ds DNA antibodies and hypocomplementemia are more specific serologic markers of SLE.

    2. In **scleroderma,** limitation of motion is usually related to skin and periarticular involvement, although a chronic inflammatory polyarthritis may exist.

C. Seronegative spondyloarthropathies. Ankylosing spondylitis (AS), psoriatic arthritis (PA), Reiter syndrome (RS), and the enteropathic arthropathies can all present as chronic polyarthritis. While they can be RA-like, they generally involve large, lower extremity joints in an asymmetrical fashion. In AS, as many as one-third of patients exhibit peripheral joint involvement at some stage; the diagnosis is based on the characteristic spine and sacroiliac disease. The other syndromes are diagnosed on the basis of other clinical findings (e.g., skin rash, urethritis, and bowel disease). Further diagnostic information is found in the chapters concerning these diseases.

D. Chronic crystal-induced disease

    1. Chronic gout. One-third of patients with gout can present with polyarticular involvement. When appropriate treatment is not instituted, a pattern of chronic (rather than episodic) polyarticular arthritis may result. The diagnosis is confirmed by the presence of hyperuricemia, synovial fluid urate crystals, and tophi.

    2. Pseudogout (calcium pyrophosphate crystal deposition disease) may present as a progressive chronic polyarthritis of the hips and knees that is indistinguishable from osteoarthritis. Involvement of more distal joints may mimic chronic RA. The diagnosis is based on radiographic demonstration of chondrocalcinosis and the demonstration of the characteristic calcium pyrophosphate crystals in synovial fluid. Acute pseudogout attacks may be superimposed on a chronic disease pattern.

    3. Osteoarthrosis. Although osteoarthrosis can be erosive and inflammatory in some cases, it generally is not. This degenerative disease most commonly involves the distal interphalangeal joints of the fingers, hips, knees, and lower lumbar and cervical vertebrae. It is further characterized by lack of systemic features and inflammatory signs, development in the elderly, and the presence of Heberden (distal interphalangeal) and Bouchard (proximal interphalangeal) nodes.

E. Sarcoidosis. Sarcoid arthritis may be acute, recurrent, or chronic. Despite chronic or recurrent episodes, the arthritis is usually nondestructive. The diagnosis is based on the demonstration of noncaseating granulomas on synovial biopsy.

8. Muscle Pain and Weakness

J. Robert Polk

Muscle pain and weakness are commonly encountered in clinical medicine. Evaluation of a patient with these symptoms and signs begins with a careful history and thorough physical examination. Family history and medication history are important and should be verified personally by the primary physician. Proximal weakness is the usual symptom and sign of myopathy. Muscle pain may also be present but is experienced less often than weakness. Syndromes of muscular pain and weakness can be divided into neurologic and myopathic categories.

Neurologic Causes

I. **Upper motor neuron disease.** These entities include brain and brainstem hemorrhages, infarctions, and neoplasms. Some demyelinating diseases may present in this category. Spasticity, increased deep tendon reflexes, pathologic reflexes, sensory abnormalities, and impaired cerebral functions may be noted.

II. **Lower motor neuron disease.** Brainstem lesions such as progressive bulbar palsy and poliomyelitis may present with weakness but usually have other features, such as cranial nerve dysfunction, that lead to the correct diagnosis. Anterior horn cell lesions can cause muscle weakness. There is segmental involvement of muscles, which are flaccid; fasciculations and loss of deep tendon reflexes are seen. Sensory abnormalities do not occur. Muscle atrophy occurs early.

III. **Nerve root disease.** These lesions present with muscle weakness if the ventral root is involved. Loss of deep tendon reflexes and muscle atrophy also occur. Muscles are hypotonic. Atrophy is less pronounced than in anterior horn cell lesions. Fasciculations do not occur. Pain and sensory loss may occur with dorsal root dysfunction.

IV. **Peripheral nerve disease.** These entities present with loss of deep tendon reflexes, no fasciculations, and hypotonia. Sensory abnormalities may or may not occur. Characteristically, several peripheral nerves are involved simultaneously. Distal weakness occurs early. These diseases can easily be confused with primary myopathies, especially during later stages when a primary myopathy may have proximal and distal weakness, muscle atrophy, and loss of deep tendon reflexes.

V. **Myoneural junction disease.** Myasthenic syndromes resemble myopathies more than neuropathies. Muscle weakness is often more proximal than distal, without early reflex changes or sensory abnormalities. Myasthenia gravis is characterized by increased muscle fatigue with continued exertion. Improvement occurs with rest. Ocular muscles are frequently involved. An edrophonium test along with electromyography (EMG) can be used to confirm the diagnosis. The Eaton-Lambert syndrome may present with similar features, but repetitive electrical stimulation on EMG causes augmented muscle response at higher frequencies. Drugs that induce a myasthenic syndrome include D-penicillamine and the aminoglycoside antibiotics.

Myopathic Causes

The major causes of myopathy are drugs, toxins, metabolic disturbances, inflammatory syndromes, endocrinopathies, infections, and muscle dystrophies.

I. **Toxin- and drug-induced myopathy**

   A. **Steroid myopathy.** The insidious onset of proximal muscle weakness in a patient on steroids should suggest steroid myopathy. Myopathy may occur while on low- or high-dose steroids, frequently after a recent increase in dosage. Duration of steroid treatment does not correlate with the time of onset. Patients with steroid myopathy frequently have at least two other steroid side effects, such as osteoporosis, Cushingoid facies, hyperglycemia, hypertension, or psychiatric disorders. Concomitant hypokalemia has not been seen. Serum muscle enzymes—creatine phosphokinase (CPK), aldolase, and serum glutamic oxalacetic transaminase (SGOT)—are not increased; urinary creatine excretion, however, is increased. Electromyographic studies give conflicting results and are not helpful. Muscle biopsy in patients with Cushing syndrome has shown predominantly type II fiber atrophy, but biopsy in steroid myopathy has given conflicting results and has not been helpful. Inflammation is not present. Treatment is to reduce the steroid dose to as low as possible or to discontinue the drug.

B. Hypokalemic myopathy. Any drug or pathologic condition causing hypokalemia can probably cause muscle weakness. Several drugs have been implicated, some with better substantiation than others. An acute syndrome of muscle pain, tenderness, and weakness of proximal and axial muscles may be seen. More generalized weakness may also occur. Serum muscle enzymes are elevated and muscle biopsy may show vacuolar myopathy, with or without fiber necrosis and regeneration. EMG may show myopathic changes of polymyositis (see Chap. 33). Reflexes may be depressed or absent. Chronic hypokalemia can result in a painless proximal or generalized myopathy, also with depressed or absent reflexes. As in the acute syndrome, serum muscle enzymes are elevated and muscle biopsy shows vacuolar myopathy. Diagnosis is based on demonstration of hypokalemia and identification of the offending drug.

Drugs usually implicated are diuretics and cathartics. Treatment is restoration of the normal serum potassium level.

C. Alcoholic myopathy. Alcohol has been shown to be a direct hepatotoxin; proof of its muscle toxicity still rests largely on clinical interpretations. Three types of myopathy caused by alcohol are seen.

1. Acute. This form presents with cramps and, at times, with fulminant rhabdomyolysis and myoglobinuria, which usually occur together with swelling and tenderness of proximal muscles. Muscle enzymes are markedly elevated. Muscle biopsy shows necrosis and phagocytosis with little regeneration. Recovery occurs with abstinence.

2. Chronic. This form is least common and may occur even in the absence of a history of the acute clinical variety, described in the preceding section. Proximal muscles are weak, atrophic, and mildly tender. Unless alcoholic neuropathy is also present, distal muscle strength remains intact. Muscle enzymes are moderately elevated and EMG shows myopathic changes. Lower extremities are affected more prominently than distal extremities, with both atrophy and tenderness. Histopathologic findings include fiber necrosis, a mild increase in fibrous tissue, focal fat infiltration, a large variability in muscle fiber size, and regeneration of fibers.

3. Subclinical. In this form, muscle enzyme elevation occurs without clinical weakness, and is quite common in confirmed alcoholics. Diagnosis of alcoholic myopathy is based on the standard tests mentioned previously (enzymes, EMG, and muscle biopsy), but it should be remembered that a coexistent peripheral neuropathy caused by nutritional deficiency or other toxin may be present.

D. Drug-induced rhabdomyolysis and myoglobinuria. Features include severe muscle pain with swelling and tenderness, markedly elevated serum muscle enzymes, and gross (dark red-brown) pigmenturia. The urine is positive by "dipstick" (benzidine or orthotolidin). If hemolysis is suspected, the urine is reddish; the serum is pink; and a low serum haptoglobin is present. Immunoassays and electrophoresis can definitively differentiate hemoglobin and myoglobin and, in doubtful instances, should be done. Renal failure is the worst consequence of myoglobinemic states. Emphasis from the outset should be placed on maintaining urinary output with furosemide and mannitol, as needed. Other acute lab abnormalities are hypocalcemia and hyperkalemia.

There are several drugs and toxins that can induce acute rhabdomyolysis: Included are heroin, amphetamines, alcohol, plasmocid (an antimalarial drug), anesthetics, and other drugs that cause hypokalemia. Other causes of myoglobinuria not related to drugs include McArdle disease, phosphofructokinase deficiency, exertion, crush injury, ischemia, and malignant hyperthermia syndrome.

II. Metabolic myopathies

A. **Disorders of glycogen metabolism.** This is a group of closely related disorders characterized by an inborn error of glycogen metabolism. There are eight distinct enzyme abnormalities, five of which cause myopathic symptoms. Three of these disorders present solely as myopathies.

1. **Acid maltase deficiency.** The infantile form (Pompe disease) presents a few months after birth with diffuse muscle weakness, severe hypotonia, and cardiomyopathy with congestive heart failure. Death caused by cardiorespiratory failure occurs within two years. The adult or late-onset form is caused by a partial deficiency of acid maltase activity. The late-onset form presents in childhood or adult life with gradually progressive limb-girdle weakness. The pelvic girdle muscles are more involved than the shoulder muscles. Clinical heart or liver involvement has not been seen. Respiratory muscles are involved in 25% to 50% of cases, leading to chronic respiratory insufficiency. The late-onset may be mistaken for polymyositis, limb-girdle dystrophy, or spinal muscular atrophy.

   Serum CPK is increased, and the EMG changes are similar to those of polymyositis. Muscle biopsy shows a vacuolar myopathy. Biochemical assay revealing decreased or absent activity in muscle confirms the diagnosis. Also useful in diagnosis is decreased urinary excretion of acid maltase. There is no proven effective therapy for the infantile or late-onset forms.

2. **Muscle phosphorylase deficiency (McArdle disease).** This inherited deficiency of skeletal muscle phosphorylase is more common than acid maltase deficiency or phosphofructokinase deficiency; 60 cases have been reported. The male-female ratio is 4 : 1. Childhood symptoms of fatigue are usually overlooked. A characteristic pattern of exercise-induced muscle pains, stiffness, and weakness, which resolve with rest, occurs after puberty. Prolonged exercise results in severe cramps of the exerted muscles. Myoglobinuria and muscle necrosis may occur if exercise is strenuous; however, there may be improved exercise tolerance after a nonstrenuous warm-up period (i.e., the "second wind phenomenon"). As the result of recurrent attacks of myoglobinuria, some patients have a persistent proximal myopathy. The muscle cramps are actually contractures which may last several hours. Serum CPK is increased. Venous lactic acid levels do not rise with the ischemic forearm exercise test. Muscle biopsy shows PAS-positive vacuoles beneath the sarcolemma and scattered necrotic or regenerating muscle fibers. There is no long-term effective treatment.

3. **Muscle phosphofructokinase deficiency.** Phosphofructokinase (PFK) deficiency results in a syndrome similar to McArdle disease. Easy fatigability occurs during childhood. Later, exercise-induced muscle pain or cramps with myoglobinuria occur. However, unlike those of McArdle disease, PFK's exercise-induced symptoms often include nausea and vomiting. It is an autosomal recessive disease. Serum CPK is increased. Venous lactate levels do not rise after the ischemic forearm exercise test. A mild hemolytic anemia occurs when PFK is absent from erythrocytes; this occurrence may be helpful diagnostically. Diagnosis is confirmed by absence of PFK activity on direct measurement in muscle biopsy by biochemical or histochemical methods. Therapeutic attempts have not been reported as yet; glucose infusions or glucagon would not help acutely as happens in McArdle disease.

B. Disorders of lipid metabolism. Glycogen provides energy for short duration work while fatty acids provide energy for periods of rest, low intensity prolonged exercise, and fasting. This knowledge allows prediction of the symptoms of abnormal fatty acid metabolism in muscle.

1. **Carnitine palmityltransferase (CPT) deficiency** is inherited as an autosomal recessive disorder with a male preponderance. Patients with CPT deficiency tolerate short periods of exercise normally. However, after prolonged exercise or fasting, patients develop muscular pains and myoglobinuria. Muscle strength is normal between attacks. There is no second wind phenomenon. Serum CPK is normal at rest but elevated during attacks. There is a normal rise in venous lactate with ischemic forearm exercise test. Hypertriglyceridemia, which is probably related to the impaired fatty acid utilization of CPT deficiency, may be found. The muscle biopsy may be normal or show intrafiber lipid droplets. A screening test is a 38-hour fast which will cause an elevation in serum CPK. Diagnosis is confirmed by biochemical assay of CPT activity in muscle. Therapy consists of avoiding prolonged exertion and eating regular meals. A diet high in carbohydrates and low in fats is effective in reducing the incidence of acute attacks.

2. **Carnitine deficiency** is probably inherited in an autosomal recessive pattern. It occurs as an isolated muscle carnitine deficiency and as a systemic carnitine deficiency. The muscle carnitine deficiency is characterized by childhood onset of a slowly progressive limb-girdle weakness. Fascial and pharyngeal muscles may be involved. Deep tendon reflexes are decreased or absent. Serum CPK is moderately increased. EMG reveals a myopathic pattern. Serum carnitine levels are normal or slightly decreased. Muscle biopsy shows prominent intrafiber lipid droplets, especially in type I fibers. Carnitine levels in muscle are reduced one-tenth to one-fifth of normal. Preferred long-term treatment is oral administration of carnitine with a medium chain triglyceride diet. Prednisone is effective but not desirable in long-term treatment. The systemic carnitine deficiency presents with the myopathy and hepatic insufficiency. Hepatic encephalopathy and attacks of lactic acidosis occur. Death occurs usually by age 20. In the systemic deficiency, patients uniformly have decreased levels of serum carnitine. Treatment with oral carnitine resulted in improved strength and normalization of hepatic function in a single patient so treated.

C. Disorders associated with abnormal serum potassium. These interrelated syndromes of muscular weakness are associated with either hypokalemia or hyperkalemia. The exact pathogenetic role of potassium in the disorders is largely unknown.

1. **Familial periodic paralysis.** An autosomal dominant disease, this disorder is characterized by attacks of intense weakness of limb muscles that progress to complete paralysis. Attacks begin in adolescence or early adulthood and occur less frequently with age. There is marked hypotonia and absent to decreased tendon reflexes during attacks. Strenuous exercise or a high carbohydrate intake may precipitate attacks. Chronic myopathy after repeated attacks may occur. Serum CPK is elevated during attacks. Muscle biopsy shows vacuolar changes. The serum potassium is low during the attacks. Treatment is with oral potassium (2 to 8 gm potassium chloride until the attack resolves) or intravenous potassium (50 mEq over several hours). Hyperaldosteronism, exogenous diuretics or cathartics, and hyperthyroidism with periodic paralysis may mimic the syndrome.

2. **Adynamia episodica hereditaria (Gamstorp disease).** This autosomal dominant disease is characterized by attacks of weakness or paralysis of skeletal muscle, similar to those of familial periodic paralysis. The onset is between ages 5 and 10 years. The disease is most active during adolescent years, after which it subsides. Attacks are precipitated by prolonged exertion or by administration of 2 to 5 gm potassium chloride. During attacks the serum potassium

is elevated, although high normal values have been noted. Between attacks the patient is asymptomatic and serum potassium is normal, although persistent weakness may last for several days after an attack. Serum CPK is elevated. Therapy with potassium-lowering agents such as hydrochlorothiazide 50 to 100 mg PO daily is effective in preventing attacks.

III. Endocrine myopathies

A. Hypothyroid myopathy. The most commonly recognized endocrine myopathy occurs as a feature of hypothyroidism; it may antedate the diagnosis of hypothyroidism by several months. Symptoms and signs of this entity range from mild aches and pains, muscle cramps, and proximal weakness to apparent muscle hypertrophy and the mounding phenomenon, or myoedema (a transient focal ridging of muscle in response to percussing or pinching the muscle). In the usual form, proximal weakness may be observed, although atrophy is rare. Hypertrophic muscles may exhibit myotoniclike contractions that are electrically silent on EMG. Serum CPK is often markedly elevated. A variety of EMG changes have been noticed, most of which indicate a myopathic process. Muscle biopsy may show focal necrosis, regeneration, and vacuolization of fibers, but is usually normal. Fiber size is quite variable. Sarcolemma nuclei are numerous, enlarged, and centrally placed. Mucoprotein deposits occur in one-third of patients. Histochemical staining has shown a decrease in type II fibers which is directly proportional to disease severity and serum CPK levels. CPK levels are not increased in hypopituitarism, and a myopathy has not been reported with hypopituitarism; nonetheless, for a patient with hypothyroidism, hypopituitarism should be ruled out. Treatment of hypothyroidism is thyroid hormone replacement. With proper therapy, serum CPK levels will return to normal over several months.

B. Thyrotoxic myopathy. The manifestations of this disorder range from complaints of diffuse weakness, easy fatigability, and mild atrophy to severe proximal muscle weakness with pronounced atrophy. Laryngeal and pharyngeal muscles are not involved. Serum muscle enzymes are not elevated, even in the severe form; creatinuria, however, is present. EMG may show myopathic changes. Muscle biopsy may reveal only small fiber size or atrophy of fibers with replacement of fat and lymphocyte infiltrates. (Less common myopathies in association with hyperthyroidism are exophthalmic ophthalmoplegia, thryotoxic periodic paralysis, and the association of Graves disease in 5% of patients with myasthenia gravis.)

C. Acromegalic myopathy. Proximal muscle weakness and easy fatigability occur in up to 50% of patients with acromegaly. Myalgias and cramps may occur in a few patients. Muscle mass, however, is increased. Serum CPK and aldolase are usually normal but may be slightly elevated. EMG shows myopathic findings. Muscle biopsy shows no consistent pattern, but there is some evidence that type II fiber hypertrophy is specific for acromegaly. With treatment of the pituitary tumor, recovery of strength occurs gradually over months or years.

IV. Muscular dystrophy.
This group of primary muscle diseases is characterized by degeneration of muscle fibers, which occurs on a genetic basis. Although there is no specific treatment for these disorders, it is important to distinguish them from treatable forms of myopathy. Genetic counseling is suggested for patients and their families.

A. Duchenne pseudohypertrophic muscular dystrophy. This sex-linked disease has a usual onset in early childhood and is characterized by pelvic girdle involvement, manifested by frequent falls, difficulty in climbing stairs, difficulty in rising from the floor, and a peculiar gait. Onset is insidious and progression is slow. Gradually the trunk and shoulder muscles become involved, causing the patient to require a wheelchair by age 12. Patients usually die in their twenties of either pulmonary infection or the cardiomyopathy associated with the disease. Physical examination early in the disease reveals enlarged, firm (pseudohypertrophic), but weak calves and sometimes quadriceps and deltoids. Facial and distal muscles usually retain normal strength. Serum muscle enzymes are increased. Elevated creatinuria is present. Muscle biopsy shows fiber size variation and fat infiltration, depending on the stage of the disease. EMG reveals low amplitude potentials of short duration. Electrocardiographic abnormalities such as prolonged PR interval, slurred QRS complex, ST segment depression or elevation, and usually right bundle branch block are seen late in the disease. Female carriers may have mild abnormalities in serum CPK, muscle biopsy, and EMG, but are clinically asymptomatic.

B. Fascioscapulohumeral dystrophy. This is an autosomal dominant disease which affects males and females equally. The usual age of onset is between 9 and 20 years, although adult onset has been recognized. The symptoms vary in severity; thus diagnosis may be difficult. Shoulder girdle weakness and a winged scapula are usually the first findings. Facial muscles are always involved and may be the earliest muscles affected in some patients. The face is flattened and the mouth moves asymmetrically, unable to pucker or whistle. Axial and pelvic muscles may become involved late in the disease; however, distal muscles are usually spared. Cardiac disease is rare, and patients usually live a normal life span. Serum muscle enzymes may be elevated slightly, and elevated urinary creatine is common.

C. Limb-girdle dystrophy. This disease is inherited in an autosomal recessive form and affects males and females equally. Its onset occurs during the second or third decades. Shoulder or pelvic girdle muscles are involved first, with gradual progression to other muscle sites over years, although facial muscles are spared. Cardiac disease due to limb-girdle dystrophy is rare. Serum muscle enzymes are slightly elevated and creatinuria is present. Muscle biopsy shows fibrous and fatty replacement with necrosis of single fibers. Sarcolemmal nuclei are increased in number, forming chains centrally in the fibers. These changes may also be seen in Duchenne dystrophy and fascioscapulohumeral dystrophy.

D. Myotonic dystrophy. Myotonia is an inability to relax a muscle normally after its contraction. It may be elicited by grasping with the hand or by direct percussion of muscle groups such as the forearm, tongue, or thumb adductors. Myotonic dystrophy is an inherited disease that begins early in adult life. It is manifested by distal muscle weakness and atrophy. Deep tendon reflexes are reduced. Ptosis may be present and closure of the eyelids is also weak. Atrophy of temporalis muscles and sternocleidomastoids is severe. Other clinical features include early frontal alopecia, cataracts, blepharitis, conjunctivitis, and testicular atrophy. Mental retardation is common. Dystrophic cardiac disease occurs late. The disease can be quite variable, and some patients and affected family members may manifest only one or two features. EMG reveals myopathic changes and characteristic afterpotentials of myotonia. Serum muscle enzymes are usually normal, and creatinuria is rare. Histopathologic features are similar to other dystrophies; however, there may be prominent rows of sarcolemmal nuclei, spirals of myofibrils, and areas of clear sarcoplasm, devoid of myofibrils. Type I fiber atrophy is present. Peripheral nerves and anterior horn cells are normal. Quinine, 300 to 600 mg orally every 6 hours, can relieve the myotonia; however, there is no known treatment. Supportive therapy and physical therapy may prolong mobility and prevent contractures.

E. Congenital myopathies. This group of myopathies are rare, inherited diseases that begin during infancy. Progression may be quite insidious. Diagnosis rests on muscle biopsy.

V. Inflammatory myopathy. This group of myopathies is characterized by inflammation of unknown etiology within the muscles. For full discussions of idiopathic polymyositis, dermatomyositis, myositis of other rheumatic diseases, and myositis of carcinoma, refer to Chapter 33.

A. Sarcoid myopathy. Random muscle biopsies in small numbers of sarcoid patients without symptoms of muscle pain or weakness have revealed noncaseating granulomas typical of the disease. The occurrence of asymptomatic muscle involvement has clouded the issue of whether or not a true sarcoid myopathy exists. Nonetheless, there are sarcoid patients with symptomatic muscle involvement. Muscle pain and tenderness are most often seen in acute sarcoidosis with erythema nodosum. A symmetric proximal muscle weakness can be seen in chronic sarcoid. EMG shows a nonspecific myopathic pattern. Muscle biopsy shows noncaseating granulomas, surrounding lymphocytic infiltrates, muscle fiber necrosis, and fiber regeneration. Response to prednisone, 20 to 40 mg daily, has been effective in about half of patients. It should be noted that similar granulomatous reactions have been seen in various malignancies, leprosy, syphilis, tuberculosis, Crohn disease, drug reactions, and several fungal infections.

VI. Infectious myositis and myopathy. Several microorganisms have been implicated in the onset of myositis. Both diffuse and proximal myopathies have been reported. This group of myopathies are to be distinguished from isolated muscle involvement such as tropical pyomyositis, streptococcal myositis, and clostridial myonecrosis.

A. Trichinosis. This disease is caused by the nematode *Trichinella spiralis*. It is transmitted by ingestion of uncooked or poorly cooked pork or bear meat. Within two days of ingestion of the cysts, diarrhea, nausea, abdominal pain, and fever occur. By the end of the first week, patients may have fever, periorbital edema, conjunctivitis, muscle pain and tenderness, and an erythematous maculopapular rash. Muscle weakness may be mild but is often quite severe. Muscle invasion may last six weeks. Myocarditis and encephalitis may occur during this stage of illness. The larvae invade only skeletal muscle, not the central nervous system or myocardium. The most commonly invaded muscles are the muscles of the diaphragm, eye, tongue, shoulder, and calf. Deltoid or gastrocnemius muscle biopsy, revealing uncalcified larvae, should be done during the third or fourth week of illness. Pressing the tissue between glass slides will reveal the larvae. Calcified cysts represent former infection. The muscle shows a severe myositis with neutrophilic, eosinophilic, and lymphocytic infiltrates. Fiber degeneration and necrosis are present. Serum muscle enzymes are characteristically elevated. By the end of the second week, there is a 15% to 50% eosinophilia. Serologic tests become positive by the end of the third week. The best single serologic test is the bentonite flocculation test; since any single test may be falsely negative, however, either a complement fixation test or indirect fluorescent antibody test should also be done. Treatment is with thiabendazole, 25 mg/kg twice daily for 7 days. Patients with myocarditis, encephalitis, or severe hypersensitivity manifestations should be treated with prednisone, 40 mg daily, during thiabendazole administration.

B. Toxoplasmosis. *Toxoplasma gondii* has been proven to cause myositis in an occasional patient. A recent case report of a patient with polymyositis and cerebellar ataxia is an example of this problem. The patient had severe muscle cramps, coarse fasciculations, and no weakness or muscle tenderness. Serum CPK was markedly elevated. EMG indicated a chronic peripheral neuropathy. Muscle biopsy showed chronic interstitial myositis, fiber necrosis, and encysted *T. gondii*. Toxoplasma organisms were grown in mice injected with a suspension of the muscle biopsy.

Serologic evidence of toxoplasma infection in patients with polymyositis consists of elevated complement fixation titers and Sabin-Feldman dye tests in a subgroup of polymyositis, not dermatomyositis, patients. These patients had none of the common manifestations of *T. gondii* infection.

C. Viral myositis. A number of different viruses may cause an illness similar to polymyositis. Often there is a prodromal illness caused by the virus. It is unclear if the myositis is a postinfectious immune phenomenon or a true infection of muscle. Viral-like particles have been found in muscle in some cases. Serum muscle enzymes are elevated. Muscle biopsy shows myositis with fiber necrosis and regeneration. Myoglobinuria may occur, especially with influenza and herpes group myositis. Viruses implicated are hepatitis B, ECHO virus, coxsackievirus, herpes zoster, herpes simplex, and influenza. Late atrophy of muscles may occur. In addition, muscle biopsy at times may be normal.

D. Miscellaneous infections causing myopathy. It should be noted that numerous other microorganisms have been implicated as etiologic agents in myositis. Some have been noted to occur only in immunocompromised patients. Agents found include *Candida tropicalis, Mycoplasma pneumoniae, Trypanosoma cruzi,* and *Echinococcus alveolaris.*

VII. Fibromyalgia. Fibromyalgia presents as variable muscle pain with normal muscle strength. Concomitant anxiety or depression is common. The sedimentation rate and muscle enzymes are normal. It is a diagnosis of exclusion. (See Chap. 22 for a full discussion.)

VIII. Polymyalgia rheumatica (PMR). PMR presents with symptoms of muscle pain. It occurs usually in females and rarely before age 50. The sedimentation rate is very high. It should be noted that Westergren sedimentation rates up to 20 mm/hr in males and 30 mm/hr in females over 50 years of age are normal. Anemia is common. (See Chap. 32 for a full discussion.)

IX. Miscellaneous disorders presenting as myopathy. These disorders may present with muscle pain:

A. Primary amyloidosis.

B. Stiff man syndrome.

C. Cervical and lumbar spondylosis.

D. Parkinson disease.

E. Paget disease of bone.

Laboratory Aids to Diagnosis

I. Serum chemistries. As a result of the association of hypokalemia, hyperkalemia, hypocalcemia, hypercalcemia, hypomagnesemia, and hypophosphatemia with muscle weakness, tetany, and sometimes cramps, it is prudent to obtain serum chemistry values if clinical suspicion so indicates. Muscle enzymes commonly measured are creatine phosphokinase (CPK), aldolase, lactic dehydragenase (LDH), and serum glutamic oxalacetic transaminase (SGOT). CPK is probably the most reliable indicator of muscle damage since skeletal muscle, compared to other tissues, contains more of it. However, heart, brain, and smooth muscle also contain CPK. SGOT and LDH activities can arise in the liver, following damage and hemolysis, as well as in other damaged tissues. Aldolase originates in skeletal muscle. Strenuous physical exertion may increase CPK up to four times its normal level. Intramuscular injections may increase CPK sevenfold and cause elevated values for a week. Serum myoglobin has been looked for in polymyositis, where it is elevated in 75% of patients. Immunoassay and electrophoresis should be done to detect myoglobinemia. Plasma cortisol, growth hormone, and thyroxine values are indicated if one of these endocrine myopathies is suspected. CPK may also be elevated in amyotrophic lateral sclerosis (ALS).

II. Hematologic studies. The erythrocyte sedimentation rate may be elevated in any inflammatory myopathy. It is useful when following patients but is not an absolute test for any myopathy. Atypical lymphocytosis may occur in viral illness or toxoplasmosis. Eosinophilia may occur in infections and polymyositis. Cold agglutinins may indicate mycoplasma infection.

III. Urinary studies. Steroid myopathy and some muscular dystrophies may have elevated creatine-creatinine urinary excretion ratios with normal muscle enzymes:

$$\% \text{ creatinuria} = \frac{\text{creatine (mg/24 hr)}}{[\text{creatine} + \text{creatinine}] \text{ (mg/24 hr)}} \times 100$$

This ratio is calculated on at least two 24-hour urine collections as a result of collection and day-to-day variability. Greater than 6% ratio in adults is elevated.

Urinary studies for heavy metals may be useful if a peripheral neuropathy is suspected. Myoglobinuria occurs in several diseases of muscle. Both hemoglobin and myoglobin give positive reactions to orthotolidin and benzidine. Immunoassay and electrophoresis techniques can measure myoglobin. The ammonium sulfate test has often proven unreliable or difficult to interpret. Excretion of acid maltase is decreased in acid maltase deficiency.

IV. Provocative studies

A. Ischemic forearm exercise test. This test is of value in detecting myophosphorylase deficiency (McArdle disease) and phosphofructokinase deficiency. The test is done with the patient at rest and fasting. After obtaining a baseline venous lactate level through an indwelling catheter, a blood pressure cuff on the upper arm is inflated above systolic pressure. The patient exercises this arm for one minute to produce lactic acid. Sufficient work can be generated by compressing another blood pressure cuff at a rate of one stroke per second; a rise in the mercury column can then be observed. After 1 minute of exercise, the cuff is deflated and serial lactate levels are obtained at 1, 3, 5, 10, and 20 minutes after work. A normal peak occurs at 3 minutes. Patients with myophosphorylase deficiency will not show a rise in venous lactate. However, a decreased lactate production is also seen in debrancher deficiency, phosphofructokinase deficiency, and following alcohol ingestion in alcoholics and normals. In addition to decreased lactate production, patients with myophosphorylase deficiency will develop a progressive contracture of forearm muscle which is electrically silent on EMG.

B. Edrophonium (Tensilon) test. This test is used to diagnose myasthenia gravis. It should be done in a double-blind fashion. Edrophonium, 10 mg, is prepared in a syringe. Atropine is also prepared in case a cholinergic crisis caused by edrophonium arises. Edrophonium, 2 mg, is given IV as a test dose. If no adverse reaction (cholinergic crisis) occurs, then 1 minute later the remaining edrophonium, 8 mg, is given IV. By observing previously weak muscles gain strength within 1 to 5 minutes, the diagnosis of myasthenia gravis is confirmed. Effects will wear off in 5 minutes.

V. Electromyography and electroneurography.
Nerve conduction velocities are an informative way to detect peripheral neuropathies. Diseases such as infectious polyneuritis (Landry-Guillain-Barré syndrome), Charcot-Marie-Tooth disease, and several others characteristically show slowed nerve conduction velocity.

EMG abnormalities are helpful in the diagnosis of polymyositis, myasthenia gravis, myotonic dystrophy, Eaton-Lambert syndrome, and McArdle disease. Characteristic findings in polymyositis are mentioned in Chapter 33. Note, however, that trichinosis and several muscular dystrophies may cause a myopathic EMG pattern similar to that of polymyositis. In myasthenia gravis, repetitive stimulation gives a characteristic decremental conduction, which is opposite to the pattern seen in Eaton-Lambert syndrome. In myotonic dystrophy, electrical silence after a brief voluntary contraction does not occur; instead, there is a burst of electrical activity which subsides in minutes. In McArdle disease, the muscular cramping which occurs is electrically silent.

VI. Muscle biopsy.
This procedure is of major diagnostic value in inflammatory muscle disease, steroid myopathy, muscular dystrophy, and infectious myositis. It is also valuable in the diagnosis of myopathy associated with various connective tissue diseases, including vasculitis. The site for a muscle biopsy should be the deltoid or quadriceps in most cases. EMG abnormalities identify areas of pathology. The contralateral muscle should be biopsied. The EMG needles may produce artifactual change; therefore, muscles used in the EMG study should not be biopsied. The muscle chosen for biopsy should not be atrophic or severely weak.

Bibliography

Askari, A., Vignos, P. J., and Moskowitz, R. W.   Steroid myopathy in connective tissue disease. *Am. J. Med.* 61:485, 1976.

Bland, J. H., et al.   Rheumatic syndromes in endocrine disease. *Semin. Arthritis Rheum.* 9:23, 1979.

Bosch, E. P., and Munsat, T. L.   Metabolic Myopathies. In W. K. Hass (Ed.), *Medical Clinics of North America*. Philadelphia: Saunders, 1979.

Gamboa, E. T., et al.   Isolation of influenza virus from muscle in myoglobinuric polymyositis. *Neurology* 29:1323, 1979.

Lane, R. J. M., and Mastaglia, F. L.   Drug-induced myopathies in man. *Lancet* 2:562, 1978.

Perkoff, G. T.   Alcoholic myopathy. *Ann. Rev. Med.* 22:125, 1971.

Phillips, P. E., Kassan, S. S., and Kagen, L. J.   Increased toxoplasma antibodies in idiopathic inflammatory muscle disease. *Arthritis Rheum.* 22:209, 1979.

Rubin, E.   Alcoholic myopathy in heart and skeletal muscle. *N. Engl. J. Med.* 301:28, 1979.

Tang, T. T., Sedmak, G. V., Siegesmund, K. A., and McCreadie, S. R.   Chronic myopathy associated with coxsackievirus type A9. *N. Engl. J. Med.* 292:608, 1975.

9. Enteropathic Arthritis

Allan Gibofsky

Enteropathic arthritis refers to the particular pattern of joint manifestations that occurs in association with, or as a complication of, particular chronic inflammatory bowel syndromes, notably ulcerative colitis (UC) and regional enteritis (RE). Both these conditions are of unknown etiology, but while the anatomic portions of the intestinal tract are primarily distinct for each, their similar clinical features, notably the patterns of joint involvement, permit their grouping in this chapter. Also included are the rheumatic syndromes that occur in conjunction with intestinal bypass, pancreatic disease, and Whipple disease, as well as so-called reactive arthritis, which follows episodes of acute dysentery. The reader is referred to any standard textbook of medicine for discussion of these diseases.

I. Inflammatory bowel syndromes

A. Pathogenesis

1. Both UC and RE have been associated with two patterns of arthritis, **peripheral** and **axial**, the latter indistinguishable from idiopathic ankylosing spondylitis.

   a. Peripheral arthritis is seen in 12% of UC patients and 20% of RE patients; axial disease occurs in approximately 6% of both groups.

2. **Seronegativity for rheumatoid factor** is a consistent feature in both forms, occurring in nearly all patients; other extraarticular manifestations (e.g., erythema nodosum, uveitis) have been seen in both.

3. **Sex incidence** is approximately equal for peripheral arthritis in both UC and RE; slight increased male predominance is reported in axial disease.

4. 75% of patients with axial disease are positive for HLA-B27; no altered frequency of any human leukocyte antigen (HLA) occurs in peripheral disease.

B. Diagnosis

1. **Peripheral arthritis**

   a. Begins abruptly; follows an oligoarticular (usually three joints or less), often migratory, pattern.

   b. Knees and ankles most common joints affected.

   c. Duration of individual attacks usually less than 2 months in 75% of patients.

   d. Most attacks and flares occur in conjunction with flares of underlying bowel disease (75%) or other extraenteric manifestations. Alternately, joint symptoms may be delayed in onset up to ten years following bowel symptoms (25%).

   e. **Laboratory data**

      (1) Synovial membrane often indistinguishable from that in rheumatoid arthritis (RA): fluid, cell counts variable 4,000 to 40,000 per cubic millimeter, usually 70% to 90% polymorphs; protein is low; CH50, normal.

      (2) Erythrocyte sedimentation rate (ESR) and white blood cell (WBC) count increased, in proportion to bowel disease; Hgb correspondingly decreased.

      (3) Radiographic findings are nonspecific for most patients. Usually soft tissue swelling or mild periostitis with juxtaarticular osteoporosis is seen.

f. Differential diagnosis

(1) Migratory pattern may be confused with that of rheumatic fever.

(2) Monoarticular presentation may suggest gout, pseudogout, or infectious arthropathy.

(3) RA, although usually seropositive, may coexist with inflammatory bowel disease; can sometimes exclude by degree of joint deformity and temporal association with underlying bowel symptoms.

2. Spondylitis

a. Clinically indistinguishable from idiopathic ankylosing spondylitis.

b. Often antedates appearance of underlying bowel disease by several months to many years.

c. No correlation between intensity of bowel disease and spinal symptoms exists.

d. Laboratory and radiographic features are indistinguishable from those of ankylosing spondylitis.

e. Differential diagnosis

(1) Given temporal dissociation from bowel disease, other causes of low back syndrome should be excluded (see Chap. 15).

C. Therapy

1. Therapy should be directed against underlying bowel disease, since symptoms may abate with control.

2. Conservative management of arthritis should be attempted; salicylates and nonsteroidal antiinflammatory drugs (e.g., indocin, phenylbutazone) may be contraindicated during acute bowel episodes.

3. Intraarticular steroid administration may be useful; systemic steroid therapy is rarely indicated for control of joint symptoms alone.

4. Resection of diseased bowel may prevent recurrence of acute attacks of peripheral disease; it will have little, if any, effect on axial disease.

D. Prognosis

1. Peripheral form prognosis usually good, even with repeated attacks; 25% of patients have minor limitation or contracture.

2. Axial disease prognosis similar to that of idiopathic ankylosing spondylitis; spinal symptoms and activity of bowel disease tend to be independent.

II. Intestinal bypass arthritis

Jejunoileal bypass, which is performed as a last resort in therapy of morbid obesity, has been associated with a particular symmetric erosive polyarthritis at an approximate frequency of 33%. Symptoms may occur within a few weeks following surgery, or as long after as three years, and are not related to amount of weight lost or other complications. Spontaneous remission of symptoms, often experienced within one year, is the rule, and relapse is uncommon. Routine laboratory studies of blood, synovial fluid, and stool, including culture, have been unrewarding; radiographs of affected joints are similarly nondiagnostic. Circulating levels of cryoproteins and immune complexes may parallel disease activity in selected patients. Joint symptoms have been successfully managed in certain patients with nonsteroidal antiinflammatory drugs (see Appendix G) in usual dosages.

III. Arthritis of pancreatic disease.
Although uncommon, pancreatic carcinoma or chronic pancreatitis may be associated with nodular subcutaneous fat necrosis, and is clinically indistinguishable from erythema nodosum. In almost half of this group, a nonarticular or oligoarticular nondeforming arthritis involving primarily the large

joints of the lower extremity is a feature. The synovial fluid aspirated from affected joints is generally noninflammatory. Elevated levels of the pancreatic enzymes amylase and lipase have been reported in serum and in aspirated body fluids, suggesting that the lesions seen are manifestations of enzyme activity. The severity of arthritis is seemingly related to the severity of the underlying pancreatic condition; if the patient recovers, no further joint symptoms will develop.

IV. **Whipple disease.** A peripheral, episodic, migratory, nondeforming polyarthritis has been reported in 65% to 90% of patients with this unusual condition, thought to occur in middle age as a result of infection of the lamina propria of intestinal mucosa by characteristically rod-shaped organisms. Spondylitislike symptoms are rarely observed. In most cases, joint symptoms occur several months or even years before the onset of gastrointestinal manifestations, thus obscuring diagnosis. Indeed, joint symptoms may actually improve with the onset of bowel symptoms. Treatment with tetracycline, 1 gm PO daily for 1 year, results in improvement of all symptoms, including arthralgia, usually within 1 month of starting therapy.

V. **Reactive arthritis.** A classical Reiter syndrome may occur following infectious diarrhea caused by *Shigella, Salmonella*, or *Yersinia enterocolitica*. Symptoms are more likely to develop in the HLA-B27 positive individual, thus supporting the concept of genetic predisposition to infection and its sequellae (see Chaps. 5 and 35).

Bibliography

Ferguson, R. H.   Enteropathic arthritis. In D. J. McCarty (Ed.), *Arthritis*. Philadelphia: Lea & Febiger, 1979.

McEwen, C., et al.   A comparative study of ankylosing spondylitis and spondylitis accompanying U.C., regional enteritis, psoriasis and Reiters disease. *Arthritis Rheum.* 14:291, 1971.

Moll, J. M. H., and Wright, V.   *Seronegative Polyarthritis*. Amsterdam: Elsevier, 1976.

10. Rash and Arthritis

Michael I. Jacobs

The differential diagnosis of rash and arthritis is complex. Knowledge of the plethora of cutaneous manifestations of the arthritic diseases is important in making a correct diagnosis. A complete examination of the body surface is essential, because it may reveal lesions of psoriasis or discoid lupus erythematosus (DLE) that are hidden in the scalp, psoriatic pitting of the nails, or infiltration of old scars secondary to sarcoidosis.

The purpose of this chapter is to provide the physician with diagnostic information about specific cutaneous findings in each disorder. Where applicable, the newer immunofluorescent techniques, which may help confirm the diagnosis, will be described.

I. **Behcet syndrome.** Originally described as the triad of iritis and recurrent oral and genital ulcerations, Behcet syndrome is a multisystem disease involving the eyes, mucous membranes, skin, blood vessels, joints, bowel, kidneys, and nervous system.

   A. **The oral lesions** resemble aphthous stomatitis, and begin as small areas of macular erythema that then develop into superficial grey ulcers. Larger, deeper ulcerations occasionally occur.

   B. **Genital ulcerations** are most frequently located on the scrotum and labia, but may also be found on the penis or in the vagina.

   C. **Other cutaneous manifestations** of Behcet syndrome are erythema nodosumlike lesions on the lower extremities, folliculitislike lesions, pustules, furuncles, and superficial phlebitis.

II. **Dermatomyositis/polymyositis.** The cutaneous manifestations specific for dermatomyositis are heliotrope rash and Gottron papules. Additional cutaneous findings common to other connective tissue diseases are seen.

   A. **Heliotrope rash** is a violaceous discoloration of the upper eyelids accompanied by edema. It develops early in the course of the disease and often coincides with a similar violaceous eruption on the butterfly area of the face, neck, anterior chest, and other sun-exposed regions. On the extremities, the rash characteristically involves the extensor surfaces of both large and small joints, in contrast to lupus erythematosus, which involves the skin between the joints on the dorsum of the hand.

   B. **Poikiloderma**, which consists of speckled hyperpigmentation and hypopigmentation, telangiectasis, and cutaneous atrophy, appears later in the course of the disease.

   C. **Gottron papules**, which are violaceous, flat topped, and appear on the extensor aspect of the interphalangeal joints, are a late manifestation.

   D. **Calcification** of skin, fascia, and muscle occurs in patients, especially children, with severe muscle involvement.

   E. **Other findings** seen in dermatomyositis are Raynaud phenomenon, erythema, papules, and ulcerations or leukoplakia of the mucous membranes. There is generally no correlation between the extent of cutaneous involvement and the severity of the myositis. Correlation exists between the degree of nail fold capillary abnormality, as viewed with a widefield microscope, and the number of organ systems involved by the disease process.

III. **Erythema nodosum (EN).** EN appears as crops of discrete, tender subcutaneous nodules that are erythematous and whose centers are slightly raised. Lesions are usually 2 cm or more in size and are characteristically located on the shins and ankles, but may occur symmetrically on the extensor aspect of the extremities and, infrequently, on the face. Prodromal symptoms may include fever, chills, malaise, and polyarthralgia. Lesions heal without scarring or ulcerations, and undergo color changes similar to those of bruises.

A. Etiology. EN is a hypersensitivity reaction involving the vasculature of the subcutaneous tissue, and should alert the physician to search for an underlying disease process. Specific etiologies follow.

1. Infectious

    a. Beta-hemolytic streptococci. EN may appear within three weeks of an upper respiratory infection (URI).

    b. Tuberculosis. This disease was once a common cause of EN. Skin lesions appear three to eight weeks after the primary infection.

    c. Deep fungal. Coccidioidomycosis, histoplasmosis, and North American blastomycosis may produce EN lesions.

    d. Lepromatous leprosy. When accompanied by EN, iritis, orchitis, lymphadenopathy, and polyneuritis, the disease is referred to as erythema nodosum leprosum.

2. Sarcoidosis. Lofgren syndrome, consisting of bilateral hilar adenopathy and EN, is probably a benign form of sarcoidosis.

3. Drug. Allergy to sulfonamides, bromides, iodides, oral contraceptives, and other drugs has been associated with EN.

4. Inflammatory bowel disease. Both ulcerative colitis and regional enteritis produce EN in about 10% of cases.

5. Behcet syndrome. EN is seen in association with other cutaneous manifestations of this disease.

B. Differential diagnosis. Diseases to be considered in the differential diagnosis of EN are erythema induratum, Weber-Christian disease, subcutaneous nodular fat necrosis in association with pancreatic disease, recurrent thrombophlebitis, cutaneous arteritis, and lupus profundus.

IV. Juvenile rheumatoid arthritis. The characteristic rash of juvenile rheumatoid arthritis is seen in approximately 30% of patients, mostly those with systemic onset disease. It is more common in patients under the age of two years. Lesions are erythematous and flat or very slightly raised; they vary in size from 3 to 10 mm in diameter and have diffuse borders. Lesions occur on the trunk, extremities, and face, and may become confluent. The rash is evanescent, often associated with fever spikes, and occurs most frequently in early evening. It may be pruritic. The Koebner phenomenon is common.

The cutaneous eruption does not correlate with presence of rheumatoid factor in the serum, although the rash is often present during periods of active systemic disease. Skin nodules are rarely found in younger patients. Older patients with rheumatoid factor may have subcutaneous nodules similar to those in patients with adult rheumatoid arthritis.

V. Lupus erythematosus

A. The lupus band test (LBT) demonstrates deposits of immunoglobulin and complement at the dermal-epidermal junction by direct immunofluorescent staining of the skin. Biopsy of cutaneous lesions in discoid or systemic lupus erythematosus yields a positive LBT in about 90% of patients.

Clinically normal skin of patients with DLE demonstrates a negative LBT. The LBT in clinically normal skin of patients with systemic lupus erythematosus (SLE) varies with sun exposure. Approximately 50% of patients with systemic lupus erythematosus have a positive LBT in clinically normal sun-protected skin, whereas 80% have a positive LBT in clinically normal sun-exposed areas. The value of the LBT as a reflection of disease activity and as a marker for renal involvement is undetermined.

B. Discoid lupus erythematosus. The characteristic lesion of DLE is a scaly plaque that ranges in color from red to violaceous, with sharply defined borders, central atrophy, telangiectasia, and areas of hypopigmentation or hyperpigmentation. Keratinous plugging of the hair follicles can sometimes be detected as tiny rough projections across the lesion. Lesions may be multiple and asymmetric, and are most commonly found on the head and neck, particularly in the malar areas, ears, and scalp. When the scalp is involved, hair loss with scarring at the site of the lesion results. Lesions on the oral and nasal mucosae may ulcerate. Lesions of DLE produce scarring; those that result in severe scarring may, infrequently, produce skin cancer.

When discoid lesions are present below the neck, the term *generalized* or *disseminated* DLE is used. Less than 5% of patients who present with lesions of DLE will develop SLE.

C. Systemic lupus erythematosus. Cutaneous manifestations of SLE comprise six of the fourteen preliminary criteria for the classification of SLE by the American Rheumatism Association. These six criteria are facial erythema, DLE lesions, Raynaud phenomenon, alopecia, photosensitivity, and oral or nasopharyngeal ulceration.

1. **Facial erythema.** The classic butterfly rash of SLE occurs in up to 40% of patients. It begins as a transient erythematous, edematous eruption across the bridge of the nose and malar areas. It is often exacerbated by sun exposure and may accompany a flare of systemic disease. If the rash is persistent, atrophy, telangiectasia, and scaling will develop.

2. **Discoid lesions** seen in SLE are identical to those of DLE and occur in approximately 20% of patients.

3. **Raynaud phenomenon** is seen in up to 30% of cases.

4. **Alopecia** can be of two types in SLE. **Scarring** alopecia is produced when discoid lesions affect the scalp; these lesions are easily recognized. More subtle is the **reversible** (diffuse or patchy) alopecia that may arise. Diffuse alopecia is more common than patchy alopecia. It may accompany a clinical flare of SLE and is sometimes elicited only by specifically questioning the patient about increased hair loss. The frontal hairline may consist of short, broken hairs, as in traction alopecia.

5. **Photosensitivity** will often precipitate butterfly pattern erythema, the rash of subacute lupus erythematosus, and lesions of DLE. The active spectrum is ultraviolet light of 280 to 320 nm ultraviolet B (UVB), which normally produces sunburn erythema. Sunlight may also cause a flare of systemic disease.

6. **Oral or nasopharyngeal ulcerations** are shallow and have gray bases with red borders. They are often painful and usually seen in patients with severe cutaneous disease.

7. **Subacute lupus erythematosus** is a nonscarring eruption with papulosquamous and annular-polycyclic patterns. The distribution is over the malar area, nose, ears, upper trunk, and extensor aspect of the arms. The axillae, lateral aspect of the trunk, and knuckles are spared. The **papulosquamous** eruption is composed of confluent and discrete scaly erythematous papules and plaques. The **annular-polycyclic** type has scaly erythematous borders surrounding central areas of subtle hypopigmentation and telangiectasia.

8. **Vasculitis**

   a. Arteritis may result in focal areas of gangrene on the fingers or toes.

   b. Livedo reticularis is a purple, netlike, deep vascular discoloration that is most common on the lower extremities.

c. All manifestations of leukocytoclastic vasculitis (see sec. **XIV.A.2.**) may be observed.

d. Painful ulcers may develop over the forearms, hands, fingers, and near the malleoli.

9. **Periungual telangiectasia** occur on the fingers. This disorder commonly occurs in scleroderma, dermatomyositis, and, less frequently, rheumatoid arthritis.

10. **Urticaria** may be the presenting cutaneous manifestation of SLE.

11. **Lupus profundus** is characterized by firm vasculitic nodules in the subcutaneous fat. Erythema of the overlying skin sometimes occurs. The nodules may be found on the forehead, cheeks, buttocks, and upper arms.

VI. Lyme arthritis. This multisystem inflammatory disorder is caused by the bite of an ixodid tick. A rapidly expanding annular erythematous lesion, termed *erythema chronicum migrans*, develops at the site of the bite. The rash appears approximately three days to three weeks after the bite, and is frequently accompanied or followed by arthritis. The nervous system and heart are sometimes involved by the disease. Systemic manifestations may be mediated by immune complexes.

VII. Psoriasis. This chronic disease involves the skin and joints, and may present at any age. There is a family history of the disease in approximately 30% of cases. Psoriasis has been estimated to affect about 2% of the United States' population.

Psoriasis is characterized by increased epidermal proliferation. The typical skin lesion is a well-delineated, raised erythematous plaque covered by a loosely adherent silvery scale. As the scale accumulates, the lesion may even appear white. Lesions vary in size from small papules to extensive plaques, and occasionally assume an annular or gyrate configuration. Although psoriasis usually has a *symmetric* distribution, a solitary lesion is sometimes seen. **Sites of predilection** include the elbows, knees, scalp, and lumbosacral region. Lesions of psoriasis heal without scarring.

Any clinical pattern of psoriasis may be associated with psoriatic arthritis. However, **nail involvement** is seen in 80% of patients with arthritis and in only 30% of patients without joint involvement.

Medications that may cause psoriasis to flare include chloroquine and lithium; withdrawal of systemic corticosteroids is also a possible cause.

The **Koebner phenomenon** refers to the appearance of new lesions at sites of trauma such as scratching, sunburn, or physical injury. Bluntly scraping off the scale to reveal punctate bleeding points underneath produces the **Auspitz** sign.

A. **Chronic plaque type** is seen on sites of predilection noted in **VII.**, and on the trunk and extremities. Lesions may become confluent.

B. **Inverse psoriasis** is localized to intertriginous areas.

C. **Guttate psoriasis** is characterized by teardrop-shaped lesions on the trunk and proximal extremities; it is often precipitated by a beta-hemolytic streptococcal infection.

D. **Palmar psoriasis** is characterized by scaly, erythematous patches on the palms and fingers. This form may be mistaken for a dermatophyte infection.

E. **Pustular psoriasis** may present as localized sterile pustules of the palms, soles, or paronychial skin, or as severe generalized pustules accompanied by fever, arthralgia, and leukocytosis, known as pustular psoriasis of von Zumbusch.

F. **Exfoliative erythroderma**, in which the skin of the entire body is thickened, erythematous, and scaly, may be precipitated by an infection, drug allergy, sunburn, or severe contact dermatitis.

G. **Nail changes** include surface pits, yellow discoloration of the nail plate, lifting of the nail bed, subungual keratotic accumulation, thickening, crumbling, grooving, and splitting.

VIII. Pyoderma gangrenosum. This disease is commonly associated with ulcerative colitis and regional enteritis, and rarely with rheumatoid arthritis, myeloproliferative disorders, multiple myeloma, and leukemia. It begins as a tender pustule which rapidly expands, resulting in a large ulcer many centimeters in diameter with a bluish, undermined border and a necrotic, purulent center. Lesions most frequently occur on the legs and trunk, and heal with scar formation. Cutaneous trauma may exacerbate existing ulcers or cause the formation of new lesions.

Skin biopsy of pyoderma gangrenosum is not diagnostic. The diagnosis can be made only when other causes of cutaneous ulcerations such as vasculitis, syphilis, tuberculosis, bacteria, fungi, and protozoa are excluded.

IX. Reiter syndrome. This disorder consists of the tetrad of arthritis, urethritis, conjunctivitis, and mucocutaneous lesions. The mucocutaneous lesions, present in about 80% of cases, may be divided into the following categories.

    A. Mucosal lesions. The penis is commonly affected by superficial ulcerations around the urethral meatus. Eroded red papules involving the corona and glans become confluent and are referred to as *balanitis circinata*. Erosion, erythema, and purpura are seen frequently in the mouth and pharynx.

    B. Cutaneous lesions

        1. Red macules may develop on the palms and soles, then form pustules and progress to thick hyperkeratotic plaques called *keratoderma blennorrhagica*.

        2. Psoriasiform plaques, which may pustulate, are sometimes found scattered on the scalp, trunk, extremities, and scrotum.

        3. Nail changes include subungual hyperkeratosis and thickening of the nail plate.

        4. Generalized exfoliative erythroderma may be seen in severely ill patients.

X. Rheumatic fever. Three types of skin lesions are observed in rheumatic fever. They are listed in decreasing order of frequency.

    A. Subcutaneous nodules are usually less than 0.5 cm in diameter and are found over bony prominences of the elbows, knuckles, ankles, and occiput. Nodules may persist up to a month or recur over several months, and are frequently associated with carditis.

    B. Erythema marginatum is most commonly seen on the trunk, extremities, and the axillary vault. These flat or slightly raised polycyclic and annular lesions begin as small erythematous macules or papules that rapidly spread peripherally. The outlines of the lesions may become irregular. Usually associated with carditis, the lesions often erupt soon after the onset of arthritis and may recur for months.

    C. Erythema papulatum, an extremely rare manifestation of rheumatic fever, is characterized by indolent papules that are found over the flexor and extensor surfaces of large joints.

XI. Rheumatoid arthritis. Rheumatoid nodules and manifestations of vasculitis are the major cutaneous findings in rheumatoid arthritis, and are observed primarily in patients with rheumatoid factor.

    A. Rheumatoid nodules are found in approximately 20% of patients. They are firm, up to several centimeters in diameter, and most frequently located subcutaneously, although they can involve tendon sheaths and periosteum. They are found in skin subjected to repeated minor trauma, such as the juxtaarticular region of the elbows, the Achilles tendons, the ischial tuberosities, the scapular areas, and the hands and feet. If they occur on the sclera, scleromalacia with possible globe perforation may result. Rheumatoid nodules may rarely soften and ulcerate.

    B. Vasculitic lesions are commonly found on the digits. They present as tiny red or purpuric macules or papules that can progress to painful subcutaneous nodules or ulcers, 2 to 3 mm in diameter. In severe cases of digital arteritis, gangrene of the finger pulp can ensue. Vasculitis frequently affects the dependent lower extremities, manifesting itself as purpuric macules and papules, urticarial lesions, hemorrhagic bullae, painful ulcers, and livedo reticularis.

C. **Other cutaneous features** of rheumatoid arthritis are palmar erythema, skin atrophy of the hands, Raynaud phenomenon and, infrequently, periungual telangiectasia.

XII. **Sarcoidosis.** All cutaneous manifestations of sarcoidosis, except erythema nodosum and transient maculopapular eruptions, show histologic evidence of sarcoid granulomas on skin biopsy.
Circulating immune complexes may be responsible for both erythema nodosum and transient maculopapular eruptions, either of which may be a presenting sign of the disease.

A. **Erythema nodosum** is a panniculitis that appears as painful, erythematous, slightly raised, rounded lesions symmetrically distributed on the extensor aspect of the extremities, often localized to the shins. Fever and polyarthralgias may occur. When healing, the lesions assume the color of a bruise. Recurrent lesions appear in crops. Erythema nodosum is not specific for sarcoidosis, but the condition is termed *Lofgren syndrome* when accompanied by bilateral hilar adenopathy.

B. **Transient maculopapular eruptions** occur on the trunk, face, or extremities, and may be accompanied by acute uveitis, peripheral lymphadenopathy, and parotid enlargement.

C. **Granulomatous cutaneous lesions** of sarcoidosis include:

   1. **Papules.** Translucent, reddish brown; they are found on the periorbital area, ala nasi, and upper torso.

   2. **Annular lesions.** Formed from papules coalescing in rings.

   3. **Nodules.** Rarely found on the extremities or trunk.

   4. **Plaques.** Purple to reddish brown in color; they are symmetrically located on the extremities and buttocks. Plaques present on the face, ears, fingers, or toes are referred to as *lupus pernio*.

   5. **Ichthyosislike lesions.** Large scales which are usually located on the lower extremities.

   6. **Generalized erythroderma.**

   7. **Infiltration of old scars.** A phenomenon peculiar to sarcoidosis; scars become purple and raised.

XIII. **Scleroderma and variants.** Scleroderma may present as a disease localized to the skin or as a systemic process.

A. **Localized scleroderma**

   1. **Morphea** is a discrete, well-defined plaque of scleroderma that is smooth, indurated, yellow white in color, and has a violaceous halo when the disease is active.

   2. **Generalized morphea** is comprised of numerous large plaques that may involve almost the entire body, usually sparing the face. Underlying muscle atrophy is often prominent on the extremities.

   3. **Guttate morphea** consists of small, white, sclerotic lesions usually located on the chest and shoulders.

   4. **Linear scleroderma** generally begins during childhood, is unilateral, and may result in joint contractures secondary to involvement of muscle and bone.

      a. **Facial hemiatrophy** may be associated with facial linear scleroderma.

      b. **Coup de sabre** refers to linear scleroderma that involves the face and scalp.

B. Systemic scleroderma (progressive systemic sclerosis, PSS). Skin involvement in PSS may be classified by type of onset and presence or absence of Raynaud phenomenon.

1. Acrosclerosis is the predominant type, accounting for 90% of cases. It is characterized at an early stage by edema of the hands, fingers, feet, and legs and by Raynaud phenomenon. Later, the skin of the hands and feet becomes indurated, thick, taut, smooth, and bound down. The process may extend onto the extremities. The face, neck, and trunk are commonly involved. Cutaneous manifestations include the following.

    a. Sclerodactyly. Smooth, shiny, tapered fingers with taut, bound down skin.

    b. Joint contractures occur principally over small joints, and may involve large joints as well. Hand contractures result in "claw hand" deformity.

    c. Ulcerations usually occur over the fingers, toes, malleoli, and knuckles, and may result in infection.

    d. Facial involvement may result in either a waxy, expressionless facies or in pinched facies with thin lips, radial furrows about the mouth, sunken cheeks, and a beaklike nose.

    e. Pigment alterations appear as three types. The most common type is **postinflammatory hyperpigmentation** or **hypopigmentation** in sclerotic areas. Areas of normal skin may develop **complete pigment loss** dotted centrally by perifollicular pigment resembling vitiligo. Rarely, generalized **hyperpigmentation** similar to that seen in Addison disease occurs.

    f. Mat-like telangiectases may occur on the face, lips, hands, oral mucosa, and upper trunk. There is a high correlation between the degree of nailfold capillary abnormality, as viewed with a widefield microscope, and the extent of internal organ involvement in scleroderma.

    g. Bullae may, rarely, occur in areas of sclerosis.

    h. Calcinosis cutis generally occurs late in the course of scleroderma, and is usually limited to skin over joints. The **CREST syndrome** consists of calcinosis, **R**aynaud phenomenon, **e**sophageal dysfunction, **s**clerodactyly, and telangiectasia. It identifies a group of PSS patients with a more favorable prognosis.

2. Diffuse systemic sclerosis often begins on the trunk and rapidly spreads to involve the extremities and face. Raynaud phenomenon and sclerodactyly are absent.

3. The differential diagnosis of fibrotic skin includes:

    a. Eosinophilic fasciitis.

    b. Graft-versus-host disease.

    c. Porphyria cutanea tarda.

    d. Scleredema.

    e. Carcinoid syndrome.

    f. Scleromyxedema.

    g. Lichen sclerosis et atrophicus.

    h. Bleomycin-induced sclerosis.

    i. Chlorinated hydrocarbon–induced sclerosis (polyvinyl chloride).

    j. Occupational trauma.

    k. Primary amyloidosis.

    l. Melorheostosis with linear scleroderma.

     m. Progeria.

     n. Werner syndrome.

     o. Phenylketonuria.

C. Eosinophilic fasciitis can usually be distinguished from systemic scleroderma by skin examination. The trunk and proximal extremities develop localized areas of induration which are firmly bound to underlying tissues. A cobblestone or puckered surface is formed secondary to involvement of the subcutaneous fibrous tissue, and is most obvious upon overhead extension of the upper extremities. Raynaud phenomenon and development of internal organ involvement do not occur. A biopsy that includes skin, fascia, and muscle is necessary for diagnosis. Fibrotic thickening and a cellular infiltrate, often including eosinophils, is found in the deep fascia, and may also be present in the lower dermis, fat, and muscle. Laboratory abnormalities include blood eosinophilia in 30% of patients, increased erythrocyte sedimentation rate, and hypergammaglobulinemia.

D. Undifferentiated connective tissue syndrome (UCTS), also known as mixed connective tissue disease, denotes combined clinical features of SLE, scleroderma, and polymyositis. High titers of antibody to the ribonuclease-sensitive component of extractable nuclear antigen (ENA) occur in many of these patients. Some authorities feel that UCTS represents a prodrome of systemic lupus or scleroderma in most patients (see Chap. 40). Raynaud phenomenon and swollen hands are the most frequent skin manifestations.

Direct immunofluorescent studies of clinically normal skin in UCTS patients reveal subepidermal immunoglobulin deposits in approximately one-third of patients. In addition, speckled epidermal nuclear IgG deposition may be found. This latter finding also occurs in patients with SLE and high titer Sm antibodies.

XIV. Vasculitis, cutaneous (See also Chap. 42.)

    A. Classification. Cutaneous vasculitis includes septic and leukocytoclastic categories.

      1. Septic vasculitis. Skin manifestations of the **gonococcal arthritis-dermatitis syndrome** occur during the initial bacteremic phase, and are accompanied by fever, rigor, tenosynovitis, and polyarthralgia. The skin lesions are usually tender, few in number, and located on the distal extremities. They may present as petechiae, small ecchymoses, hemorrhagic papules, vesiculopustules on a hemorrhagic base, or hemorrhagic bullae. It is difficult to culture gonococci from skin lesions. Fluorescent antibody tests may help identify organisms in a biopsy of a lesion.

      2. Leukocytoclastic vasculitis. Lesions of "palpable purpura" on the lower extremities may be easily recognized. The morphologic expression of the immune complex vasculitis that involves the postcapillary venules of the skin is manifold. Lesions are usually concentrated on the legs and are distributed symmetrically. They may begin as erythematous macules or urticarial papules. These lesions then become purpuric. The vasculitis may rapidly progress to form hemorrhagic vesicles and bullae, nodules, or superficial ulcers covered by eschars. Such lesions are painful and may appear in recurrent crops, which may last for weeks. Three important syndromes manifested by leukocytoclastic vasculitis follow.

        a. Henoch-Schönlein purpura occurs primarily in children and young adults following an upper respiratory tract infection. Purpuric lesions develop over the extensor surfaces and the buttocks. Edema of the lower legs is common; edema of the hands, scalp, and periorbital areas occurs in young children. Arthritis, abdominal pain, gastrointestinal bleeding, and renal involvement presenting as proteinuria and hematuria are other features. Serum complement levels are usually normal. Immunofluorescent staining of skin biopsies of early lesions reveals mainly IgA and complement deposition in the walls of affected vessels.

b. **Hypocomplementemic vasculitis** is characterized by recurrent attacks of urticarial skin lesions accompanied by arthritis and hypocomplementemia. The urticarial lesions may last for days and small purpuric lesions may occasionally be present. Abdominal pain, edema of the face and larynx, and mild renal disease may occur. Biopsy and immunofluorescent staining of early skin lesions reveal immunoglobulin and complement deposition in vessel walls.

c. **Mixed cryoglobulinemia** demonstrates the spectrum of cutaneous manifestations of leukocytoclastic vasculitis and is accompanied by immune complex renal disease (often severe), hepatosplenomegaly, and lymphadenopathy. The presence of mixed cryoglobulinemia, positive rheumatoid factor, and hypocomplementemia help to define this disease. Immunofluorescent staining of early skin lesions reveals immunoglobulins and complement in the walls of affected vessels.

B. **Differential diagnosis**

1. **Infectious agents.** Gonococcus, meningococcus, *Staphylococcus aureus*, beta-hemolytic streptococcus, hepatitis B virus, *Mycobacterium leprae*, endocarditis-producing bacteria.

2. **Drugs.** Penicillin, sulfonamides, thiazides, phenothiazines, aspirin, phenylbutazone, allopurinol.

3. **Rheumatic diseases.** SLE, rheumatoid arthritis, sicca syndrome, Henoch-Schönlein syndrome, hypocomplementemic vasculitis, mixed cryoglobulinemia, hyperglobulinemic purpura.

4. **Malignancies.** Lymphoproliferative disorders, Hodgkin disease, carcinoma.

5. **Systemic diseases.** Serum sickness, ulcerative colitis, chronic active hepatitis, primary biliary cirrhosis, Goodpasture syndrome, retroperitoneal fibrosis.

6. **Genetic disorders.** C2 deficiency.

Bibliography

General
Braverman, I. M. *Skin Signs of Systemic Disease.* Philadelphia: Saunders, 1970.

Moschella, S. L. Connective Tissue Disease. In S. L. Moschella, D. M. Pillsbury, and H. J. Hurley, Jr. (Eds.), *Dermatology.* Philadelphia: Saunders, 1975. P. 913.

Behcet Syndrome
Tokoro, Y., et al. Skin lesions in Behcet's disease. *Int. J. Dermatol.* 16:277, 1977.

Dermatomyositis
Callen, J. P. Dermatomyositis. *Int. J. Dermatol.* 18:423, 1979.

Erythema Nodosum
Blomgren, S. E. Erythema nodosum. *Semin. Arthritis Rheum.* 4:1, 1974.

Moore, C. P., and Willkens, R. F. The subcutaneous nodule: Its significance in the diagnosis of rheumatic disease. *Semin. Arthritis Rheum.* 7:63, 1977.

Mullin, G. T., et al. Arthritis and skin lesions resembling erythma nodosum in pancreatic disease. *Ann. Intern. Med.* 68:75, 1968.

Lupus Erythematosus
Monroe, E. W. Lupus band test. *Arch. Dermatol.* 113:830, 1977.

Sontheimer, R. D., Thomas, J. R., and Gilliam, J. N. Subacute cutaneous lupus erythematosus. *Arch. Dermatol.* 115:1409, 1979.

Lyme Arthritis
Hardin, J. A., Steere, A. C., and Malawista, S. E. Immune complexes and the evolution of lyme arthritis: Dissemination and localization of abnormal Clq binding activity. *N. Engl. J. Med.* 301:1358, 1979.

Psoriasis
Guilhou, J. J., Meynadier, J., and Clot, J.   New concepts in the pathogenesis of psoriasis. *Br. J. Dermatol.* 98:585, 1978.

Moll, J. M. H., and Wright, V.   Psoriatic arthritis. *Semin. Arthritis Rheum.* 3:55, 1973.

Pyoderma Gangrenosum
Lazarus, G. S., et al.   Pyoderma gangrenosum, altered delayed hypersensitivity, and polyarthritis. *Arch. Dermatol.* 105:46, 1972.

Rheumatic Fever
Bywaters, E. G. L.   Skin Manifestations of Rheumatic Disease. In T. B. Fitzpatrick, et al. (Eds.), *Dermatology in General Medicine.* New York: McGraw-Hill, 1979. P. 1316.

Rheumatoid Arthritis
Hurd, E. R.   Extraarticular manifestations of rheumatoid arthritis. *Semin. Arthritis Rheum.* 8:151, 1979.

Sarcoidosis
Jones, J. V., et al.   Evidence for circulating immune complexes in erythema nodosum and early sarcoidosis. *Ann. N.Y. Acad. Sci.* 278:212, 1976.

Scleroderma and Variants
Chubick, A., and Gilliam, J. N.   A review of mixed connective tissue disease. *Int. J. Dermatol.* 17:123, 1978.

Fleischmajer, R., Jacotot, A. B., Shore, S., and Binnick, S. A.   Scleroderma, eosinophilia, and diffuse fasciitis. *Arch. Dermatol.* 114:1320, 1978.

Jablonska, S., and Rodnan, G. P.   Localized forms of scleroderma. *Clin. Rheum. Dis.* 5:215, 1979.

Maricq, H. R., Spencer-Green, G., and LeRoy, E. C.   Skin capillary abnormalities as indicator of organ involvement in scleroderma (systemic sclerosis), Raynaud's syndrome, and dermatomyositis. *Am. J. Med.* 61:862, 1976.

Vasculitis, Cutaneous
Ackerman, A. B.   Vasculitis. In A. B. Ackerman, *Histologic Diagnosis of Inflammatory Skin Diseases: A Method by Pattern Analysis.* Philadelphia: Lea & Febiger, 1978, P. 333.

Brogadir, S. P., and Schimmer, B. M.   Spectrum of the gonococcal arthritis-dermatitis syndrome. *Semin. Arthritis Rheum.* 8:177, 1979.

McDuffie, F. C., et al.   Hypocomplementemia with cutaneous vasculitis and arthritis. *Mayo Clin. Proc.* 48:340, 1973.

Sams, W. M., Jr., et al.   Leukocytoclastic vasculitis. *Arch. Dermatol.* 112:219, 1976.

11. Raynaud Phenomenon

Mary Kuntz Crow

Raynaud phenomenon (RP) is characterized by episodic ischemia of the digits. A typical attack consists of sequential well-demarcated pallor, extending from the distal digits proximally, followed by cyanosis, and finally by rubor, often associated with pain. An attack may last from several minutes to hours. The upper extremities are most frequently involved but 40% of patients have symptoms in the lower extremities. Episodes are usually precipitated by exposure to cold or by emotional stress.

This disorder was first described by Maurice Raynaud in 1862 when he wrote of a young woman, otherwise entirely healthy, who experienced episodic transient pallor of her fingers in the presence of moderate cold. It later became apparent that the syndrome described by Raynaud was a primary idiopathic process (now referred to as primary RP). In 1932, Allen and Brown defined criteria for diagnosing primary RP.

1. Appearance of symptoms with exposure to cold or emotional upset.
2. Bilateral, symmetrical involvement of the hands.
3. Presence of normal pulses.
4. Absence of, or only superficial, digital gangrene.
5. Absence of an underlying disorder commonly associated with the symptom complex.
6. Symptoms present for at least two years without the appearance of an underlying cause.

These guidelines for diagnosis remain valid; however, some patients followed for presumed primary RP have been noted to develop systemic disease many years after the onset of symptoms.

Raynaud phenomenon is a common disorder. There is a strong female predominance (5:1), and the first episode commonly occurs between the second and fourth decades. Apparent primary RP accounts for 50% to 90% of cases that manifest the syndrome.

I. Pathogenesis

A. **Primary RP** may be precipitated by direct exposure of the extremities to low temperature, or by stress. Although the pathogenesis of primary RP is unknown, among the mechanisms that have been postulated to contribute to the ischemia occurring in this disease are increased activity of the digital vasomotor nerves and heightened vascular tone of digital arteries. A generalized increase in sympathetic nervous system tone may initiate or prolong attacks. The pallor phase of the classic syndrome is felt to be secondary to spasm of the dermal arterioles and arteries; cyanosis occurs when blood pools in the digital capillaries; and hyperemia is noted when vasospasm resolves and a reactive vasodilation follows.

B. **Secondary RP** may be associated with a systemic illness or with neurologic or vascular abnormalities.

1. **Collagen vascular disease**

a. **Progressive systemic sclerosis (scleroderma).** Among those patients diagnosed as having progressive systemic sclerosis, 80% to 90% have RP. It is the presenting symptom in 30% of those who ultimately develop progressive systemic sclerosis. Progressive sclerodactyly and ulceration of the skin of the digits occur, and calcium may be deposited in the skin and subcutaneous tissue. Histologically, intimal hypertrophy and thrombosis in the medium-sized digital arteries occur.

RP also occurs in patients with a scleroderma variant known as the CREST syndrome (calcinosis, RP, esophageal dysfunction, sclerodactyly, and telangiectasis). Less extensive systemic involvement appears in this disorder, and the prognosis is better than that of progressive systemic sclerosis.

b. **Systemic lupus erythematosus.** RP occurs in 10% to 35% of cases of systemic lupus erythematosus. Pathologic study of digital vessels shows microangiopathy with intravascular fibrin deposition.

c. **Rheumatoid arthritis.** Vascular spasm and obliterative intimal proliferation of digital arteries may be seen.

d. **Systemic vasculitis.**

e. **Polymyositis.** 25% of patients may manifest RP; such patients often show other features of mixed or undifferentiated syndromes.

2. **Traumatic vasospastic disease.** Persons who are exposed to repetitive trauma are at increased risk of developing RP. It has been postulated that chronic stimulation of the pacinian corpuscles in the hands may result in digital artery vasospasm through a reflex that involves the sympathetic nervous system. Typists, pianists, and those who work with sewing machines or pneumatic hand tools are at risk.
Frostbite or prolonged exposure to cold may also predispose to the development of RP.

3. **Peripheral vascular disease.** Atherosclerosis and arteriosclerosis obliterans may result in RP in the distribution of the narrowed blood vessels. Aneurysms or thrombosis of the ulnar artery, digital artery thrombosis, and arterial emboli may precede the development of RP.

4. **Nerve compression.** A thoracic outlet syndrome (caused by abnormalities of the cervical spine or cervical ribs, or by the shoulder girdle compression syndrome) may lead to the symptoms of RP. Compression of the sympathetic fibers of the brachial plexus or of the subclavian artery is implicated in these disorders. RP may also be seen in patients with the carpal tunnel syndrome.

5. **Drugs and chemicals.** Ergot alkaloids have a direct vasoconstrictive action in blood vessels. Methysergide may cause intimal fibrosis. Polyvinyl chloride or arsenic exposure may also predispose to the development of RP. Beta blockers and bleomycin have recently been implicated as the responsible agents in some patients with RP.

6. **Hematologic abnormalities.** RP has been reported in cryoglobulinemia, cold agglutinin disease, polycythemia, and macroglobulinemia.

7. **Other disorders.** Immune complex deposition may be the mechanism of the RP observed in the setting of malignancy or hepatitis.

II. Diagnosis

A. **Symptoms.** The diagnosis of RP is based on a history of the classic triad of sequential digital pallor, cyanosis, and rubor in response to cold exposure or emotional stimuli. Occasionally only pallor or rubor will occur, without cyanosis. Primary RP must be differentiated from secondary RP by undergoing a thorough history to discover associated systemic disease, collagen vascular disease, blood dyscrasias, malignancy, vascular or anatomic abnormalities, occupational factors, or drug exposure.

B. **Physical examination.** Examination is unlikely to reveal abnormalities of the digits in patients with RP, but sclerodactyly, trophic changes, and digital ulcers should be looked for. An episode can sometimes be initiated by cold challenge (immersion of the hand in water at 15°C for 15 minutes).
The presence of hypertension, skin rash, telangiectasia, mucosal lesions, lymphadenopathy, loud pulmonic heart sound, abnormal peripheral pulses, arterial bruits, hepatosplenomegaly, arthritis, or neurologic abnormalities may suggest an underlying rheumatic disease, atherosclerosis, or a malignancy. Maneuvers to detect thoracic outlet compression or carpal tunnel syndrome should be performed.

C. Laboratory data. A complete blood count with differential, a platelet count, erythrocyte sedimentation rate, microscopic urinalysis, antinuclear antibody, rheumatoid factor, serum protein electrophoresis, cryoglobulin, and chest x-ray comprise a screening laboratory evaluation for a patient who presents with the symptoms of RP. Any abnormalities in these tests should be carefully followed up with appropriate studies such as anti-DNA antibody or serum complement studies, cervical spine films, urine immunoelectrophoresis, electromyogram, or nerve conduction studies.

Doppler study of vessels is a noninvasive way to demonstrate a large vessel occlusion that is secondary to atherosclerosis or embolus and could resemble RP.

D. Differential diagnosis. RP, which is an *episodic* disorder, must be differentiated from processes characterized by persistent vasospastic ischemia.

1. **Acrocyanosis,** like RP, is exacerbated by low temperatures and by emotional stress.

2. **Livedo reticularis,** characterized by a persistent purple or blue mottling of the skin, predominantly involves the extremities; it is usually a benign condition but can be a prominent feature of cutaneous vasculitis syndromes.

III. Therapy. Since no specific treatment of primary RP exists, therapy is limited to reassurance and palliation. Therapy of secondary RP should be aimed at correction of the underlying disorder.

A. General measures. Patients with primary RP should be reassured that their prognosis is good. Avoidance of a cold environment and the use of warm clothing and gloves should be emphasized. Tobacco smoking must be discontinued. Repetitive traumatic injury to the extremities should be avoided. Beta-blocker drugs must not be used since they may induce arteriolar spasm.

B. Drug therapy of vasospasm. These agents are not helpful if a significant occlusive component to the peripheral vascular disease exists. Even when the disease process is purely vasospastic, such drugs are of only moderate efficacy.

At our institution, the sequence of therapy is guanethidine followed by prazosin. If these agents fail to relieve symptoms, trials of alternative agents in each drug class below can be undertaken.

1. **Presynaptic sympathetic inhibitors**

   a. **Guanethidine** prevents release of norepinephrine from sympathetic nerve terminals. Major adverse reactions are orthostatic hypotension, diarrhea, and edema. Dosage is 30 to 50 mg daily. Supplied as 10- and 25-mg tablets.

   b. **Methyldopa** inhibits sympathetic tone by an undefined central nervous system mechanism. Side effects include drowsiness and edema. Dosage is 250 to 500 mg QID.

2. **Alpha blockers and direct vasodilators**

   a. **Prazosin.** Syncope may occur with the first dose but can be prevented by giving the drug at bedtime and limiting the dose to 1 mg. Subsequent doses are better tolerated. Dosage may be increased to as much as 20 mg daily in gradual increments, but most patients can be managed on 2 mg QID. Supplied as 1-, 2-, and 5-mg capsules.

   b. **Phenoxybenzamine** dilates cutaneous arterioles by blocking alpha-adrenergic receptors. This drug is indicated as an adjunct to guanethidine if single drug therapy does not control symptoms. Orthostatic hypotension and reflex tachycardia are the major side effects. Dosage is 10 mg daily initially which is increased to a maintenance of 20 to 60 mg daily as required. Supplied as 10-mg capsules.

   c. **Tolazoline** may be used alone or in combination with a sympathetic inhibitor. Major adverse reactions are headache and hypotension. Dosage is 80 mg BID. Supplied as 80-mg timed-release capsules.

3. **Experimental drugs.** Verapamil, a calcium antagonist, and captopril, which blocks angiotensin conversion, are promising drugs under investigation.

C. **Sympathectomy.** This procedure is rarely indicated since it provides infrequent long-term benefit. Lumbar sympathectomy for episodic lower extremity vasospastic disease is more effective than cervicodorsal sympathectomy for upper extremity disease.

D. **Exercises** to strengthen the shoulder muscles are indicated when a thoracic outlet syndrome is present. Surgical decompression of the thoracic outlet may be necessary.

E. **Behavioral therapy.** Recent studies have demonstrated that biofeedback methods may, at least temporarily, help patients abort the initiation of a vasospastic episode when they are exposed to cold; however, such techniques remain experimental.

IV. **Prognosis.** Primary RP has an excellent prognosis. Only 1% of patients progress to partial digital loss. The prognosis of secondary RP depends on the character of the underlying disease.

Bibliography

Birnstingl, M. Raynaud's syndrome: Diagnosis and management. *Br. J. Hosp. Med.* 21:602, 1979.

Coffman, J. D., and Davies, W. T. Vasospastic diseases: A review. *Prog. Cardiovasc. Dis.* 18:123, 1975.

Halperin, J. L., and Coffman, J. D. Pathophysiology of Raynaud's disease. *Arch. Intern. Med.* 139:89, 1979.

12. Neck Pain

Thomas P. Sculco

I. **Anatomic considerations.** The cervical area is composed of an integrated complex of structures whose dysfunction singly or in combination can cause neck or radicular pain. They include:

  A. Vertebrae.

  B. Intervertebral discs.

  C. Apophyseal and uncovertebral joints.

  D. Vertebral arteries.

  E. Spinal cord and nerve roots.

  F. Ligamentous complex.

   1. Anterior and posterior longitudinal ligaments.

   2. Interspinous and supraspinous ligaments.

  G. Paracervical musculature.

II. **History**

  A. **Mode of onset**

   1. A history of neck trauma can provide information about structures injured.

   2. If unrelated to trauma, acute severe restriction of motion can indicate paracervical muscle spasm ("wry neck").

   3. If symptoms began after frequent neck rotation, neck pain can indicate cervical disc degeneration and osteoarthritis.

  B. **Duration and localization of pain**

   1. **Acute onset** of pain usually suggests muscle spasm or nerve root irritation; radiation to the occiput or interscapular area may occur.

   2. **Chronic neck pain,** which occurs intermittently with or without radicular symptoms, may be seen in cervical osteoarthritis.

   3. If **radiculitis** is severe, pain radiation to shoulder and arm indicates either nerve root compression by a disc herniation or foraminal encroachment by the osteophytes of osteoarthritis.

   4. **Primary shoulder pain** can be referred proximally and lead to neck and trapezial pain.

  C. **Relief and aggravation of pain.** Rest in the supine position usually relieves local neck pain produced by muscle spasm, but may have little or no effect on processes primarily involving osseous structures.

  D. **Neurologic signs and symptoms**

   1. **Paresthesias** radiating from the neck to the arm are an important indicator of nerve root irritability.

   2. **Numbness and weakness of the arm or hand** indicate more severe nerve root compromise; the cervical nerve root involved can be localized by careful neurologic examination (See Appendix E).

   3. Patients with **vertebral artery** compromise may complain of dizziness, visual dysfunction, and syncopal episodes.

4. Cervical myelopathy can be seen in cases of severe cervical osteoarthritis; patients may have only mild complaints of difficulty with walking or holding objects.

E. Past medical history should be thoroughly explored. History of malignancy, associated musculoskeletal disorders, metabolic bone diseases, and smoking habits should be pursued.

F. Occupational history may provide inciting cause of patient's pain. Patients who do extensive overhead work such as painting or hanging wallpaper may have increased pain after work.

III. Physical examination. The patient should disrobe fully to allow visualization of the neck and thoracic spine.

A. Patient standing

1. Observe the position in which the neck is held. With severe **unilateral paracervical spasm,** the head may be flexed laterally to that side and rotated to the opposite side.

2. Severe **paracervical muscle spasm** can be visualized posteriorly.

3. Evaluate the presence of neck or paracervical **muscle atrophy.** Also compare trapezial and shoulder musculature symmetry.

4. Examine shoulder range of motion and palpate for localized shoulder tenderness.

B. Patient sitting

1. Record active and passive **neck range of motion.**

   a. Normal **flexion** is from chin to chest; normal **extension** is from occiput to approximately C7.

   b. Normal **rotation** approaches 70 degrees bilaterally; normal **lateral bending** approaches 50 to 60 degrees.

2. Examine for **supraclavicular lymphadenopathy** and **carotid artery pulses.**

3. **Neurologic examination** of upper extremities.

   a. **Sensory examination** with pin and cotton ball as well as tuning fork.

   b. **Motor testing,** particularly of deltoid, biceps, triceps, wrist extensors and wrist flexors, finger extensors and flexors, and interossei.

   c. **Reflex examination** should include biceps, triceps, and brachioradialis.

C. Patient prone, forehead on pillow

1. Palpate paracervical area and spinous process for specific areas of tenderness or trigger points.

2. Evaluate deep percussion sensitivity in interscapular area.

IV. Laboratory studies

A. Radiographs should be taken in anteroposterior (AP), oblique, and lateral views. An open-mouth view of the odontoid may be used to supplement these films. Flexion–extension films are often helpful when instability is suspected.

1. **Alignment of the spine** in the AP and lateral projection should be evaluated.

   a. The distances between spinous processes should be approximately equal on the AP film.

   b. Alignment of the posterior bodies of the vertebral bodies should form a gentle curve.

2. **Narrowing of the disc space** is best seen on the lateral view and most commonly occurs at the C5 to C6 level.

3. The oblique view best demonstrates the **neural foramina** through which the cervical nerve roots pass.

4. The **uncovertebral joints** (joints of Luschka) are best seen on the AP view; these may be narrowed with cervical osteoarthritis.

5. The presence of a **cervical rib** should also be noted.

6. **Congenital fusions of cervical vertebrae,** or other bony anomalies, may be present.

B. Further diagnostic studies

1. **Myelography** is indicated in patients with intractable neck pain and radiculopathy to localize spinal cord or nerve root compromise by disc, osteophyte, or neoplasm.

2. **Electromyography** may be useful in demonstrating subclinical neurologic deficits.

3. **Computerized axial tomography** is useful in determining spinal stenosis and osteophytic areas of nerve root compression.

4. **Bone scan** may demonstrate osseous involvement by neoplasm in the cervical spine.

V. Differential diagnosis

A. Neck pain without radiculopathy. Referral to occiput and upper back may or may not be present.

1. Vertebrae

a. Primary or metastatic tumor.

b. Fracture. Traumatic or osteoporotic (rare).

c. Septic spondylitis.

2. Intervertebral disc

a. Herniated cervical disc.

b. Disc space infections. Rare in the cervical area but may present with severe neck pain and torticollis.

c. Degeneration of disc.

3. Apophyseal and uncovertebral joints

a. Degenerative osteoarthritis.

b. Rheumatoid arthritis may lead to destruction of these joints with resultant pain and instability, particularly at the C1 to C2 level.

4. Soft tissues.

a. Ligamentous injury to neck resulting in pain and cervical instability.

b. Acute muscular spasm can produce acute pain and torticollis (wry neck). Wry neck may arise after trauma (whiplash), prolonged exposure to cold, and other activities that strain and require considerable neck rotation or positioning.

c. Tension and anxiety can produce severe spasm in paracervical musculature.

5. Surrounding structures. Neck pain may be referred from the shoulder or periscapular structures. Cervical lymphadenopathy, if painful, can produce severe restriction in neck motion. Occipital headaches may produce secondary neck pain and muscle spasm.

B. Neck pain with radiculopathy. Objective neurologic deficit may or may not be present.

    1. Vertebra. Tumors or infections may produce radicular symptoms and signs.

    2. Intervertebral disc. Herniation or degeneration of an intervertebral disc may produce specific radicular patterns, depending on level of involvement. Considerable overlap among the patterns outlined below exists. C5 to C6 and C6 to C7 are far more common levels of involvement than C7 to T1 or C4 to C5.

        a. C5 to C6 (C6 nerve root). There will be pain either to the shoulder or lateral arm and dorsum of forearm. Paresthesias and numbness may be present in the thumb and index finger. Weakness, if present, will involve the biceps and wrist extensors. The biceps reflex is often decreased or absent.

        b. C6 to C7 (C7 nerve root). The pain pattern is similar to that of the C5 to C6 level. Paresthesias and numbness, when present, involve the index and long fingers. Weakness, if present, is noted in the triceps muscle, wrist flexors, and finger extensors. The triceps reflex may be decreased or absent.

        c. C7 to T1 (C8 nerve root). Pain may occur along the medial aspect of the upper arm and forearm. Parasthesias and numbness involve the ring and small fingers. Weakness, if present, is noted in the finger flexors and intrinsic musculature of the hand. The triceps reflex may be reduced.

    3. Apophyseal and uncovertebral joints. Degenerative arthritis affecting these joints in the cervical area can lead to secondary encroachment of the cervical intervertebral foramina with nerve root irritation (see sec. **V.B.2**).

    4. Surrounding structures

        a. Thoracic outlet syndrome. Radicular symptoms with or without neurologic deficit can occur with compression of the subclavian vessel by a cervical rib or tight scalenus anterior muscle.

        b. Brachial plexus injuries can lead to marked neurologic deficits with retrograde pain to cervical area.

        c. Pancoast tumors of the lung apex may occasionally produce neck pain and neurologic deficits.

VI. Therapy

A. Rest is the cornerstone of therapy for patients with neck pain, whether or not radiculopathy is present.

    1. The patient should be advised to avoid activities that are particularly stressful to the neck; examples are driving, overhead lifting, athletic activities such as tennis and golf, and sitting at a desk for prolonged periods reviewing papers or books.

    2. The neck should be supported by a firm cervical collar, fitted so that cervical motion is limited 60% to 70% and the patient is comfortable. Soft foam collars provide little, if any, cervical immobilization, but may be useful at night during sleep if the firm collar is uncomfortable. Initially the collar should be worn full time; as symptoms recede, the patient may be weaned from the collar approximately one-half hour daily.

B. Moist heat generally relaxes tight spastic musculature. A moist warm towel can be wrapped around the neck as a collar; as the towel cools, this action can be repeated. A hydroculator or a hot water bottle wrapped in a moist towel can also be used.

C. Medications may be useful depending on the underlying cause of the neck pain.

    1. If there is inflammation or cervical radiculitis, **aspirin** 650 to 975 mg PO QID may be used.

    2. If muscle spasm is severe, **diazepam** 5 to 10 mg PO QID can be used.

    3. If pain is severe, **codeine** 60 mg PO every 4 hours is used as needed.

D. Physical therapy is useful if an osseous spur is compromising the intervertebral foramina, thus causing nerve root entrapment.

    1. Three to five sessions per week of **intermittent cervical traction,** each lasting 20 to 30 minutes and reaching a maximum of 20 to 25 pounds, may be used.

    2. Traction may be preceded by **ultrasound** or **diathermy** to the upper neck and upper back.

    3. If pain is severe, travel to the therapy center should be minimized. For these individuals, **home cervical traction** may be prescribed.

    4. Patients who improve during supervised cervical traction should also obtain home traction units for use twice daily, gradually decreasing length of sessions as symptoms resolve.

E. Exercises should be encouraged only if they do not exacerbate the pain. Active range of motion can be easily performed in a shower or sauna. As the patient improves, isometric exercises in various positions of neck rotation and lateral bending may be prescribed (see Appendix A). If weakness remains after cervical pain has diminished, exercises while swimming in a pool may prove useful.

13. Shoulder Pain

Russell F. Warren

The diagnosis and treatment of problems of the shoulder region require an understanding of the anatomy and function of this joint.

I. **Anatomy and function.** The shoulder consists of three joints and two gliding planes which allow an exceedingly large range of motion at the expense of glenohumeral stability. As a result, the glenohumeral joint is the most commonly dislocated joint in the body. The gliding planes consist of the scapulothoracic surface and the subacromial space. The three joints are the acromioclavicular, sternoclavicular, and glenohumeral articulations. Elevation of the arm is caused by the combined rotation between the scapula and chest wall as well as by the glenohumeral joint. The rotator cuff consists of four muscles: the supraspinatus, the infraspinatus, the teres minor, and the subscapularis. In addition to assisting in internal and external rotation, these muscles act as a depressor on the humeral head during shoulder elevation. In this manner a fulcrum that allows the deltoid to elevate the arm is established. As long as some depressor action of the rotator cuff remains, surprisingly large tears of the rotator cuff may be compatible with full elevation of the arm.

II. **Types of pain.** Pain may be related to intrinsic lesions of the shoulder or it may be referred from other sites.

   A. **Cervical spondylosis** of C5 to C6 often results in a referred type of pain to the shoulder. If the radiculopathy includes weakness of shoulder abduction and external rotation, it may closely mimic a torn rotator cuff. Cervical types of shoulder pain are usually increased by neck motion, particularly extension with rotation to the involved side.

   B. **More than one basis** for pain may be present; for example, patients with cervical spondylosis and referred pain to the shoulder may also develop limitation of shoulder motion secondary to adhesive capsulitis (see sec. II.C.2.).

   C. **Intrinsic shoulder pain** is generally worse at night and is increased by lying on the shoulder. Shoulder motion will generally aggravate the pain, particularly full elevation in the forward flexed position or abduction to 90 degrees. Tears of the rotator cuff may also cause pain radiating into the forearm and, rarely, the hand. Specific problems of the shoulder region tend to occur at certain age intervals.

      1. From age **20 to 30 years,** the impingement syndrome and instability problems may present as a painful shoulder.

      2. From age **40 to 50 years,** the impingement syndrome, calcific tendinitis, and adhesive capsulitis become more common.

      3. From age **60 to 70 years,** the impingement syndrome may progress to a full thickness rotator cuff tear. In addition, adhesive capsulitis is common. Degenerative lesions of the acromioclavicular, sternoclavicular, and occasionally the glenohumeral joints become more frequent. Pain from metastatic disease should be considered.

III. **Physical examination.** On examining the shoulder region, one should note that the musculature of the dominant extremity may be somewhat hypertrophied about the shoulder and arm, particularly in athletic individuals.

   A. **Observation**

      1. The **position of the shoulder** relative to its contralateral side should be noted. Elevation or dependency of shoulder may be related to scoliosis, Sprengel deformity, or simply athletic activity.

81

2. **Swelling** about the shoulder region may be secondary to inflammation of a bursa or may be associated with rotator cuff tears.

3. View the shoulder from both the **anterior and posterior aspects.** Observe the **range of motion** as elevation of the arm occurs to note the scapulohumeral rhythm.

4. **Specific muscle atrophy** may indicate either rotator cuff tears or neurologic involvement.

B. Palpation

1. The **supraclavicular fossa** should be carefully palpated for lesions as well as for tenderness of the brachial plexus, which is seen in thoracic outlet syndrome.

2. **Local tender spots** indicative of trigger points should be sought along the interscapular region and overlying musculature of the shoulder. If pressure is applied to these spots, radiation of pain into the upper arm may be observed.

3. Specific sites of tenderness should be noted: anteriorly over the biceps tendon, laterally over the subdeltoid bursa and rotator cuff.

4. The **acromioclavicular and sternoclavicular joints** should be carefully examined for tenderness.

C. Motion

1. In examining the shoulder, one should observe the full range of **active** and **passive** motion, noting any discrepancy such as that sometimes seen in a rotator cuff tear.

2. Shoulder motion is recorded as **abduction,** 180 degrees, and **forward flexion,** 180 degrees. External rotation of the humerus is noted with the arm at the side as well as in the abducted position of 90 degrees. Internal rotation is recorded by placing the hand behind the back and noting which spinous process the thumb will reach.

3. The **impingement sign** is positive in patients with rotator cuff inflammation and is performed by flexing the arm forward to the full overhead position. Pain is present during the last 10 degrees of passive elevation. Passive abduction to the 90-degree position with internal rotation will similarly produce pain.

4. The **adduction** test consists of fully adducting the humerus across the chest. This test stresses the acromioclavicular joint and will cause pain if degeneration of the joint is present.

5. In cases where **instability of the glenohumeral joint** is a possibility, the joint should be carefully stressed in the following manner. The patient is placed in the supine position and, after maximal muscle relaxation is achieved, the shoulder is adducted and internally rotated with pressure placed in the posterior direction. If **posterior instability** is present, a click or a clear-cut subluxation may be noted during this maneuver. To evaluate **anterior instability,** the shoulder is placed in the abducted, externally rotated position with gentle pressure placed in an anterior direction behind the humeral head. In some patients, clear-cut apprehension is observed, preventing the completion of the test.

D. Neurovascular examination

1. A complete **neurologic examination** should be performed. Weakness may be the result of intrinsic shoulder lesions, as in a cuff tear, or of nerve lesions of the brachial plexus or cervical roots.

2. The pain of a **carpal tunnel syndrome** may be referred proximally to the shoulder region.

3. Because **thoracic outlet syndrome** may be present, the circulation of the arm and the hand must be carefully evaluated.

a. **Adson test,** which may be positive, consists of palpating the radial pulse while the patient's head is turned to the involved side, and performing a Valsalva maneuver. A positive test, decrease in the pulse, is not diagnostic; it occurs in a significant percentage of asymptomatic subjects. Reduction of radial pulse with testing should be compared to the pulse on the contralateral side.

b. In the arterial type of thoracic outlet syndrome, **auscultation** of the supraclavicular region may demonstrate a bruit with the arm in both the adducted and abducted positions. The blood pressure in these two positions may be significantly reduced as well.

IV. Radiographs

A. **Standard views** of the shoulder generally have included internal and external rotation which, although helpful in the diagnosis of calcific tendinitis, provide little information regarding the anteroposterior (AP) alignment of the shoulder or the width of the glenohumeral joint. Since the scapula lies on the chest wall at approximately a 40-degree angle, x-rays should be taken at a right angle to the scapula and glenohumeral joint rather than to the chest.

B. **Lateral and axillary views** of the scapula are useful in identifying degenerative changes of the glenohumeral joint and calcification of the rotator cuff; they are particularly important in evaluation of acute injuries to the shoulder.

V. Common shoulder problems. The most common shoulder problems are impingement syndrome with rotator cuff tears, calcific tendinitis, adhesive capsulitis, acromioclavicular joint pain, thoracic outlet syndrome, and shoulder instability.

A. The **impingement syndrome** represents a constellation of findings that occur over a wide age range; **inflammation of the rotator cuff** is the basic pathology. **Tears of the rotator cuff** may also be seen.

1. During the **second and third decades,** shoulder pain is frequent in the athletic population since repetitive use results in progressive rotator cuff inflammation. This problem is commonly seen in young tennis players, swimmers, and baseball players.

   a. **Pain** generally has a gradual onset and is increased by activity. Initially the pain will follow the particular activity but, in time, pain will develop during the athletic activity.

   b. Pain is generally aggravated by elevating the arm to the full overhead position. Careful evaluation of shoulder motion will demonstrate some **loss of forward flexion and internal rotation.**

   c. The **impingement sign** (see sec. III.C.3.) is positive; further pain is produced with abduction and internal rotation to the 90-degree position.

   d. Careful palpation of the rotator cuff will demonstrate **tenderness** of the anterior superior humeral head and the proximal biceps tendon.

   e. **X-rays** are generally negative.

   f. In evaluating these patients, one should be careful that **shoulder instability** is not present.

   g. A useful test consists of subacromially injecting 5 to 6 cc of 1% lidocaine, then noting if pain is reduced on performing overhead elevation of the arm.

   h. **Therapy** is based on activity modifications and temporary avoidance of the offending positions.

      (1) Any contractures about the shoulder region must be eliminated by a stretching program.

      (2) Oral antiinflammatory agents may be helpful, particularly indomethacin 25 mg QID for 7 to 10 days.

(3) A muscle-strengthening program must be established since shoulder pain will often lead to weakness, particularly of the rotator cuff. In carrying out this program of exercise, the pain-producing positions should be avoided.

(4) Subacromial injection of 40 mg methylprednisolone acetate (Depo-Medrol) is administered if the previous methods have failed, but should be limited to one or two injections over a three-month period.

(5) If no significant improvement is noted after six months, surgical resection of the coracoacromial ligament may be warranted. On occasion, resection is combined with excision of the inferior surface of the anterior edge of the acromion to provide further clearance for the rotator cuff during shoulder motion.

2. During the **fourth or fifth decade** a similar picture is noted, particularly in the middle-aged tennis player who will often complain of pain while serving or hitting an overhead shot.

   a. X-rays may show some sclerosis of the greater tuberosity or of the acromion.

   b. Management is similar to that in the younger group.

3. During the **sixth or seventh decade,** further rotator cuff degeneration develops as a result of decreased vascularity of the supraspinatus tendon.

   a. The rotator cuff becomes attenuated as well as inflamed, with subsequent partial tearing which may progress to full thickness in some patients.

   b. The findings are similar to those of the younger patient but increase in severity. Crepitation of the subacromial space from an inflamed thickened subacromial bursa may be present. In this age group, **biceps tendinitis** and **subacromial bursitis** are rarely separate entities and form part of the impingement syndrome.

   c. Atrophy of the infraspinatus and supraspinatus regions will increase in severity, particularly if a cuff tear is developing.

   d. When a small tear of the rotator cuff is present, shoulder motion may initially be normal, but as the tear increases, elevation will gradually be replaced by a shoulder-shrugging movement.

   e. Loss of external rotation may develop; however, it is seen only in patients with large extensive tears that involve both the supraspinatus and the infraspinatus.

   f. In patients with large tears of the rotator cuff, a **drop sign** will be positive. This sign is elicited by having the patient elevate the arm either actively or passively into the full overhead position, then lowering it in the plane of the scapula. At approximately the 90-degree position, marked weakness is noted, and the arm will drop 30 to 40 degrees, often with pain.

   g. Shoulder x-rays will demonstrate sclerosis of the acromion with a reversal of the normal convexity of the inferior surface of the acromion.

   (1) Occasionally a large spur will develop at the anterior inferior edge of the acromion.

   (2) If a cuff tear is suspected or if the patient does not respond to treatment, an arthrogram should be obtained which, if positive, demonstrates extravasation of dye from the glenohumeral joint into the subacromial bursa.

   (3) For older patients, surgical treatment consists of acromioplasty and, if a tear is present, rotator cuff repair.

   h. The conservative management of older patients is similar to that of younger patients, unless a rotator cuff tear is obvious.

(1) Stretching, strengthening, and antiinflammatory agents can often be beneficial.

(2) Injection of the subacromial space on one or two occasions may be helpful in allowing the patient to restore shoulder function; a long, repeated course of injections, however, will only lead to further degenerative changes of the rotator cuff.

B. Calcific tendinitis may present in either an acute or chronic form.

1. In the **acute** process the patient notes the sudden occurrence of severe shoulder pain and will present holding the arm carefully at the side to avoid all shoulder movement.

   a. A distinct swelling may be seen overlying the humeral head, and gentle **palpation** reveals a well-localized area of extreme tenderness.

   b. All movements of the shoulder are resisted by pain.

   c. Shoulder x-rays will generally show a fluffy calcific deposit within the rotator cuff tendons, most commonly the supraspinatus.

   d. Therapy of the acute situation consists of injecting the deposit with 2 to 3 cc of 1% lidocaine and 40 mg Depo-Medrol. After achieving some local anesthesia, the deposit should be needled in an attempt to break it up, thus allowing the deposit to migrate into the subacromial bursae where it will be absorbed. Occasionally, spontaneous rupture of the calcific deposit will occur, with prompt resolution of the patient's pain.

      (1) Because pain may be temporarily increased following the injection of the calcium deposit, ice should be applied to the shoulder for 20 to 30 minutes on several occasions over the next 24 hours.

      (2) In addition, indomethacin 25 mg QID is given for 3 to 4 days.

      (3) When pain is improved, full shoulder motion should be encouraged to avoid developing a contracture.

2. In the **chronic** situation, the calcific deposit becomes indurated within the rotator cuff.

   a. There is a chronic history, often of multiple attacks of shoulder pain. Complaints will often mimic those of the impingement-type syndromes.

   b. Therapy is similar to that of acute tendinitis. Oral antiinflammatory agents (indomethacin 25 mg QID) and exercises are prescribed. Injections of 40 mg Depo-Medrol are administered if no improvement is seen following conservative management. If pain persists or repeated attacks occur, operative removal of the calcium may be required.

   c. It should be noted that many patients of 40 or more years of age have asymptomatic calcium deposits in the shoulder.

C. Adhesive capsulitis (frozen shoulder), frequently seen during the fifth and sixth decades, may develop as a result of intrinsic shoulder pathology or occur secondary to extrinsic causes, particularly cervical spondylosis. Often, no specific etiologic factor can be found.

1. In addition to varying losses of shoulder motion, **pain** is present, particularly at the extremes of motion and at night.

2. On occasion, a large **loss of shoulder motion** will develop so slowly that the patient is unaware of the magnitude of the problem. Conversely, the onset may be sudden and severe with nearly complete loss of glenohumeral motion and a restriction of abduction to the 70- to 80-degree range.

3. **Tenderness** is present but poorly localized.

4. A history of **diabetes** may be obtained.

5. **X-rays** will often be negative in the early stage but, with time, will show osteoporosis.

6. The cervical spine region, and chest and diaphragmatic lesions, should be carefully evaluated. Complete radiographic evaluation, including cervical spine, chest, and shoulder views, may be required.

7. **Metastatic lesions** involving the shoulder, spine, or brachial plexus may present as an adhesive capsulitis.

8. **Therapy** is directed solely to achieving an improved range of motion. Injections and oral antiinflammatory agents may be required depending upon the severity of the pain. A vigorous program of physical therapy is instituted both actively and passively at home and with a therapist. Improvement in range of motion is variable but may require up to two years.

D. **Acromioclavicular joint.** Pain secondary to pathology of acromioclavicular joint is frequently overlooked. The joint lies directly over the rotator cuff and thus any alterations of the inferior surface will result in inflammation of the supraspinatus tendon deep to this joint.

1. **Degenerative lesions** of this joint may result in thickening and swelling and create an impingement syndrome.

2. **Pain** will occur with overhead activity of the arm and be aggravated by adduction of the arm across the chest. Pain occurs at night and is often increased by lying on the shoulder.

3. **Tenderness** is well-localized to the involved joint.

4. **Radiographs** demonstrate narrowing of the joint with sclerosis and marginal osteophytes. Specific views taken at a 15-degree cephalic tilt allow better visualization of the acromioclavicular joint.

5. **Therapy** of the chronic situation consists of antiinflammatory medication, lidocaine injected locally, and Depo-Medrol. The degree of relief obtained from these injections confirms the diagnosis.

   a. In the posttraumatic condition, muscle-strengthening exercises, particularly for the deltoid and trapezius, will result in improvement if significant degenerative changes are not present.

   b. In the chronic situation where pain persists despite 1 or 2 injections, resection of the outer 2 cm of the clavicle may be warranted.

E. **Subluxation of the shoulder** is an important cause of pain in the younger population. Often the patient will state that the shoulder "comes out," although some patients will complain only of shoulder pain, particularly in the posterior humeral region.

1. **Specific testing** for shoulder instability (see sec. **V.A.1.g.**), noting any positions associated with apprehension, should be performed.

2. **Radiographic evaluation** may provide confirmatory evidence of shoulder instability.

3. In those patients who have subluxation of the shoulder without dislocation, **rotation exercises** may be helpful. If symptoms persist despite this approach, surgical stabilization may be required.

F. **Additional shoulder conditions.** Although the more common causes of shoulder pain have been discussed, a wide variety of conditions may affect the shoulder.

1. The **thoracic outlet syndrome** with vascular or brachial plexus involvement may be the basis for extremity pain or fatigue.

2. Any type of **arthropathy,** including rheumatoid arthritis, degenerative joint disease, and syndromes such as polymyalgia, may be expressed as rheumatic

shoulder pain; however, in contrast to the conditions reviewed in this chapter, such problems are part of more generalized rheumatic syndromes.

3. **Avascular osteonecrosis** commonly affects the humeral head and should be considered in the differential diagnosis of shoulder pain (see Chap. 29).

4. The **shoulder-hand syndrome (sympathetic reflex dystrophy),** a poorly understood but common basis for shoulder pain, is associated with diffuse swelling, pain, and vasomotor changes in the distal upper extremity (see Chap. 36). The problem occurs in elderly subjects, is sometimes related to myocardial infarction or other cardiopulmonary conditions, and, when bilateral, may be difficult to distinguish from acute rheumatoid arthritis.

   Unless there is vigorous institution of an exercise program, supported by the use of analgesics and antiinflammatory drugs, **adhesive capsulitis** may be the outcome. If agents such as indomethacin (100 to 150 mg/24 hr) do not control pain sufficiently to permit exercise, a short course of prednisone (25 mg/24 hr for 3 to 4 days) may be instituted.

5. A variety of **intrathoracic problems** (including coronary ischemia, pulmonary embolus, pleuritis, and pneumonitis) and **diaphragmatic irritation** from abdominal lesions should be considered in the differential diagnosis of pain referred to the shoulder region.

14. Hand Disorders

Gary M. Gartsman

Disorders of the hand are common; the primary physician is frequently called upon to diagnose, evaluate, treat, or refer these conditions. The diagnosis of hand disorders can generally be made by appropriate history, physical examination, laboratory data, and radiographs. A knowledge of basic anatomy and physiology, together with a systematic approach to examination, will enable the practitioner to plan a rational therapeutic regimen.

I. **History.** Since hand function is integral to all activities of daily living, the patient will usually be able to describe accurately duration and degree of disability.

   A. **General history** should include patient's occupation, hand dominance, age, medical history, and hobbies and activities which might use the hand.

   B. **Specific history** regarding dysfunction of the hand itself should include duration of disability, precipitating cause, and specific loss of function.

      1. **Pain** location and pattern are important; questions such as does pain radiate from the neck, does it awaken the patient, what relieves the pain, and are analgesics required should be asked.

      2. Symptoms of **numbness, weakness,** or **paresthesias** may indicate neurologic dysfunction.

      3. The patient should be questioned in detail about dysfunction of the neck or any of the other joints of the upper extremity.

II. **Physical examination**

   A. The patient should be sitting and the entire upper extremity unclothed.

      1. **Surrounding joints.** Begin at the **neck;** check range of motion and palpate for areas of tenderness.

         a. Shoulder and elbow should also be fully examined since either may be a source of hand disorder.

         b. Closely evaluate shoulder and forearm musculature for evidence of atrophy.

      2. **Wrist.** Evaluate both active and passive range of motion, and palpate for localized areas of swelling or tenderness.

      3. **Hand.** Observe the resting posture of the hand and record specific areas of muscle atrophy, discoloration, abnormal swelling, or deformity.

         a. Always compare to contralateral hand as a control.

         b. Evaluate and record active range of motion at metacarpophalangeal (MCP), proximal interphalangeal (PIP), and distal interphalangeal (DIP) joints.

         c. Grossly evaluate grip strength, pinch, and five-finger coordination.

         d. Passively flex and extend joints of fingers and record fixed contractions.

         e. To test for flexor tendon function activity, ask the patient to flex DIP joint while holding PIP joint in extension. This action evaluates the flexor digitorum profundus. To test flexor digitorum sublimus function, hold other fingers in extension at MCP joint and ask patient to flex digit. Flexion should occur at PIP joint, and DIP joint should be flaccid.

         f. The ulnar and radial **pulses** should be palpated and capillary refill tested in each digit.

    g. Sensation is best tested with cotton and two-point discrimination, using the prongs of a paper clip. Measure the distance where distinction is not accurate, and compare to the contralateral hand.

III. Diagnostic studies

A. Radiographs should include anteroposterior, lateral, and oblique views of the involved digit.

B. Nerve conduction and electromyographic studies should be performed if neurologic basis for weakness or atrophy is suspected.

IV. Painful conditions

A. Pain in the finger

1. **Felon.** This is a painful infection and swelling of the **distal pulp.** Initial treatment includes elevation, splinting with aluminum or plaster, and dicloxacillin 500 mg every 6 hours. If there is no resolution of pain within 24 hours, or if fever develops during that time, surgical drainage is necessary.

2. **Paronychia.** An infection around the base of the nail, this condition usually occurs as the result of rough manicuring or ill-advised picking of a hangnail. Severe pain, swelling, and erythema limited to the **base of the nail bed** occur. Therapy regimen follows that of felon (see sec. **IV.A.1.**).

3. **Subungual hematoma.** This extremely painful condition usually results from trauma to the distal finger (e.g., car door slam, hammer blow). Immediate elevation and immersion in ice water may reduce the nail pain and bleeding. Relief of pain is dramatic if the nail bed is carefully punctured over the hematoma area with a paper clip prong that has been inserted in a flame until red hot. Soak the finger in antiseptic solution and then apply a band-aid.

4. **Flexor tendon rupture.** Pain in the palmar aspect of the finger can be caused by rupture of the flexor digitorum profundus tendon from its insertion into the distal phalanx. A history of sudden pain in the finger while grabbing an object (e.g., a football jersey, a stumbling child) is classic. Methodic testing of flexor digitorum profundus function (see sec. **II.3.e.**) establishes the diagnosis. Surgical repair is the treatment of choice.

5. **Mallet finger.** Similar trauma may rupture the terminal extensor tendon, producing a flexed distal phalanx and an inability to actively extend the DIP joint. The pain here is localized over the dorsum at the joint. X-rays of the affected finger are necessary since avulsion fractures of the distal phalanx may occur as the tendon ruptures. Therapy consists of an aluminum foam splint applied to the dorsal surface of the finger, immobilizing only the DIP joint in extension (avoid hyperextension). A dorsal splint spares the palmar tactile surface and allows PIP joint motion during the necessary six weeks of splinting.

B. Pain in the finger or palm

1. An infected **tenosynovitis** most commonly presents as pain in the palm or palmar aspect of the finger. The finger is generally swollen and throbbing, and there is often a history of a puncture wound. As a result of the venous and lymphatic drainage pattern and the loose tissue on the dorsum of the hand, dorsal swelling is common. Remember **Knavel's** four cardinal signs.

    a. Flexed posture of the digits.

    b. Pain on palpation of the flexor tendon sheath.

    c. Pain on passive extension of the digit.

    d. Painful and limited voluntary flexion. Aspiration of the tendon sheath under sterile conditions should be performed, and Gram stain and bacteriologic cultures should be obtained before beginning antibiotics. This is a potentially destructive infection of the tendon sheath. Early surgical debridement and decompression is necessary.

2. **Trigger finger.** Occasionally the first presentation of trigger finger can be pain in the palm or palmar surface of a digit. This represents a tenosynovitis of the flexor tendon sheath with a nodular enlargement on the flexor tendon itself. It may be seen in diabetics and patients with rheumatoid arthritis. Attempted passage of the nodule is blocked by the unyielding pulleys, and the patient describes a painful "locking" of the finger in flexion. Extension often is possible only by using the contralateral hand to forcibly extend the finger. Physical examination demonstrates a tender, palpable nodule in the flexor tendon in the palm, and passive flexion and extension will reproduce the "catching sensation." Injection of methylprednisolone acetate (Depo-Medrol) 20 mg (0.5 cc) into the tendon sheath may diminish the inflammatory response around the nodule and allow normal motion. Surgical release of the flexor pulley is sometimes required.

C. **Pain in the palm.** Infection is a common cause of pain in this region of the hand, and is usually the result of a direct puncture wound or extension of an infected flexor tendon sheath. These conditions are serious and usually necessitate surgical drainage and parenteral antibiotics.

D. **Pain in the thumb**

1. **Disorder of the carpometacarpal joint** of the thumb may produce pain caused by synovitis, degenerative arthritis, or subluxation. Actions such as pinching may be difficult or impossible. X-rays will often reveal joint destruction. Therapy modalities include:

   a. Antiinflammatory medication, indomethacin 25 mg QID.

   b. Intraarticular injection of steroid Depo-Medrol 10 mg.

   c. Immobilization.

2. **DeQuervain tenosynovitis.** Pain in the area of the anatomical snuffbox usually results from inflammation of the tendon sheaths of abductor pollicis longus and extensor pollicis brevis tendons. A history of chronic, repetitive movements of the wrist and thumb will usually be elicited. Diagnosis is confirmed by tenderness and pain over the area when the thumb is enclosed in the palm and the wrist deviated (Finklestein test). Therapy includes immobilization by splinting, antiinflammatory medication (indomethacin 25 mg QID), or injection of Depo-Medrol 10 to 20 mg into the tendon sheath. Refractory cases may require surgical release of the tendon sheath.

E. **Painful joints**

1. **Infection.** Pyarthosis of the MCP joints is most commonly caused by a human bite or tooth abrasion to a clenched fist. These infections usually present as severe pain and joint swelling, fever, and marked limitation of motion. Admission to the hospital for debridement, immobilization, and intravenous antibiotics is recommended.

2. **Arthritis.** The synovitis of osteoarthritis and rheumatoid arthritis commonly causes pain in the wrist and small joints of the fingers. Therapy includes antiinflammatory medications (nonsteroidal or steroidal) and immobilization during periods of acute symptoms. Intraarticular steroid can be administered if symptoms persist. Aids to improve range of finger motion, and grip and pinch strength include a spring grip, a small rubber ball or sponge, and clay or putty.

V. **Hand deformities**

A. **Dupuytren contracture.** In this condition, part or all of the palmar fascia undergoes painless thickening and contracture, drawing the MCP, PIP, and DIP joints into flexion. The condition is more common in males (90% of patients) than females, is often bilateral, and is often seen in patients with a history of diabetes, epilepsy, or alcoholism. These individuals complain of inability to open their hands fully and are unable to grasp large objects. The diagnosis is confirmed by the flexion posture of the digit or digits, the presence of palpable nodules, and thickened longitudinal cords in the palm extending into the digit. Similar bands may also be present in the plantar fascia. Surgical excision is recommended if the deformity impairs hand function.

B. Swan neck. This abnormality consists of hyperextension of the PIP joint and flexion of the DIP joint. It may occur following trauma or, more commonly, rheumatoid arthritis. Anatomically, synovitis causes erosion of the volar-stabilizing elements, allowing dorsal displacement of the extensor apparatus. With contracture of the joint and extensor apparatus, PIP flexion is impossible and deformity can be severe. In the early posttraumatic condition, splinting may be attempted with the deformity reversed (PIP flexed and DIP extended) for a six-week period. Surgical correction is necessary if hand function is sufficiently impaired.

C. Boutonnière. Disruption of the extensor mechanism over the PIP joint from trauma, laceration, or synovitis will produce flexion of the PIP joint and extension of the DIP joint. The deformity is not as functionally disabling as swan neck deformity since grasp function is still possible. Acute therapy consists of splinting the finger with the PIP joint extended and the DIP joint flexed. Surgical reconstruction may be necessary if disability is marked.

D. Extensor tendon ruptures without laceration are uncommon except in patients with chronic rheumatoid arthritis. Rupture probably results from multiple factors, notably compromise of the tendon blood supply as a result of florid tenosynovitis. The ring and little fingers are most commonly affected. The presenting complaint of inability to extend the thumb or finger should alert the examiner. Examination of the resting posture of the hand will demonstrate increased flexion of the digit or digits; active extension of digits will not be possible. These extensor tendon ruptures are usually painless and may go unnoticed by the patient. Early surgical consultation is advised since a single extensor tendon rupture puts more strain on the remaining tendons and often heralds a chain of tendon ruptures across the dorsum of the hand.

VI. Swelling

A. Ganglions are the most common soft tissue tumors in the hand, most commonly presenting as painless, firm dorsal swellings around the wrist. They may also be located over the volar wrist and in the hand near the metacarpophalangeal flexion crease. Although their etiology is unknown, ganglions are cystic swellings containing mucinous material that are closely connected to joints or tendon sheaths.

Ganglions rarely interfere with hand function, but on occasion, particularly after strenuous activity, they may become painful. Aspiration, if attempted, should be with a 14-gauge needle since the ganglionic fluid is extremely viscous. Recurrence is common; if symptomatic, surgical excision is recommended.

B. The **carpometacarpal boss** is a bony prominence involving the carpometacarpal joints of the index and long fingers. It may appear similar to a ganglion. Pain may be produced on wrist extension, but excision is rarely required.

C. Synovitis of rheumatoid disease may present as swelling over the PIP, MCP, and wrist joints as well as over the dorsum of the hand. Swelling over the dorsum of the hand should not be confused with an infectious process. Motion of fingers and wrist may be limited. Aspiration may be attempted if the diagnosis is doubtful but care should be taken not to convert a synovial swelling into an iatrogenic infection. Immobilization by splinting, together with an appropriate antiinflammatory medication, is indicated for therapy of the acute attack. Tenosynovectomy may be indicated in selected patients with refractory dysfunction.

D. Swelling of disuse. Normal active hand motion is essential to promote venous and lymphatic drainage. Any condition that produces an absence or decline of hand motion will promote the collection of edema and lead to diffuse hand swelling, stiffness, and, ultimately, loss of function. Bed rest and inactivity resulting from an unrelated condition (myocardial infarction, skeletal traction, sciatica) may lead to this potentially disabling condition. Physician awareness of problem and the services of a trained therapist are essential in management of the problem (see Chap. 36).

VII. Abnormalities of sensation

A. **Carpal tunnel syndrome.** This condition is produced by compression of the median nerve at the wrist. As the nerve passes through the unyielding carpal tunnel, it is at risk for compression by the transverse carpal ligament. In most patients no specific etiology can be determined, but thickening and proliferation of the peritendinous synovium are seen. This condition, which is very common in rheumatoid arthritis, is also seen in postmenopausal women as well as the myxedema of thyroid disease.

1. **History** of wrist pain and paresthesias in the thumb, index, and long fingers (the median nerve distribution), which frequently occur at night, is fairly typical. The patient may report being awakened by the pain and paresthesias, needing to shake the hand for relief. The lack of muscle activity at night allows fluid accumulation, and the wrist flexion posture during sleep is thought to account for this exacerbation of symptoms. Patients may also report daytime paresthesias, clumsiness or dropping of objects, and weakness of pinch or grasp.

2. **Physical examination** may demonstrate a mild flattening of the thenar eminence. Light touch with a cotton applicator along the radial border of the ring finger and both sides of the index finger and thumb will demonstrate a decrease in sensation. Care must be taken to apply the applicator along the palmar surface of the digit as the dorsa of the fingers are supplied by the radial and ulnar nerves. A decrease in two-point discrimination occurs later in the neuropathy. Thumb opposition, the ability to draw the thumb away from the palm and oppose the thumb pulp to the pulp of the little finger, may be diminished. Tapping the volar surface of the wrist over the median nerve may produce the **Tinel sign,** which appears as shooting pain in the long or index finger and indicates median nerve compression. **Phalen sign** is also helpful and is performed by flexing both wrists for 30 to 60 seconds, eliciting median nerve numbness in the affected hand.

3. **Electromyography (EMG) and nerve conduction studies** may confirm a delay in nerve conduction across the carpal canal and denervation of thenar musculature.

4. **Therapy**

   a. **Splints** to hold the wrist in slight extension during sleep.

   b. **Depo-Medrol** 40 mg may be injected into the area of the carpal canal and provides some relief in early cases. Care must be exercised to avoid injuring the median nerve and flexor tendons during injection.

   c. **Surgical release** of the transverse carpal ligament is indicated if response to local measures is poor or if neurologic deficit progresses.

B. **Ulnar nerve entrapment.** This condition may recur at the wrist as the ulnar nerve passes through the tight canal (of Guyon). It may be seen after wrist trauma, in rheumatoid arthritis, as well as with jackhammer workers. Symptoms include weakness of the intrinsic muscles of the hand and numbness in the ulnar nerve distribution. Diagnosis is confirmed with nerve conduction and EMG studies. Therapy is usually by local injections of Depo-Medrol and surgical decompression if symptoms persist or neurologic findings progress.

15. Low Back Pain

Thomas P. Sculco

The low back region is defined as the area of the spine inferior to the L-1 level. Low back pain is one of the most common conditions seen by the practitioner and results in an annual loss of 1,400 work days per 1,000 workers in the United States.

I. **Etiology.** The lumbosacral complex is composed of diverse components, any of which may be a factor in low back pain.

   A. Vertebrae.

   B. Intervertebral discs.

   C. Apophyseal joints.

   D. Nerve roots.

   E. Ligamentous complex

      1. Anterior and posterior longitudinal ligaments.

      2. Interspinous and supraspinous ligaments.

      3. Iliolumbar ligaments.

   F. Paraspinal and abdominal musculature.

II. **History.** Past medical history may give important information concerning trauma, previous malignancy, rheumatoid arthritis, ankylosing spondylitis, a visceral source for the patient's pain, or metabolic bone disorder.

   A. Character of pain. The following features of pain help formulate a specific diagnosis.

      1. Mode of onset and timing

         a. If **trauma** was involved, the patient may have bony or ligamentous injury.

         b. If pain followed **lifting,** it may indicate a ligamentous sprain or herniation of an intervertebral disc.

         c. If chronic and **activity-related,** the pain may result from muscle fatigue or apophyseal joint arthritis.

      2. Localization of pain

         a. If **only lumbar** and of rapid onset, usually indicates ligamentous sprain, although herniated nucleus pulposus can only give midline pain.

         b. If **radicular,** usually indicates nerve root irritation by herniated disc.

      3. Aggravating and relieving factors

         a. If radicular, pain aggravated by coughing, sneezing, or straining may indicate herniated disc.

         b. If aggravated by sitting and relieved with recumbency, significant muscular spasm is likely.

         c. The efficacy of analgesic medications can provide information regarding pain severity.

   B. Neurologic complaints. The patient should be questioned carefully concerning the presence of neurologic signs.

      1. Paresthesias present in a dermatomal distribution can indicate the level of nerve root involvement (see Appendix E).

2. A history of **weakness** or **numbness** similarly helps identify the affected lumbosacral level.

3. **Bowel or bladder dysfunction** with sacral or perineal numbness suggests the presence of a cauda equina lesion.

III. **Physical examination.** The patient should be completely disrobed.

A. **Patient standing**

1. Note the **alignment** of the spine. A tilt to one side may indicate asymmetric paravertebral muscle spasm. Reversal of normal lumbar lordosis is seen in severe paravertebral muscle spasm.

2. A **structural scoliosis** may be present and contribute to the patient's pain.

3. Evaluate the standing **posture** of the patient.

4. Have patient flex the spine, and record distances of hands from floor. Lateral bending and spinal rotation are also measured (see Chap. 1 for normal values).

5. **Toe and heel walking** help assess function of ankle dorsiflexors and plantar flexors.

B. **Patient supine**

1. Elevate each leg in turn with knee extended (**straight leg–raising test**) and record angle where pain begins. Note if pain radiates into posterior thigh and calf or is limited to the buttock, indicating nerve root irritation (sciatica).

2. Evaluate **hip and knee motion** to eliminate these areas as source of pain.

3. Perform thorough **muscle testing** and **sensory examination** to evaluate neurologic function (see dermatome chart in Appendix E).

C. **Patient prone**

1. Palpate **lumbosacral area** and identify specific zones of tenderness.

2. Perform **neurologic examination** of posterior leg.

3. Extend knee and hip if pain was elicited anteriorly in thigh. L-4 radiculopathy is indicated by this positive **femoral nerve stretch sign.**

4. Sciatic notch tenderness may be present.

D. **Patient sitting**

1. Compare a sitting **straight leg–raising test** to that from the supine examination. If significant disparity is present, it may indicate malingering.

2. Test **tendon reflexes** of patellar (L3-L4), posterior tibial (L4-L5), and Achilles tendons (L5-S1) for symmetry.

IV. **Laboratory studies**

A. **Radiographs.** Anteroposterior, lateral, and oblique views may help determine the diagnosis.

1. Evidence of **narrowing of the intervertebral disc space** can indicate a degenerative process of long standing. Complete disc space obliteration with rarefaction of subchondral vertebral end plates indicates septic spondylitis.

2. **Congenital and developmental defects**

a. **Spondylolysis** (defect in the pars interarticularis).

b. **Spondylolisthesis** (forward displacement of one vertebra over a lower one).

c. **Transitional vertebrae** with complete or incomplete sacralization of L5 or lumbarization of S1.

d. Scoliosis (lateral spinal curvature).

e. Vertebral anomalies include hemivertebrae, butterfly vertebrae, and bony vertebral bars.

3. Apophyseal joint degenerative changes, indicative of osteoarthritis, may be seen.

4. Destructive lesions of the vertebral bodies suggest a metastatic process or infection.

B. Further diagnostic studies

1. Myelography is indicated when symptoms are severe and do not resolve with conventional treatment. Both intradural and extradural abnormalities may be seen.

2. Electromyography may identify nerve root disease not detected by clinical examination.

3. Discography. Injecting dye into the disc may reveal evidence of disc degeneration. Reserved for patients with persistent symptoms and an equivocal or negative myelogram.

4. Computerized axial tomography is useful to evaluate patients in whom spinal stenosis may be the cause of back pain. Spinal stenosis may be secondary to osteoarthrosis, causing dural and foraminal encroachment.

5. Bone scan is useful if a malignant lesion or infection is suspected and routine radiographs are normal.

V. Differential diagnosis. Diagnosis is discussed according to anatomic site of involvement.

A. Low back pain without radiculopathy

1. Vertebrae

a. Primary or metastatic tumor.

b. Fracture, traumatic or osteoporotic.

c. Congenital or developmental abnormalities (see sec. **IV.A.2.**).

d. Coccydynia.

2. Intervertebral disc

a. Disc herniation, particularly if protrusion is midline.

b. Degenerated disc results in an increased load on the supporting soft tissues.

c. Infection results in acute, severe pain with secondary vertebral body infection. In contrast to osteomyelitis in other areas, septic spondylitis is commonly produced by gram-negative organisms and is seen with urinary tract infection.

3. Apophyseal joints

a. Osteoarthritis causes recurrent chronic pain.

b. Rheumatoid arthritis.

c. Ankylosing spondylitis and other seronegative spondyloarthropathies.

4. Soft tissues

a. Ligamentous sprain.

b. Postural abnormality leading to muscle fatigue and back pain.

c. Poor muscle tone caused by inactivity, obesity, or neuromuscular disease.

5. Visceral causes

   a. Aortic aneurysm.

   b. Uterine disorders.

   c. Renal stone.

   d. Prostate disorders.

   e. Retroperitoneal neoplasm.

B. Low back pain with radiculopathy. Radicular symptoms or objective neurologic deficits may be present.

   1. Vertebrae. Spondylolisthesis and spondylolysis can produce radicular pain (usually without neurologic deficit) by applying tension to the nerve root.

   2. Intervertebral disc. Herniation or degeneration of the disc often causes symptoms at the following neurologic levels.

   a. L3-L4 level. Patients present with posterolateral thigh or anterior leg pain. Sensation is decreased over the anteromedial aspect of the leg, and knee extension is weak. The patellar reflex may be diminished or absent.

   b. L4-L5 level. These patients complain of classic sciatic pain distribution, posterior thigh and calf pain. Decreased sensation may be present over the lateral leg and dorsum of the foot including the big toe. Weakness of the extensor hallucis longus as well as other toe extensors and ankle dorsiflexors may be present.

   c. L5-S1 level. Patients present with posterior thigh, calf, and heel pain. Decreased sensation is present over lateral leg and foot, particularly the lateral three toes. There may be weakness of ankle and toe plantar flexion and gluteus maximus–controlled hip extension. The Achilles tendon reflex is diminished or absent.

   3. Apophyseal joints. Patients with hypertrophic apophyseal joints secondary to osteoarthritis may develop stenosis of the neural foramina, which can cause radicular pain or neurologic deficit. The patients are generally elderly and the radicular pain is increased by walking.

   4. Soft tissue lesions rarely cause radicular symptoms.

   5. Vascular occlusive disease can cause claudication pain in buttocks and calves.

VI. Therapy

A. Acute low back pain with or without radiculopathy

   1. Bed rest with knees and hips flexed. A pillow is placed under knees. When lying on side, the patient should assume a fetal position.

   a. Mattress should be firm or supplemented with a ⅜-inch thick plywood board.

   b. Patient may lie on floor with hips and knees flexed by resting the feet on a chair.

   c. Bed rest should be strictly enforced until symptoms improve (7 to 14 days). Patient is allowed out of bed only for toilet purposes during acute phase of pain.

   2. Physical therapy

   a. Moist heat should be used to relieve muscular spasticity. A wet towel wrapped around a hot water bottle or a hydroculator pack delivers the heat effectively.

b. **Gentle massage** to the low back BID is recommended.

3. **Medication** includes muscle relaxants, analgesics, and antiinflammatory preparations. The goal is to achieve a painless state while at bed rest.

a. Either diazepam 5 mg QID or cyclobenzaprine 10 mg TID can be used as a **muscle relaxant.**

b. Codeine 60 to 120 mg every 3 hours is used as an **analgesic.**

c. Indomethacin 25 mg QID is an effective **antiinflammatory drug** which is prescribed for 7 to 10 days.

d. Injections of local anesthetics or corticosteroids into the lumbar area are usually ineffective and are not recommended.

B. **Convalescent phase**

1. As pain recedes, **ambulation** is allowed as tolerated.

2. A lumbosacral **corset** may help by limiting lumbar mobility.

3. Initially, a low back **exercise program** performed twice daily is encouraged. As recovery progresses, three daily exercise sets with five repetitions should be performed. Low back exercises are illustrated in Appendix C.

a. **Pelvic tilt.** Buttocks are tightened and lumbar spine is flattened isometrically for 5 seconds.

b. **Knee-chest.** Both knees are brought to the chest and held with arms for 5 seconds; knees are then extended. Knees can be brought up separately or together.

c. **Modified sit-up.** Knees are flexed and head is brought toward knees. The position is held for 5 seconds.

d. **Walking.** Increased amounts daily.

e. **Swimming.** Should be strongly encouraged, particularly the freestyle stroke.

4. **Weight reduction** program is mandatory in patients who are overweight.

5. **Lifestyle modifications.** Advise patient to avoid lifting objects greater than five pounds or sitting for long periods (at desk or in car). If heavy objects must be lifted, the patient should use a squatting technique rather than bending forward from the waist. Occupational alterations may be required in laborers with recurrent, intractable back pain.

C. **Failure of treatment**

1. If patient is not improved after the above measures, admission to the hospital may be required for pelvic traction and further diagnostic evaluation.

2. If a **neurologic deficit** is present, the patient should be evaluated by a neurologist. If the deficit progresses, the patient should be admitted to the hospital for observation, further diagnostic studies (myelogram, EMG), and consideration for surgery.

16. Hip Pain

Thomas P. Sculco

I. **Etiology.** The anatomic structures of both the hip joint and the hip region should be considered in evaluating the patient's pain.

A. **Hip joint**

1. Proximal femur and acetabulum.

2. Articular surfaces.

3. Synovium.

B. **Periarticular soft tissues**

1. **Bursae:** Greater trochanteric, iliopsoas.

2. **Tendons:** Hip adductor, abductor, rotator, extensor, flexor, hamstring.

3. **Herniae:** Inguinal, femoral.

C. **Referred pain**

1. Lumbosacral.

2. Visceral.

II. **History.** Patients with hip pain usually complain of limitation of hip motion and a painful limp. Past medical history may reveal a previous diagnosis of osteoarthritis, rheumatoid arthritis, gout, joint infection, malignancy, or low back pain, which may provide insight into the etiology of the hip pain. Pain response to antiinflammatory medications helps one to assess the severity of the pain.

A. **Duration and location of pain**

1. Pain of **short duration** is usually inflammatory or posttraumatic.

2. Pain that is **chronic and progressive** may indicate mechanical joint incongruity related to an underlying arthritis.

3. **Lateral hip pain** with radiation to the lateral thigh may be related to greater trochanteric bursitis or abductor tendinitis; **groin pain** with radiation to the buttock indicates hip joint dysfunction.

4. **Pain arising in buttock** and extending posteriorly to thigh and below knee suggests a lumbosacral disorder with sciatica.

B. **Relation of pain to activity**

1. **Pain arising from the hip joint** and surrounding soft tissue is usually aggravated by weight bearing and relieved by rest. However, pain from arthritis may be severe at night.

2. **Pain from an incarcerated femoral hernia** is persistent and presents as groin pain.

C. **Decreased function.** Patients complain of progressive decrease in maximum walking distance and exercise tolerance. Patients with significant loss of hip motion may be unable to clip their toenails, get into a bathtub, pull on stockings, or cross their legs.

III. **Physical examination**

A. **Gait.** Observe the patient walk without external support, and note the gait pattern.

1. **Abductor lurch.** Shifting of body weight over affected limb to unload weakened hip abductors.

2. **Coxalgic gait.** Patient quickly unloads painful leg when weight bearing.

3. **Stiff hip gait.** When limitation of hip motion is marked, the patient will walk by rotating the pelvis and swinging the legs in a circular fashion.

B. **Patient standing**

1. Measure **leg length** inequality by balancing pelvis with calibrated blocks, if necessary.

2. Evaluate **spine alignment.**

3. **Trendelenberg sign.** When weight bearing on affected side, patient will drop contralateral pelvis since hip abductor, which normally elevates pelvis, is weakened.

C. **Patient supine**

1. Record active and passive **hip range of motion,** and compare to values of opposite side (see Chap. 1 for normal values).

   a. Note flexion, extension; abduction, adduction, internal and external rotation in both flexion and extension.

   b. **Thomas test for hip flexion contracture.** Flex contralateral knee to chest and evaluate the degree of flexion assumed by the affected hip.

2. Palpate anterior hip capsule by applying pressure just inferior to the inguinal ligament over the femoral triangle and evaluate the degree of **tenderness.**

3. Palpate the groin in supine and standing positions, searching for femoral or inguinal **herniae.**

4. Measure **thigh circumference** bilaterally to assess muscle atrophy.

5. Measure **leg lengths** with a tape measure, recording from umbilicus to medial malleolus and from anterior superior iliac spine to medial malleolus. It is important that leg position be comparable if joint contractures are present.

6. Evaluate **neurovascular status** of limb.

7. Examine the **knee and ankle.**

D. **Patient lying on unaffected side**

1. Palpate greater trochanteric area for **bursal tenderness.** By adducting the leg, one can increase tensor fascia pressure on the bursa and elicit pain if bursa is inflamed.

2. Assess **abductor muscle power.**

E. **Patient prone**

1. Palpate **lumbosacral area** to evaluate low back as a potential source of pain.

2. Evaluate **hip extensor power.**

3. Palpate **sciatic notch** for tenderness.

IV. **Laboratory studies**

A. **Radiographs** should include an anteroposterior view of the pelvis, which allows comparison between hips, and a lateral view of the affected hip. If lumbosacral disease is suspected, obtain films of lumbosacral spine.

1. May demonstrate degenerative changes in the hip joint with osteophytes and subchondral sclerosis consistent with **osteoarthritis.**

2. **Rheumatoid arthritis** involving the hip joint usually produces periarticular osteoporosis and joint space narrowing as cartilage is destroyed.

3. **Infection** involving the hip joint will rapidly produce cartilage destruction. Bone destruction involving the femoral head and acetabulum may also be seen.

4. **Calcifications** may rarely be seen over the abductor tendon insertion or greater trochanteric bursa.

5. **Incongruous joint surfaces** secondary to congenital hip dysplasia, Legg-Calvé-Perthes disease, or slipped capital femoral epiphysis may be seen.

B. **Blood studies** should include sedimentation rate, white blood cell count with differential, uric acid, and rheumatoid factor if indicated by the clinical evaluation.

C. **Further diagnostic studies**

1. **Hip aspiration** and **arthrography** should be performed if infection is suspected.

2. **Tomograms** may help clarify bone abnormalities in acetabulum, pelvis, or femur.

3. **Bone scan** may demonstrate osteonecrosis of the femoral head earlier than radiography.

V. **Differential diagnosis.** Consider the anatomic structures of the hip area when formulating a working diagnosis.

A. **Hip joint**

1. **Acetabulum and proximal femur**

a. **Stress fractures** may occur in the femoral neck, particularly in runners and patients with osteoporosis.

b. **Primary or metastatic tumors** may infiltrate femoral head and acetabulum, and pathologic fractures may occur. The most common tumors that metastasize to bone are breast, thyroid, prostate, renal, lung, and gastrointestinal neoplasms.

c. **Osteonecrosis** of the femoral head with or without collapse may produce severe hip pain (see Chap. 29).

2. **Articulating surfaces**

a. **Osteoarthritis, rheumatoid arthritis, ankylosing spondylitis,** or **septic arthritis** may produce hyaline cartilage destruction with resultant hip joint incongruity and pain.

b. The articulating surfaces can also be rendered incongruent by a **segmental collapse of the femoral head** secondary to osteonecrosis, or to a fracture or dislocation that damages either the joint surface itself or the blood supply to the femoral head.

3. **Synovium**

a. **Synovitis in the hip joint** may result from inflammatory diseases such as rheumatoid arthritis.

b. **Posttraumatic synovitis** usually resolves rapidly with rest and mild analgesics.

c. Tuberculosis may lead to a **proliferative synovitis** and severe joint destruction. Diagnosis is confirmed by hip aspiration, acid-fast stain, and culture.

d. **Pigmented villonodular synovitis** may lead to cyst formation in the femoral neck or joint destruction.

B. Periarticular soft tissues

1. Bursae

a. Greater trochanteric bursitis is common and produces acute pain over the lateral thigh which usually radiates distally. Swelling and pain with weight bearing are often present, and a limp may result.

b. Iliopsoas bursitis is uncommon. It may communicate with the hip joint in 15% of patients.

2. Tendons and fascia

a. Hamstring, abductor, adductor, and rotator tendons may become inflamed at their insertions into bone.

b. The fascia lata is quite taut as it passes over the greater trochanter and may produce a snapping sensation and pain, particularly on hip flexion and adduction.

3. Herniae

a. Inguinal herniae, if symptomatic, may produce severe groin pain and limitation of hip motion.

b. Femoral herniae that prolapse may produce severe pain and limping. However, pain is intermittent until incarceration occurs.

C. Referred pain

1. Lumbosacral

a. Osteoarthritis involving the lumbosacral apophyseal joints can produce buttock pain.

b. Radicular pain from **nerve root irritation** may be manifested in the lateral thigh or groin. Disc herniations at the L3-L4 level often produce radicular pain over the upper anterior thigh.

2. Visceral origin

a. Renal colic pain can radiate to the groin.

b. Femoral vein phlebitis can present with thigh and groin pain.

c. Vascular occlusive disease of aorta can produce buttock pain.

VI. Therapy.

For therapy of specific disease entities, see the appropriate chapters. However, the following general therapy modalities are recommended for patients with hip pain.

A. Rest

1. Joint rest

may be accomplished by unloading the affected hip using various forms of external support.

a. Cane. It should be held in the contralateral hand to assist the weakened abductors and to unload the hip.

b. Crutches. Lofstrand forearm crutches or axillary crutches.

2. Bed rest

is recommended for severe pain.

B. Compresses

1.

If there is an acute inflammatory condition involving a tendon or bursa, **ice** compresses are useful.

2.

For chronic pain, **moist heat** compresses improve the local blood supply and relax spastic musculature.

C. Medications

1. **Antiinflammatory medications** are useful for arthritic problems involving the hip joint. Indomethacin 25 mg QID after meals or buffered aspirin 900 mg QID are equally effective.

2. **Analgesics.** Darvocet-N 100 (propoxyphene napsylate 100 mg and acetaminophen 650 mg) may be used in conjunction with an antiinflammatory drug. Dosage is 1 tablet every 4 hours p.r.n.

3. **Soft tissue injections.** For bursitis or tendinitis, local injection with methylprednisolone acetate (Depo-Medrol) 40 mg and 1% lidocaine 3 to 5 cc is effective. If no improvement occurs after one injection, two more weekly injections may be given.

D. Exercises

1. Attempts should be made to maintain passive and active hip motion without aggravating the underlying pain.

2. Gentle isometric exercises for the quadriceps and hamstrings, and antigravity exercises as tolerated for hip flexors, extensors, abductors, adductors, and rotators are recommended. See Appendix C for specific exercise prescriptions.

3. Swimming is an excellent activity to maintain hip motion and muscle function.

E. Weight reduction.
The prognosis in many hip disorders is guarded if aggravating factors such as obesity are not addressed. Ideal patient weights are listed in Appendix D.

17. Knee Pain

Douglas M. Joseph

I. History

A. Age. The age of the patient can provide insight into the cause of knee pain.

1. The most common causes of knee pain in **children** (under 18 years) include Osgood-Schlatter disease, osteochondritis dissecans, discoid lateral meniscus, and chondromalacia patella.

2. From **adolescence through young adulthood,** sporting injuries predominate. Trauma may result in patellar dysfunction, and meniscal and ligamentous problems. Rheumatoid arthritis and other inflammatory arthropathies also present in this age group.

3. From the **midforties onward,** degenerative diseases predominate. Osteoarthritis, osteonecrosis, rheumatoid arthritis, and degenerative meniscal tears are common problems.

B. The pattern and localization of pain are important in distinguishing various diseases; however, there may be significant overlap.

1. **Meniscal injuries** are the most common causes of pain along the joint line.

2. **Patellar dysfunction** and **primary degenerative arthritis** often present as isolated joint line pain (although patellar pain is usually more anterior).

3. **Osteonecrosis** and **osteochondritis dissecans** may present as localized pain over the involved femoral condyle or as posterior knee pain.

4. If the patient complains while **climbing** stairs or after **sitting** in a chair for a period of time, patellar disease is usually present.

5. If **squatting** or **torsional motions** produce pain, meniscal damage is usually present. If pain is present with **motion** and **at rest**, the cause is often degenerative changes in the knee joint or surrounding structures.

C. Trauma. The direction and type of knee injury can help define the cause of knee pain.

1. **Contact to the knee** may result in ligamentous or meniscal damage, fracture of the tibial plateau, or fracture of the femoral condyles.

2. **Noncontact cutting maneuvers,** with sudden changes in direction or speed, may lead directly to meniscal and ligamentous tears or patellar dislocation.

3. **Osteochondral fractures** and dislodgment of a fragment of osteochondritis dissecans may also result from such torsional motions.

D. Locking is defined as an inability to extend the knee completely. If this complaint is prominent, it may indicate a displaced tear of the medial meniscus which is blocking the knee.

E. Giving way or buckling may result either from quadriceps muscle weakness or a ligamentous injury to the knee.

F. An **effusion** noted immediately after an acute injury is usually a hemarthrosis. It often indicates a torn cruciate (either anterior or posterior) or collateral ligament, torn meniscus, or osteochondral fracture.

1. These lesions may require early surgical care, and early orthopedic evaluation should be arranged.

2. **Mild effusions,** which may not be apparent for several hours following trauma or torsion, may indicate a patellar subluxation or a torn meniscus.

3. **A chronic effusion** or, more commonly, an effusion often present during periods of acute pain suggests a chronic degenerative problem.

II. **Physical examination.** The patient should be sufficiently unclothed to allow visualization of both lower extremities.

A. **Weight bearing.** Observe the patient walking and standing: leg length inequality and alignment of the knees (varus knees, bowed; valgus knees, knock-kneed). The normal knee is in 5 to 10 degrees of valgus alignment. Have the patient attempt a squat, if possible.

B. **Supine.** Examine for an effusion by emptying the suprapatellar pouch with the heel of the hand and palpate with the opposite hand both laterally and medially to the patella.

1. The range of **active and passive motion** should be recorded; measure amount of flexion contracture, if present.

2. Stress the knee medially and laterally at the joint line for instability. By sitting on the patient's foot and pulling forward, the **anterior stability** can be evaluated; **posterior stability** is tested by pushing backward.

3. **Specific areas of tenderness** are recorded as the medial and lateral joint line is examined systematically. The patella is palpated with the knee extended, and tenderness recorded.

4. Note the **tracking alignment** of the patella as the knee is flexed.

5. **Thigh circumference** should be measured bilaterally at a mark made 10 cm above the superior pole of the patella. In lean individuals, a significant difference may indicate atrophy of the hamstring and quadriceps muscles.

6. **The McMurray test** is performed with the knee acutely flexed and the tibia rotated both internally and externally. The knee is then extended gradually, continuing tibial rotation. A click palpated over the medial joint line indicates a possible torn meniscus.

C. **Prone.** Observe and palpate for the presence of a **popliteal cyst.** Palpate for specific posterior areas of **tenderness,** particularly in the area of the hamstring tendons.

III. **Diagnostic studies**

A. **Radiographic determinations** of the knee include standing (weight-bearing) anteroposterior, lateral, and infrapatellar views.

1. **A standing anteroposterior x-ray** is essential for determination of joint space narrowing as in degenerative arthritis (osteoarthritis, rheumatoid arthritis, and osteonecrosis).

2. **Infrapatellar views** (Merchant or Hughston) must be taken to demonstrate patellofemoral alignment.

3. **X-rays taken by applying medial or lateral stress** to the joint may be helpful in determining the extent of ligament laxity.

4. **A tunnel view** that demonstrates the entire intercondylar notch may also be included with the routine series if a loose body or an area of osteochondritis dissecans is suspected.

B. Although the appropriate diagnosis is usually made following history, physical examination, and standard x-rays, certain **blood tests** may be useful in the differential diagnosis of knee pain. Tests include a complete blood count with differential, sedimentation rate, uric acid, and rheumatoid factor.

C. **Special tests** include bone scans, arthrograms, and synovial fluid analysis.

1. **Bone scans** are helpful in differentiating an arthritis (increased uptake) from an internal derangement of the knee, such as a meniscus tear. The location of the increased radioisotope uptake will help differentiate patellofemoral arthritis from tibiofemoral, medial, or lateral compartment arthritis and femoral condylar osteonecrosis.

2. **Arthrograms** are used to define damage to a meniscus. More recently this technique has been used to demonstrate tears in the anterior and posterior cruciate ligaments.

3. **Synovial fluid analysis** is helpful in the diagnosis of rheumatoid arthritis, gout, pseudogout, and joint infections (see Chap. 4).

IV. **Principles of therapy**

A. **Rest** to the painful knee joint should be provided, either by decreased activity or protected weight bearing.

1. Patients should be advised to **decrease walking distance** and to **avoid stairs or prolonged standing.**

2. **Crutches** (axillary or Lofstrand forearm) with partial weight bearing may be utilized. However, a cane in the contralateral hand is usually sufficient to unload the knee.

3. **Athletic activities** should be avoided. Swimming, if permitted, should occur under supervision.

4. In patients with acute pain on motion, a canvas knee immobilizer or bulky knee dressing should be used.

B. **Exercises** as tolerated should be prescribed to maintain quadriceps tone. These include:

1. **Quadriceps isometric exercises** in repetitions of 10.

2. **Antigravity exercises** (straight leg raises), unweighted in repetitions of 10.

C. **Medications** may be useful depending upon the cause of underlying knee pathology. Aspirin 650 to 975 mg PO QID, indomethacin 25 mg PO QID, or phenylbutazone 100 mg PO QID may be prescribed in divided doses after meals depending upon severity of the problem.

1. **Local linaments** provide transient relief.

2. Intraarticular injections of **steroid preparations** may be useful for acute or chronic synovitis (see Appendix G and Chap. 3).

D. **Compression with ice** is useful for the acutely inflamed knee.

E. A variety of **knee braces** which may assist the patient by limiting motion are available; however, they do not provide significant static stability to the joint.

V. **Common causes of knee pain**

A. **Patellofemoral chondromalacia** refers to a variety of problems of the patellofemoral articulation, characterized by anterior knee pain. Often there are no specific articular cartilage changes, and the pain is felt to be secondary to malalignment of the patellofemoral mechanism. Causes of malalignment include: an increase in the anterior torsion of the femoral neck which promotes a toeing-in type of gait, femoral condyle dysplasia, a hypoplastic high-riding patella, external tibial torsion, foot pronation, excessive genu valgum, or a combination or all of these factors. This malalignment of the patellofemoral joint produces pain and may result in patellar subluxation and dislocation.

1. History

a. **Pain is felt anteriorly,** aggravated by climbing and descending stairs or sitting for prolonged periods with the knee flexed (as in a movie theater or car). Some patients report a cracking sensation in the knee with stair climbing.

b. Pain may develop as a result of **direct trauma** (dashboard injury or fall on the knee) or **overuse syndromes** associated with sports (especially jogging). Effusion is rare.

c. The pain may not be severe while walking but may worsen with strenuous activity.

d. **Subluxation or dislocation** may result from torsional stresses with a fixed foot as in basketball, gymnastics, and dancing or from direct injury to the lateral side.

2. Physical examination

a. The important physical findings are **crepitation with flexion-extension** over the edge of the table with **pain** on compression of the patellar facets. This compression test is best done with the patient supine on the table with the knee flexed gently over the other leg (about 30 degrees). Compression against the medial and lateral facets of the femur will be painful.

b. If the patient has experienced recent patellar dislocation or has habitual patellar subluxation, attempted lateral displacement will produce significant apprehension and pain.

c. **Squatting** causes pain in patients with patellar syndrome; however, once a full squat is reached, pain lessens and may disappear.

3. Radiographic findings

a. **An infrapatellar x-ray** is important in assessing congruence of the patellofemoral articulation.

b. **A lateral x-ray** will show the patellar position relative to the femoral condyles. If the ratio of the length of the patellar tendon to the size of the patella is greater than 1.2 : 1, then a high-riding patella (*patella alta*) is present. This condition predisposes the patella to incongruence or subluxation.

c. **A bone scan** will occasionally reveal patellofemoral osteoarthritis.

4. Differential diagnosis

a. The most common differential diagnosis is between **patellar diseases** and **meniscal cartilage tears.**

b. Meniscal tears are usually associated with a traumatic history, pain with activity, associated effusion, and locking. On examination the meniscal tear is painful at the joint line on rotational tests, and a full squat is difficult.

c. Meniscal lesions may be apparent on arthrogram, which should be useful if the diagnosis is in doubt.

5. Therapy

a. The most important therapy is a program of **quadriceps muscle exercises** to develop tone in the muscle and thus diminish laxity in the patellofemoral articulation. These exercises should be done actively in an isometric or straight leg fashion (see Appendix A).

b. **Antiinflammatory medications** are used if pain is acute and disabling. Aspirin 650 mg QID is usually effective.

    c. Patients should curtail those activities that exacerbate pain.

    d. A patellar "cut-out" knee brace may be effective in limiting some patellar laxity; however, it is valuable only when used in combination with a good exercise program.

B. Patellar tendinitis. This condition is related to activity and is often referred to as *jumper's knee* because it is common in athletes, particularly basketball players. Characteristically, pain is located over the anterior aspect of the knee.

  1. Examination. Pain is elicited on direct palpation of inferior surface of the lower pole of the patella, at the origin of the patellar tendon. There may be pain with active extension against resistance.

  2. Differential diagnosis. Patellar tendinitis is a very localized condition and therefore differs from chondromalacia patella. Pain with Osgood-Schlatter disease (tibial tubercle apophysitis) presents identically to pain with patellar tendinitis; however, on examination, the pain is elicited at the tibial tubercle and not at the inferior patellar pole.

  3. Therapy

    a. Rest of the affected knee is crucial. Often a knee splint or cylinder cast with the knee in extension may be required for acute cases.

    b. Aspirin is also useful while the knee is immobilized.

    c. After the pain has subsided, a gradual **rehabilitation program** is started. Quadriceps exercises and proper stretching routines should precede a graduated running program. Reintroduction to sports should be delayed until the rehabilitation phase is over. With proper care, reinjury is rare.

    d. The injection of methylprednisolone acetate (**Depo-Medrol**) 40 mg and 1% **lidocaine** 1 cc into the tendon may relieve acute symptoms when other measures have not been successful.

C. Medial meniscus tear. Traumatic tears of the medial meniscus are a common cause of knee pain, particularly in the athletically active individual. The medial meniscus is prone to tearing when sudden rotational forces are applied to the knee because it is fixed by ligamentous and capsular attachments.

  1. History

    a. Patient usually gives a history of a **twisting injury** with sudden pain over the medial aspect of the knee.

    b. The knee may swell immediately, but more commonly an **effusion** develops over a 24-hour period.

    c. If the effusion is significant, **acute hemarthrosis** with associated ligament injury should be suspected.

    d. The patient may be unable to extend the knee fully (**locked knee**) as a result of impingement of the torn segment of meniscus.

  2. Physical examination

    a. An effusion is generally present, and the patient ambulates with a limp and a flexed knee if the joint is locked.

    b. Joint line tenderness is present medially.

    c. Range of motion will be painful, particularly flexion beyond 110 degrees. Extension may also be painful if the knee is locked or the meniscal tear is anterior.

    d. McMurray test will often be positive. Rotation of the knee is usually quite painful, particularly when the knee is flexed.

3. Diagnostic studies

a. Routine x-rays of the knee are usually normal but may show suprapatellar effusion.

b. Arthrography generally demonstrates the torn meniscus. This procedure is accurate in 90% to 95% of patients with tears of the medial meniscus.

c. Arthroscopy may be performed if arthrography is equivocal.

4. Differential diagnosis

a. Medial collateral ligament sprains may produce medial joint line pain and tenderness with a limp and an effusion. Locking is not present. Arthrography is negative or demonstrates leakage of dye in the area of the ligament injury.

b. Acute chondromalacia patella may produce anteromedial pain. An effusion is rarely present, and locking is also very uncommon. Arthrogram is negative.

c. A pes anserine bursitis presents with pain and tenderness over proximal medial tibia just below the joint line without effusion, limitation of motion, or locking. Direct tenderness is present over bursa, and arthrogram is negative.

d. Medial compartment tibiofemoral osteoarthritis may produce an effusion with medial joint line pain, tenderness, and a limp. X-rays will demonstrate sclerosis and joint space narrowing in the medial aspect of the knee joint.

5. Therapy.
In patients with a locked knee or recurrent symptoms from a torn medial meniscus, surgical removal is the treatment of choice. If the tear is longitudinal, simple excision of the injured segment may be performed.

D. Tibial tubercle apophysitis (Osgood-Schlatter disease).
This condition occurs primarily in adolescents and presents as pain located at the insertion of the patellar tendon into the tibial tubercle. Some authors believe the syndrome represents an injury to the apophysis similar to mild avulsion.

1. Diagnosis.
There is localized pain on palpation of the tubercle. X-rays often show a displaced ossicle of bone anterior to the tubercle, within the tendinous insertion.

2. Therapy.
The pain usually disappears when the ossicle fuses to the underlying tibia. Until that time, the child's activity level must be monitored. Depending on the severity of the pain, some or all athletic activity must be discontinued. A cylinder cast for four to six weeks may be necessary in resistant cases. Aspirin 650 mg PO QID may be used during the acute phase.

18. Ankle and Foot Pain

William K. P. Li

Disorders of the ankle and foot are bases for some of the most common pain syndromes. This chapter deals primarily with problems in the sphere of degenerative disease. Sports injuries, a related topic, are reviewed in Chapter 19.

I. Anatomy. The ankle and foot are subdivided into two distinct groups of joints, the hindfoot and the forefoot.

    A. Joints of the **hindfoot** include the ankle, subtalar, calcaneocuboid, and talonavicular.

    B. Joints of the **forefoot** include the midtarsal, tarsometatarsal, metatarsophalangeal, and interphalangeal (proximal and distal).

    C. Ligaments

        1. The fan-shaped **deltoid** ligament stabilizes the medial aspect of the ankle. Components of the deltoid traverse tibiotalar, tibiocalcaneal, and tibionavicular joints.

        2. The **collateral** ligament stabilizes the lateral aspect of the ankle. There are separate anterior talofibular, posterior talofibular, and calcaneofibular attachments.

    D. Muscles

        1. Ankle motion consists of dorsiflexion (tibialis anterior, extensor digitorum, communis and extensor hallucis longus), plantar flexion (gastrocnemius, soleus) inversion (posterior tibialis), and eversion (peroneal longus and brevis).

        2. The toes are flexed and extended by their respective short and long flexors and extensors.

    E. The ankle and foot are richly innervated from peripheral branches of the sacral roots (see Appendix E). Vascular channels are abundant.

II. History

    A. Pain pattern. Exact localization of pain in forefoot or hindfoot is important. The onset of pain should be recorded. Associated trauma should be noted, together with the duration of foot or ankle pain and the pain-producing activity. Activities that relieve pain (rest, removing shoes) and medications, if any, required for pain relief should be noted.

    B. Footwear. Recent alteration in footwear can lead to pain. The patient should be questioned about composition of shoes, style, and heel height, all of which provide important information.

    C. Past medical history should be thorough. Numerous conditions including gout, rheumatoid arthritis, neoplasms, peripheral vascular occlusive disease, and congenital deformity can all lead to foot and ankle dysfunction.

III. Physical examination

    A. Gait. Observe carefully as the patient walks both in shoes and barefoot, and note the presence of a limp, gait pattern (toe-in or toe-out), or other signs of associated lower extremity joint dysfunction.

    B. Weight bearing. The patient should be examined with shoes and socks removed and the leg from the knee down should be exposed. Note alignment of the ankle and forefoot. Evaluate the longitudinal arch and note forefoot deformities of the great and lesser toes. Evaluate for pelvic tilt secondary to leg length inequality. The temperature of the foot and ankle, the rapidity of capillary refill on blanching the skin, and the intensity of the dorsalis redis pulse provide data on the vascular status of the foot. Trophic changes on the leg and atrophy of the calf musculature should be recorded.

C. **Range of motion** should be compared to the contralateral foot and ankle. Grasp the calcaneus in one hand and move the ankle into dorsiflexion, plantar flexion, and inversion, as well as laterally. Both active and passive motion should be tested. Motion in the great and lesser toe metatarsophalangeal joints should be noted.

D. **Local changes.** Record bony prominences and joint and toe deformities.

1. **Hallux valgus (bunion).** Deformity of the great toe characterized by lateral deviation of the toe and medial prominence of the metatarsal head.

2. **Hammer toe.** Deformity of the lesser toes with fixed or flexible flexion of the proximal interphalangeal joint. Some hyperextension is usually present at the metatarsophalangeal joint; if severe, the term *claw toe* is used. Calluses may be present over the dorsal surface of the joints.

3. **Mallet toe.** Deformity of the distal interphalangeal joint in which this joint is fixed in flexion. Callus may be present over the distal pulp of the affected toes.

E. **Tenderness.** The presence of discrete areas of tenderness can assist diagnosis. Tenderness over the lateral collateral ligament usually indicates an inversion sprain, while sensitivity over the first metatarsophalangeal joint usually indicates degenerative joint disease or gout. Pain on compression of the forefoot or tenderness in an interdigital space suggests an interdigital neuroma. Metatarsalgia occurs when the plantar surface of the second metatarsal head is palpated.

F. **Swelling,** localized or diffuse, may be nonspecific, and systemic etiologies should be considered (dependent edema caused by dysfunction of the cardiac, venous, or lymphatic systems). Swelling over the dorsum of the foot, together with pain on weight bearing, suggest a stress fracture of a metatarsal. Swelling anterior and inferior to the fibula indicates a lateral collateral ligament sprain (anterior division).

G. **Examination of shoes.** Type of shoe should be noted. Wear pattern of heel and sole gives information on gait pattern. Toe box dimensions should be measured if forefoot deformity present. Medial collapse of the shoe can be seen with flatfoot deformity. By looking inside the shoe, the distribution of weight bearing on the foot can be seen.

IV. **Laboratory studies**

A. **Hematologic** tests may include complete blood count, erythrocyte sedimentation rate, latex fixation, and uric acid, particularly if inflammatory arthropathy is suspected.

B. **Radiographs** for ankle disorders should include anteroposterior, lateral, and mortise (true anteroposterior film of ankle taken with the ankle internally rotated 30 degrees to correct for normal external rotation) views.

1. **Foot x-rays,** anteroposterior and lateral, should be taken with the patient weight bearing. The series should also include an oblique view.

2. **Stress x-rays** can be taken if ankle instability is suspected. The degree of talar tilt can be measured when an inversion stress is applied to the ankle. Since considerable normal variability exists, both ankles should be stressed and the degree of talar tilt on the affected side should be compared to the normal side.

C. **Arthrography** of the ankle is useful if loose bodies are suspected, and may also be used acutely to measure the extent of a ligament tear.

V. Common foot problems

A. **Achilles tendinitis** characterized by heel pain, usually at the insertion of the Achilles tendon into the calcaneus or just proximal to its insertion, may be idiopathic or seen in patients with gout or other inflammatory conditions. Characteristically, dorsiflexion of the ankle elicits posterior heel pain. Swelling and erythema may be marked, and gait may be "toe-touch" only. **X-rays** may demonstrate spurring at insertion of the Achilles tendon. **Therapy** of acute tendinitis consists of rest by immobilization in a posterior plaster splint with the ankle in 30 to 45 degrees of equinus. Medications are discussed in detail in Chapter 21. Weight bearing should be avoided for several weeks, depending on severity of symptoms. As symptoms resolve, the patient may gradually resume normal ambulation. A 1½-inch heel is added to both shoes to relax tension on the tendon. Stretching and strengthening exercises may be prescribed at this point to reduce likelihood of recurrence.

B. **Heel pain** may be secondary to an inflammation of the plantar fascia at its origin from the calcaneus, and is common in patients with an atrophic heel fat pad. Swelling and tenderness may be present, often in the medial facet of the calcaneus; however, ankle and foot motion is normal. **X-rays** may demonstrate a calcified spur on the calcaneus. **Therapy** is directed at relieving pressure in this area, usually with a foam cushion or heel cup. Antiinflammatory medication or local injection may be beneficial. Surgical removal of calcaneal spurs, if present, is *not* recommended since symptoms often persist or recur after such therapy.

C. **Plantar fasciitis** is characterized by tenderness along the plantar aponeurosis, particularly when it is placed under stress. **Therapy** consists of supporting the plantar fascia with a scaphoid pad. Antiinflammatory medication can be prescribed.

D. **Pes planus (flatfoot) deformity** can be painful and disabling. The most frequent complaint is of fatigue while standing or walking. Anatomically, the heel in the weight-bearing posture is deviated laterally (valgus), and the longitudinal arch is depressed, with medial prominence of the talonavicular joint. Pain, tenderness, and occasionally acute synovitis may be palpable medially over the first cuneiform metatarsal joint. **Radiographs** confirm the loss of arch and may also demonstrate early degenerative changes in the medial tarsometatarsal joints. **Therapy** consists of wearing shoes with a firm medial border and firm instep support or scaphoid pad. Insoles to correct heel position can often decrease foot fatigue dramatically.

E. **Metatarsalgia** is characterized by pain in the area of the metatarsal heads, particularly on weight bearing. The condition is particularly common in women who wear thin-soled shoes with excessively high heels. In older patients and rheumatoid patients, the normal metatarsal fat pad atrophies, and metatarsal heads become more prone to pressure on weight bearing. Tenderness is usually present beneath some or all of the metatarsal heads, and will be further aggravated by certain forefoot deformities that increase metatarsal head prominence (claw toe, hammer toe, pes cavus). Radiographs are usually normal except in patients with a high longitudinal arch, whose x-rays show increased verticality of the metatarsal heads. **Therapy** is directed at unloading the transverse metatarsal arch. A **metatarsal pad** can be placed in the patient's shoe proximal to the metatarsal heads to relieve pressure on them. Leather **metatarsal bars** are placed on the sole of the shoe proximal to the metatarsal heads. An insole can be fabricated after a mold is taken of the patient's foot, and a metatarsal pad can be apposed to the sole. If pain is intractable and limited to one metatarsal, an osteotomy of the metatarsal can be performed and the metatarsal head shifted dorsally.

F. **Neuroma** formation on an interdigital nerve may cause a painful entrapment neuropathy. Tenderness is present between the third and fourth toes or the second and third metatarsal heads (Morton neuroma). Pain is initially present on weight bearing but ultimately occurs while at rest, and the patient characteristically removes the shoe and massages the foot for relief. Numbness and dysesthesia of the toes, together with a palpable mass, may be present. **Therapy** consists of supporting the arch and preventing hyperextension of the toes. Local injection with lidocaine or corticosteroid may provide temporary relief, but surgical excision is often necessary.

G. **Inversion sprains** usually injure the anterior division of the lateral collateral ankle ligament complex division. Swelling may be marked and is associated with inability to bear weight on the injured ankle. Ecchymosis after several days may be extensive, especially along the plantar border of the foot. The ankle is usually stable to stress testing. Tenderness is present immediately anterior and inferior to the lateral malleolus. In severe sprains tenderness and discoloration may be present over the deltoid ligament. X-rays are usually negative except for soft tissue swelling over the lateral ankle. **Therapy** begins with an Unna boot (Gelco strapping), which provides stability to the ankle and aids in reduction of the swelling. It is reapplied weekly until swelling is well controlled and weight-bearing function is improved. Advance from Unna boot to ace bandage wrap, which should be applied snugly, especially over the lateral aspect of the ankle. Gradually begin active exercise program to strengthen dorsiflexors, plantar flexors, and invertors; peroneal (evertor) exercises are particularly important. Increase weight bearing as symptoms decrease; advance from crutches to cane in contralateral hand. Swimming with a flipper and bicycle riding are good athletic methods of rehabilitating the ankle.

H. **Forefoot deformities** include hallux valgus, hammer toes, mallet toes, corns, and callositas. Footwear is important in the treatment of these patients. An ample and high toe box with a soft leather or suede front is recommended. The shoe should have a low heel and thick sole. Use fine cotton to prevent pressure from adjoining toes. If deformities are the source of intractable pain, surgical correction is recommended.

19. Sports Injuries

Mark F. Sherman

Heightened interest in personal fitness and athletic participation has resulted in a marked increase in sports-related injuries. The physician may expect to see a variety of athletic injuries and must be able to recognize these conditions in order to institute prompt and proper management. As with any general medical or surgical patient, proper history, physical examination, and utilization of laboratory data are essential to establish proper diagnosis and to then institute correct treatment for the injured athlete.

I. Ligamentous injuries of the knee

A. Basic anatomy. Stability of the knee occurs in four planes: anterior, posterior, medial, and lateral. Medial and lateral stability are determined by the medial collateral and lateral collateral ligaments, respectively; anteroposterior stability is determined by anterior cruciate and posterior cruciate ligaments. Other structures that contribute to knee stability include the capsule, menisci, and surrounding muscles.

1. **Medial collateral ligament.** Prevents medial opening of the knee with valgus stress. Anterior cruciate and posterior capsule are secondary stabilizers against medial opening with valgus stress.

2. **Lateral collateral ligaments.** Prevents lateral opening with varus stress. Secondary stabilizers against varus stress are the anterior cruciate ligament, posterior cruciate ligament, and posterolateral capsule.

3. **Anterior cruciate ligament.** Prevents anterior displacement of the tibia relative to the femur. Secondary stabilizers play a minimal role, with the medial collateral ligament being most significant.

4. **Posterior cruciate ligament.** Prevents posterior displacement of the tibia relative to the femur. Secondary stabilizers are anterior cruciate ligament, posterior capsule, and posterolateral capsule.

B. Classification

1. **Grade I (first-degree or mild sprain).** Characterized by local pain and swelling, without instability. Microscopically represented by a mild tear in the collagen fibers of the ligament; however, full continuity of the ligament is maintained.

2. **Grade II (second-degree or moderate sprain).** Characterized by pain and swelling, minimal to moderate instability. Represented by a more substantial tear of collagen fibers. There is some loss of continuity in the ligament.

3. **Grade III (third-degree or severe sprain).** Characterized by swelling, marked instability. There is complete disruption of ligament continuity.

C. History

1. History of **prior injury.** An apparent acute tear of a ligament may actually represent the last of many recurrent episodes, each of which has damaged the structure subclinically.

2. **Mechanism** of injury. Determine exactly how the patient twisted the knee. Was it a valgus stress or a hyperextension injury? If a ski injury, ask the patient in which direction his ski pointed at the time of injury. If a football injury, determine how the foot was planted at the time of impact, and the site and direction of the injury force.

3. **Pain.** Collateral ligament injuries are most painful at the site of damage;

cruciate ligament injury pain is usually related to the capsular distention of hemarthrosis.

4. **Ability** to continue sports. An athlete who, at the time of injury, could not resume activity as a result of pain or instability usually has more severe pathology than one who was able to continue.

5. **"Pop" or "snap".** A pop or snap immediately followed by swelling is characteristic of more than 50% of anterior cruciate ligament injuries.

6. **Swelling.** Swelling that occurs immediately usually indicates acute hemorrhage into the joint (hemarthrosis) and should raise the suspicion of intraarticular fracture or cruciate ligament damage. Swelling that appears over the first 24 hours is more common in grades I or II collateral ligament injuries and is characteristically serosanguinous (see Chap. 4); often no joint swelling will occur in a grade III collateral ligament injury because the complete disruption allows joint fluid to escape into the periarticular soft tissue. (**Remember:** A knee without swelling may be the worst of all knees.)

7. **Locking and "giving way"** are more typically signs of chronic ligamentous instability or meniscal problems than of acute ligamentous injury.

D. **Physical examination**

1. **Inspection**

   a. **Gait.** Patients with an acute ligamentous injury often walk with a limp and a flexed knee.

   b. **Swelling.** Is suprapatellar fullness present in either the standing or prone positions?

   c. **Ecchymosis.** Collateral ligament injuries often show external signs of hemorrhage into soft tissue, which can present along the calf or ankle secondary to gravitational flow along muscle sheaths.

2. **Range of motion** is frequently limited secondary to pain. Lack of extension secondary to effusion should not be confused with the locked knee of meniscal etiology. Palpate for intraarticular effusion by compressing the suprapatellar pouch and balloting the patella.

3. **Neurovascular status.** A knee evaluation must include an assessment of popliteal and distal pulses as well as a thorough neurologic exam. The peroneal nerve is particularly susceptible to damage, especially in varus stress injuries that stretch the lateral structures of the knee.

4. **Ligament stress testing.** The patient should be supine and must be relaxed, as spasm and apprehension can obscure the diagnosis from even the most zealous examiner. The collateral ligaments should be tested with the knee in 0 degrees of extension and 30 degrees of flexion. At 30 degrees, the test is more specific for the collateral ligaments. During full extension, secondary stabilizers tighten to stabilize the joint; if the knee should "open" in extension, the injury is severe. Occasionally 1% lidocaine injected into the site of pain, or even general anesthesia, may be needed to evaluate the knee properly.

   a. **The medial collateral ligament** stabilizes the joint against medial opening, and thus protects against a valgus stress. To test this ligament, the limb is grasped with one hand, while the femur is stabilized with the other, and a valgus stress is applied. Instability, if present, is more often sensed than seen. If the ligament has torn completely, the usual firm, abrupt, end point checking the stress will be absent. If the ligament is injured but not completely torn (grade II), the end point from the remaining intact fibers is present; however, excursion may be increased.

   b. **The lateral collateral ligament** should be tested with a varus stress in the same manner.

c. **The anterior cruciate ligament** is tested with the patient supine, the hip flexed 45 degrees, the knee flexed 90 degrees, and the foot flat on the table. The examiner sits on the foot while placing hands around the proximal tibia, immediately below the joint line. An anterior force is applied to the tibia, and the amount of excursion and the quality of end point are noted (anterior drawer sign). If the knee, following acute injury, cannot flex to 90 degrees, the **Lachman test** is performed. This test is essentially an anterior drawer sign in extension. The femur is grasped with one hand while an anterior force is applied to the tibia with the other. The amount of excursion and end point are noted.

d. **The posterior cruciate ligament** is best evaluated by the posterior drawer sign. This test is similar to the anterior drawer sign; however, force is applied to the tibia in a posterior direction.

When the knees are viewed laterally, injury to the posterior cruciate will cause the tibia to appear "dropback" in comparison to the normal condition.

E. Laboratory data

1. **Radiographs.** Standard knee radiographs are usually negative but are useful to exclude a fracture. Avulsion fractures can sometimes be seen at ligamentous insertions.

2. **Stress x-rays.** The joint opening is best viewed on anteroposterior film by applying mild stress.

3. **Arthrograms.** Arthrography is most useful for definite meniscal tears but may also demonstrate tears of cruciate ligaments and the more severe tears of the collateral ligaments. Leakage of dye from the joint usually indicates a complete collateral ligament disruption.

4. **Arthroscopy.** Allows direct intraarticular visualization in equivocal cases.

F. Differential diagnosis

1. **Meniscus tear.** The history of a twisting injury followed by swelling, locking, medial or lateral pain, and a limp suggests a collateral ligament injury; however, the ligament stress tests are negative and tenderness is usually along the joint line. The combination of meniscal damage with collateral ligament or cruciate ligament injuries commonly occurs, and should always be suspected when evaluating an acute knee injury. Arthrography will usually demonstrate meniscal pathology.

2. **Patellofemoral subluxation or dislocation.** A subluxing or dislocating patella will often present as acute knee pain. Dysplasia of the patellofemoral mechanism is the underlying cause of most patellofemoral injuries. These patients often have bilateral symptoms of anterior knee pain, clicking on squatting, and pain on stair climbing (see Chap. 17).

G. Treatment

1. **Collateral ligament** injuries without cruciate involvement are treated according to the degree of injury.

a. **Grade I** sprains are acutely treated with ice and a compression dressing. Progression to early motion is encouraged, along with symptomatic protection during normal activity.

b. Isolated **grade II** collateral ligament injuries are best treated with a cylinder cast for four to six weeks, then with a knee immobilizer splint followed by a progressive exercise and weight-training program. Arthrotomy and surgical repair are indicated if either or both cruciate ligaments are also torn.

c. An isolated **grade III** collateral ligament injury is unusual and surgical repair is indicated.

   2. Cruciate ligament injury is very difficult to grade; typically, all or none of the ligament is affected. Therapy depends on age and activity level of the patient. For active patients, surgical repair may be indicated, although simple immobilization causes some to improve. An intensive exercise program to strengthen quadriceps and hamstring muscle groups is particularly important following this injury.

H. Resumption of athletics. The patient should not be allowed to resume usual athletic activities until the knee is stable, pain minimal, and the range of motion adequate. The patient should be able to run in place, hop on the affected leg without difficulty, run figure 8 patterns in both directions, and start and stop quickly. Muscle strength should be 80% or more that of the opposite extremity, and muscle atrophy should be less than 1 cm (comparative circumference). The most common cause of recurrent injury is premature return to activity.

II. Running injuries.
The majority of running injuries to the musculoskeletal system are minor and preventable. A proper therapy program for any specific injury will include an overall conditioning program to prevent the recurrence of such injuries.

A. Causes of injury

   1. Biologic fatigue. Jogging or running requires repetitive motion that exposes the musculoskeletal system to severe stress. Even the most conditioned runner reaches a point of fatigue and biologic failure. Limitations and proper preparation are important in preventing running injuries.

   2. Improper training. The overweight, poorly muscled, "once-a-week" runner is the perfect candidate for suffering a running injury. If muscle groups are inadequately trained, they will not tolerate the repetitive forces of running, and injury is likely.

   3. Anatomic variability. Patients with increased ligamentous laxity may be susceptible to sprains while running; the abnormal distribution of stress on the foot of a flatfooted runner makes the patient prone to particular problems. The likelihood of patellar problems is increased in an individual with congenital abnormalities of the patellofemoral joint.

B. Physical examination

   1. Medical examination. A complete respiratory and cardiovascular examination is mandatory for all patients, particularly those over 40 years of age.

   2. Musculoskeletal examination. Observations during your exam should include:

   a. The presence of **swelling** or **ecchymosis.**

   b. **Joint alignment**

   (1) In runners, it is important to evaluate the foot and ankle. Flatfeet (pes planus) and high arched feet (pes cavus) will have different stress patterns, predisposing to different injuries.

   (2) Always watch the patient walk or run. Such activity will best demonstrate overall joint alignment in a functional, weight-bearing position.

   c. Point of maximum **tenderness.**

   d. **Range of motion,** both active and passive, of the involved joint compared to that of the opposite side.

   e. **Neurovascular status.**

   f. **Ligamentous laxity.** Specific tests have been devised to help determine the patient's musculoskeletal profile. Some of these complex tests are:

   (1) Ability to place palms to floor.

(2) Hyperextension of elbows.

(3) Recurvatum of knees.

(4) Ability to place thumb to forearm with wrist flexed.

(5) Amount of metacarpophalangeal hyperextension with wrist flexion.

3. **Type of shoe.** Always assess the shoe since it is the runner's main piece of equipment.

    a. **General fit.** Should be wide and long enough to allow space for the toes, thus reducing blistering and subungual hematomas.

    b. **Cushioning.** Should be thick enough to reduce impact stresses.

    c. **Heel.** Should be wide, thick, and soft. Most runners use a heel-toe gait, and impact concentrates on the heel. Increasing the width of the heel increases the contact area and thus decreases the stresses transmitted.

    d. **Rigidity** is needed for support; flexibility for foot motion. The shoe should be flexible at the metatarsophalangeal region where "push-off" occurs but rigid at the arch (midfoot).

    e. **Counter.** Must be high enough to avoid injury to the Achilles tendon.

C. **Laboratory data**

1. **Radiographs.** Most running injuries are soft tissue problems, and radiographs are negative. Stress and avulsion fractures, which occur quite frequently in runners, may be visualized on routine films. Joint alignment is best visualized with weight-bearing films.

2. **Bone scan** may afford earliest diagnosis of stress fracture, which may not be apparent on routine films for several weeks.

D. **Specific injuries**

1. **Foot and ankle**

    a. **Corns, calluses, blisters.** Painful, hypertrophic skin changes caused by abnormal pressures and stresses.

        (1) Pain on plantar surface of metatarsal heads or dorsum of interphalangeal joints of toes.

        (2) Skin changes obvious by direct observation.

        (3) Underlying foot structural deformity: pes planus (flatfeet), pes cavus (high arch).

        (4) X-ray may help delineate severity of the structural deformity.

        (5) **Therapy.** Padding to reduce stress on area; proper footwear; gradual increase in distance.

    b. **Subungual hematoma.** Traumatic hemorrhage under the nail bed with severe pain.

        (1) Clotted blood under nail causes it to lift off; produced by poorly fitting footwear with tight toe box.

        (2) **Therapy.** Acute: Relieve pressure under nail bed (use sterile hot paper clip to evacuate hematoma). Chronic: Removal of nail may be needed.

        (3) **Prevention.** Well-fitted footwear and sturdy, high, wide toe box.

    c. **Metatarsalgia.** Syndrome of pain under metatarsal heads; first to third metatarsals most commonly involved.

        (1) Pain usually follows episode of prolonged running.

(2) Tenderness directly under involved metatarsal head.

(3) Underlying structural deformity (pes cavus, hammer toes) may be present.

(4) X-ray may show underlying foot deformity.

(5) Therapy. Orthotics (shoe insert) to redistribute weight from metatarsal heads; change gait to heel-toe pattern.

(6) Prevention. Footwear must have adequate cushioning; gradual increase in distances.

d. Stress fracture. Fatigue fracture of a bone secondary to repetitive stresses.

(1) Sudden or gradual onset of pain; shafts of first to third metatarsals most commonly involved; recent change in distance or running terrain is common.

(2) Swelling and tenderness at site; swelling (secondary to fracture callus) in region of fracture is late.

(3) X-ray demonstrates periosteal callus 7 to 14 days after symptoms; bone scan may demonstrate increased uptake almost immediately.

(4) Therapy. No running until symptoms pass; resume running at gradual increments; use plaster cast if necessary to immobilize area.

(5) Prevention. Adequate stretch program; avoid hard surfaces; no abrupt changes in running technique; adequate footwear.

e. Plantar fasciitis. Inflammation of the plantar fascia, typically at its medial calcaneal origin.

(1) Ache or burn along plantar fascia; pain accentuated with activity and relieved by rest.

(2) Tenderness present at anteromedial calcaneal margin.

(3) Tightness of Achilles tendon may be present.

(4) X-ray may show calcaneal spurs, but they are not diagnostic.

(5) Therapy

(a) Achilles tendon stretch program.

(b) Phenylbutazone 100 mg QID with food for 5 to 7 days.

(c) Ice after running.

(d) Adhesive strapping.

(e) Methylprednisolone acetate (Depo-Medrol) 20 to 40 mg at site of maximum tenderness.

(6) Prevention. Good warmup and stretch program: orthotics if underlying structural deformity is present.

f. Achilles tendinitis. Inflammation of the Achilles tendon as a result of repetitive stresses.

(1) Pain present, usually near insertion of Achilles tendon, with tenderness along the length of the tendon; increased warmth and swelling often present; increased pain with passive dorsiflexion of ankle.

(2) Tightness of Achilles tendon may also be present.

(3) X-ray may show calcific deposits at tendon insertion.

(4) Therapy

(a) Limit running when acute.

(b) Phenylbutazone 100 mg QID with food for 5 to 7 days.

(c) Scaphoid pads.

(d) Gradual return to running with vigorous stretch program before and after running.

(5) Prevention. Aggressive Achilles tendon stretch program.

2. Leg problems

a. Shin splints. Inflammation of leg secondary to overuse; posterior and anterior tibial muscle-tendon units most commonly involved.

(1) Aching pain after running, usually in posteromedial aspect of leg; pain may be severe enough to prevent running.

(2) Tenderness along involved muscle unit; no neurovascular deficits on examination.

(3) Produced by poor training, abnormal foot alignment, and running on hard surface.

(4) Therapy. Ice and rest when acute; vigorous exercise program to stretch tendons; muscle strengthening of foot flexors and extensors with weights.

(5) Prevention. Avoid running on hard surfaces; warmup and stretch program; good footwear; change pattern of running, for example, convert from long distances to sprints.

b. Stress fracture. Tibia or femur.

(1) Sudden or gradual onset of pain in leg; proximal posteromedial tibia most commonly involved.

(2) Tenderness at site of fracture; some swelling not uncommon.

(3) Can be caused by poor training (seen in novice runners), abrupt change in running program.

(4) Bone scan will detect site of fracture early; periosteal callus appears on x-ray in 7 to 14 days.

(5) Therapy. Reduce activity (no running) for four to six weeks; use cast if pain is severe; resume running gradually.

(6) Prevention. No abrupt changes in running style; vigorous stretch program; orthotics for underlying structural foot problems.

c. Compartment syndrome. Progressive ischemic pain secondary to increasing pressure within a closed compartment of the extremity (anterior compartment of leg most commonly involved).

(1) Increasing and progressive pain in anterior aspect of leg, not relieved by rest; numbness and paresthesias in foot are common; paralysis may be a late symptom.

(2) Induration and swelling of anterior compartment are earliest signs; decrease in capillary filling of toes; pallor of foot; pulselessness (very late in course); neurologic deficit (very late in course).

(3) Pressure within compartment may be measured and is usually increased.

(4) Therapy. Surgical decompression (fasciotomy) of compartment is urgently needed.

3. Thigh and hip problems

a. Hamstring pull. Inflammation of one or more components of the hamstring musculotendinous unit; usually a result of a minor tear.

(1) Acute or chronic onset of pain in back of the thigh or at hamstring origin from pelvis.

(2) Tenderness present in region of hamstring; increased pain with straight leg raise.

(3) More common in patients with tight hamstrings.

(4) X-rays usually negative but may show avulsion fracture or periosteal reaction at hamstring origin site.

(5) Therapy. Acute: ice, rest, mild stretch program. Chronic: stretch program vigorously before running.

(6) Prevention. Warmup and stretch program.

b. Stress fracture

(1) Acute or insidious onset of pain in hip or pelvis; running accentuates pain.

(2) Tenderness usually present over pubis or ischium in patients with pelvic stress fracture. Pain on hip motion (particularly internal rotation) may indicate stress fracture of femoral neck.

(3) Can occur as result of abrupt change in training; common in novice runners.

(4) Periosteal callus apparent on x-ray one to three weeks following injury. Fracture line may be visible.

(5) Therapy. Reduction in activity and non–weight bearing for hip stress fracture; gradual return to normal activity after six to eight weeks.

(6) Prevention. Proper training; vigorous stretch program; no abrupt changes in technique.

III. Tennis elbow. This condition causes pain at the lateral aspect of the elbow, particularly in the region of the lateral epicondyle and extensor muscle origin. It is often present in non–tennis players as well.

A. Pathogenesis. The site of pathology is at the extensor muscle origin, particularly the extensor carpi radialis brevis in the region of the lateral epicondyle. The period of peak incidence is the fourth decade of life, which suggests a degenerative process in the tendon aggravated by repetitive stress leading to macroscopic and microscopic tears of the extensor origins. In approximately 40% of these patients, there are other sites of soft tissue degenerative problems as well (e.g., shoulder bursitis, tendinitis, and carpal tunnel syndrome).

B. Clinical history

1. Pain. The patient typically presents with the acute or chronic onset of pain in the lateral aspect of the elbow. Complaints of pain while using a screwdriver, shaking hands, making a fist, or lifting a weight are common. The pain radiates from the dorsum of the forearm to the fingers. Tennis players often complain of accentuated pain during backhand strokes.

2. Numbness or paresthesias may occur; however, these complaints should alert the physician to consider alternative causes (e.g., cervical radiculopathy) as well.

C. Physical findings

1. **Tenderness.** Point tenderness is present in the region of the extensor origin at the lateral epicondyle. Tenderness may also be present distally along the extensor muscle sheaths. The tests that clarify the diagnosis stress the extensor muscle mass. Two of these tests are:

   a. **Chair test.** With the elbow extended and the forearm pronated, the patient is asked to lift a chair with the affected extremity. Patients with tennis elbow will not be able to perform this act without lateral elbow pain.

   b. **Stress test.** The patient is asked to extend the wrist while the examiner attempts to flex it. This test stresses the extensor mass and may cause pain.

2. **Strength.** Grip strength may be decreased secondary to pain. Patients with chronic tennis elbow may have atrophy of the forearm muscles.

3. **Range of motion.** During acute episode, a mild restriction of extension may be present.

4. **Neurovascular examination.** Usually negative, but other etiologies of elbow pain must be eliminated.

5. **Swelling** may be present if there is acute tendon rupture, but it is rare.

D. Laboratory data. Blood tests are nondiagnostic and usually normal. Rarely, calcification may be seen in the region of the lateral epicondyle on x-ray, but the elbow joint itself is normal.

E. Differential diagnosis

1. **Medial epicondylitis.** This inflammatory condition leads to pathology within the flexor pronator origin.

2. **Intraarticular pathology.** A patient with elbow pathology (loose bodies, osteoarthritis) may present with lateral elbow pain. Limitation of elbow motion and x-ray changes will clarify the diagnosis.

3. **Gout.** Differentiation is not difficult since the acute, inflammatory signs of gout (erythema, swelling) are not usually present in tennis elbow.

4. Referred pain from **cervical spine disease**.

F. Therapy is symptomatic, and activities that accentuate the pain should be curtailed. Oral antiinflammatory drugs can be given acutely for pain relief. Agents include phenylbutazone 100 mg QID with food or indomethacin 25 to 50 mg QID with food. Injection of Depo-Medrol 40 mg with lidocaine 1 cc into the point of maximum tenderness usually provides relief. Exercises directed at strengthening the extensor muscle without accentuating pain should be prescribed to prevent muscle atrophy. A forearm band may reduce tension on the extensor muscle origin and provide relief in some patients. A dorsal wrist splint which prevents volar flexion may also be helpful.

Approximately 3% to 5% of patients will not respond to these conservative measures. Surgical techniques are available for excising fibrous tissue at the extensor and repairing degenerative tears of the extensor muscle origin.

G. Prognosis. The patient should be informed that tennis elbow is a self-limiting process that usually responds to conservative measures.

H. Prevention

1. **Awareness.** The middle-aged athlete or worker is at great risk and must be made aware of his or her limitations. Warmup, stretching, exercise, and weight-lifting programs serve as prophylactic measures and should be encouraged.

2. **For tennis players**

   a. **Warmup.** Abrupt physical stresses are not good for any muscle group, and the forearm extensors are no exception. The first 15 to 20 minutes of tennis ball hitting should be easy, building up gradually to full capacity.

   b. **Racquet change.** Lighter racquets, larger grip size, and less taut stringing have all been reported as helpful; however, no definitive data is available.

   c. **Instruction.** Poor technique is one of the main causes of tennis elbow. Individuals with this problem should seek professional instruction with specific attention to grip and backhand strokes.

III. Diagnosis and Therapy

20. Ankylosing Spondylitis

Eric S. Schned

Ankylosing spondylitis (AS) is an inflammatory disorder of unknown etiology that primarily affects the spine, the axial skeleton, and the large proximal joints of the body. A distinctive feature of the disease is the striking tendency toward fibrosis with secondary ossification and ankylosis of involved joints. The disease typically affects young men in the second through fourth decades, although young women can be affected. There appears to be a spectrum of clinical severity, ranging from asymptomatic sacroiliitis (identified solely by x-ray) to the classic form of immobilizing spinal encasement. An important advance of the past decade has been demonstration of the strong association between AS and HLA-B27 histocompatibility antigen.

The term *spondylitis* is borrowed from the Greek word *spondylos*, meaning vertebra. Pathologic changes consistent with AS have been recognized in human skeletons 5,000 years old. The disease was long considered indistinguishable from rheumatoid arthritis and was variously called rheumatoid spondylitis, Bechterew disease, and Marie-Strümpell disease until it was recognized in the 1930s as a distinct pathologic and clinical entity.

I. Prevalence and genetic aspects

A. Prevalence. Before the discovery of the association of AS with HLA-B27, initial population studies had already suggested that AS was a genetically determined disease. Prevalence figures differ greatly depending upon the population studied and the methods used to detect and define disease. The prevalence rate in Caucasian populations is between 1 and 10 patients per 1,000 persons (0.1% to 1.0%) with an increased male-female ratio of 2 to 10 : 1. In American blacks, the overall prevalence of AS appears to be approximately one quarter that of whites. Among native Japanese, the prevalence rate is 0.5 to 2 patients per 1,000 persons. Among North American Indians, Haidas have been found to have a very high prevalence, approaching 6% to 13% of their total male population, of sacroiliitis and presumed AS. Pimas may have a prevalence rate as high as 1 : 5 (20%).

The studies also demonstrate an increased prevalence of AS and other seronegative spondyloarthropathies (SSA) among family members of affected persons as well.

The early studies were based largely on roentgenologic detection of sacroiliitis and did not define disease expression in a standardized way. Diagnostic criteria were constructed in Rome in 1962 and revised in New York in 1966 (Table 20-1) in an attempt to provide a basis for valid clinical classification of disease.

All the above data are now being reevaluated in view of the recently discovered association between AS and HLA-B27. As discussed below, the prevalence of AS may be even greater than previously thought.

B. Genetic aspects. In 1973, Schlosstein and Brewerton independently reported an extraordinary association of HLA-B27 with clinical AS. Subsequent studies have shown the HLA-B27 histocompatibility antigen to be present in about 6% to 8% of the normal white population, with equal sex distribution, while fully 90% to 95% of spondylitics bear the antigen. Most other population studies have shown a similarly high association of B27 with clinical expression of disease. The B27 antigen is found in 1% of the Japanese population, but in 95% to 98% of spondylitics. Fully 50% of Haida Indians are B27 positive. Sacroiliitis is present in about 10% of that male population, and almost 100% of these patients are B27 positive. On the other hand, the overall prevalence of HLA-B27 antigen is lower among American blacks (less than 2%), and it appears that clinical AS is less common in this group than in white populations.

Although the bulk of the data *suggests* that the risk of disease is related roughly to the genetic risk, namely HLA-B27 positivity, this association clearly is not

Table 20-1. Clinical Criteria for Ankylosing Spondylitis

Diagnosis
    Limitation of motion of the lumbar spine in 3 planes: anterior flexion, lateral flexion, and extension
    History of the presence of pain at the dorsolumbar junction or in the lumbar spine
    Limitation of chest expansion to 1 inch (2.5 cm) or less, measured at the fourth intercostal space
Grading
    Definite AS
        Grade 3 to 4 bilateral sacroiliitis with at least one clinical criterion
        Grade 3 to 4 unilateral or grade 2 bilateral sacroiliitis with clinical criterion 1 or with both clinical criteria 2 and 3
    Probable AS
        Grade 3 to 4 bilateral sacroiliitis with no clinical criteria

Source: Adapted from J. Moll and V. Wright, *Ann. Rheum. Dis.* 32:354, 1973.

absolute; that is, the HLA-B27 antigen itself is not solely responsible for development of disease. Only 50% of American black spondylitics, for example, are B27 positive. Several reports show that there are no clinical signs or symptoms that differ between B27 positive and B27 negative spondylitics. Such evidence suggests that factors other than the B27 gene itself are also involved in the development of the disease.

Studies have shown that HLA-B27 is found in approximately 50% of first-degree relatives of B27 positive spondylitic patients. Between 4% and 20% of all first-degree relatives have clinical or radiographic AS or sacroiliitis. Among those relatives who are B27 positive, this figure may reach 40%. Calin and Fries studied a population of "healthy" persons who were B27 positive, and found that 20% satisfied criteria for definite AS. Projecting these figures to the population at large, as many as 2% of North Americans might have features of AS.

C. Sex distribution. The observed male-female ratio for the identification of AS ranges from 2 : 1 to 10 : 1. This fact suggests that the disease may be more severe, and thus more recognizable, in men. Alternatively, the diagnosis in women may be overlooked or missed for various reasons, such as attributing symptoms to other causes or reluctance to x-ray the pelvis in young women. Additionally, some early population studies were occupationally based and may have had a selection bias for males. Supporting the hypothesis that clinical disease may be underestimated in women is the finding by Calin and Fries that among carefully evaluated "healthy" B27 positive persons, men and women had evidence of sacroiliitis or spondylitis in equal numbers. Also, radiographic evidence of sacroiliitis among Pima Indians is equally prevalent among males and females.

II. Pathophysiology. The etiology of AS is unknown; however, the discovery of the association between HLA-B27 and AS in most populations studied has spawned numerous hypotheses regarding its pathogenesis.

  A. Pathogenesis

    1. Direct role of antigen. The association is strong enough to have suggested a direct role for the antigen in the expression of disease; that is, it might render the host susceptible to an infectious agent or other environmental factors. However, since not all people who are HLA-B27 positive have AS, and not all patients with AS are B27 positive, the antigen is probably not itself essential for development of the disease.

    2. Antigenic mimicry. Hypothetically, an infectious agent might interact with B27 positive cells to render them autoantigenic, leading to an autoimmune state. Alternatively, the immune response to an exogenous agent might cross-react with the B27 positive host cells to propagate autoimmunity. A recent report states that almost half of a group of black B27 negative spondylitics possessed the HLA-B7 antigen, which belongs to the same serologically cross-reactive group as B27. This finding tends to support the possibility that certain properties of the HLA antigen itself may be instrumental in disease susceptibility.

3. **Linkage to an immune response (IR) gene.** Recent attention has focused on the possibility that the gene coding for the B27 antigen is closely linked to an IR, or disease susceptibility, gene. Linkage to an IR gene would help explain the occurrence of AS in B27 negative individuals, the occasional family member of an AS proband who develops a SSA but is B27 negative, and the overlapping clinical features of the several other SSAs that are also associated with B27. This hypothesis does not exclude an epistatic role for the HLA-B27 gene or gene product in modulating IR gene expression. It also permits the possibility that disease expression by the putative IR gene requires interaction with other gene products or environmental factors.

B. **Search for environmental causes.** An intensive search for triggering infectious agents has yielded several as yet unconfirmed observations. Associations of active spondylitis with the presence of *Klebsiella* species in feces, chronic prostatitis, and urethral chlamydial organisms have all been reported. Other evidence marshalled in support of an infectious etiology is the development of spondyloarthritis in patients with Reiter syndrome following urethritis or gastroenteritis. It may be that the impaired surface or mucosal defenses in patients with psoriasis and inflammatory bowel disease might expose them to infectious agents that can lead to spondyloarthritis.

C. **Pathology**

1. **Skeletal sites** of inflammatory involvement in AS and their pathologic findings are:

   a. **The axial skeleton** (including sacroiliac joints, intervertebral disc spaces, and the apophyseal and costovertebral joints).

   b. **The anterior central joints** (such as the manubriosternal joint, sternoclavicular joint, and symphysis pubis).

   c. **Large, proximal synovial joints** (hips, knees, shoulders). Small peripheral joints are seldom involved.

   d. **Pathologic findings.** Fibrocartilage is the primary site of inflammation in articular tissues. Other areas of inflammation include subchondral bone (osteitis), joint capsule (capsulitis), the annulus fibrosis of intervertebral discs, perispinal ligaments, periarticular ligamentous-bony junctions (enthesopathy), periosteum (periostitis), and, occasionally, synovial membranes (true synovitis). The synovitis of AS resembles that of RA, including pannus formation, but is less necrotic.
   In all these tissues, the initial cellular inflammatory changes are promptly followed by fibrosis and often impressive calcification and ossification, leading ultimately to characteristic bony ankylosis.

2. **Extraskeletal sites** of inflammation include the uveal tract, aortic root wall, and apical lung parenchyma. Postinflammatory fibrous tissue occasionally extends below the valve and can invade tissue, including electrical conduction pathways. A distinctive form of upper lobe pulmonary parenchymal fibrosis and bullous change is now recognized. The acute iritis seen in AS is pathologically nonspecific.

III. **Clinical presentation**

A. **Symptoms.** Recent clinical studies using HLA typing have permitted recognition of a broad clinical spectrum of disease.

1. **The classic presentation** occurs in a young man between 15 and 40 years old, with the insidious onset of intermittent or persistent low back pain and stiffness that is often **worse in early morning hours and after prolonged rest.** The pain is typically **relieved by physical activity.** The patient will often report rising from bed at night to walk around in order to find relief. The pain is usually centered in the lumbosacral spine but may also be present in the buttocks and hips and occasionally may radiate into the thighs, mimicking sciatica.

2. **Chest pain.** The patient may complain of thoracic spine, neck, or shoulder pain and stiffness. Thoracic involvement can lead to anterior chest pain that mimics angina pectoris, esophageal disorders, or mediastinal disease. The pain can also have a pleuritic quality that mimics pericardial or pleural disease. Manubriosternal and sternoclavicular inflammation are other causes of chest pain in the AS patient.

3. **Peripheral arthritis** occurs in one half of patients during the course of AS. Involved joints are usually large and proximal, such as the hips, shoulders, and knees. Asymmetric involvement is typical. **Hip** involvement is the major cause of disability in AS. Although low back pain is usually the initial symptom, peripheral arthritis may simultaneously occur, and occasionally precedes spinal involvement. **Heel pain** may occur secondary to local enthesopathy of the calcaneus.

4. **Subsets of AS**

   a. **Juvenile AS.** In childhood, AS usually presents in older boys as an asymmetric **oligoarticular arthritis** of the lower extremities, often antedating back symptoms. **Heel pain** is a common complaint. It can mimic juvenile rheumatoid arthritis (JRA), especially since radiographic sacroiliitis is often delayed. However, with time, the child develops more typical features of adult AS. Almost all children affected are B27 positive.

   b. **Pauciarthritis in rheumatoid factor negative, B27 positive, middle-aged men.** Although a few of these patients have subtle radiographic changes of sacroiliitis, it is apparent that some such patients may have predominantly **peripheral arthritis** with minimal sacroiliitis or spinal involvement.

   c. **Asymptomatic sacroiliitis.** Among relatives of probands with AS, the presence of asymptomatic radiographic sacroiliitis has been recognized for some time. In recent surveys of individuals who are B27 positive, including healthy, asymptomatic populations, 20% or more have had unequivocal radiographic sacroiliitis. Also, among patients with idiopathic acute anterior uveitis, almost half will have subtle clinical or radiographic evidence of sacroiliitis. An important question awaiting further study is whether and how often radiographically identified sacroiliitis in such individuals progresses to overt clinical disease.

5. **Extraskeletal manifestations of AS**

   a. **Aortic valve regurgitation** is present in 3% to 5% of patients. Occasionally it can lead to severe aortic incompetence. More often it is hemodynamically insignificant or causes only minimal symptoms. Electrical conduction abnormalities including various **heart blocks** can occur, usually, but not always, in association with aortic valve disease. Pacemakers are rarely required.

   b. **Pulmonary involvement**

      (1) **Restriction of the thoracic cage** during respiration, caused by fusion of costovertebral joints, can result in reduced lung volumes but rarely leads to impaired gas exchange.

      (2) **Apical lobe fibrobullous disease** of unknown pathogenesis occurs in

patients with advanced AS. It sometimes leads to striking bilateral radiographic changes including cavitation and fibrosis. The bullae are susceptible to the development of **aspergillomas.**

c. **Acute iritis** will occur in 25% of patients at some time in the course of AS. Some patients experience recurrent episodes with scarring and even secondary glaucoma. Studies have shown a high independent association of idiopathic acute iritis with HLA-B27, and subtle clinical, radiographic, or bone scan changes of AS can be demonstrated in many patients.

d. **Osteoporosis** is an early, common finding, particularly in the spine. It contributes to the susceptibility of patients to spinal fracture.

e. **Amyloidosis** may develop, especially in juvenile AS and occasionally in the adult form.

6. **Complications of AS**

   a. **Cervical spine** involvement can lead to **atlantoaxial subluxation** and **spinal cord compression.** Patients with ankylosed spines have increased susceptibility to **vertebral fractures,** especially in the cervical region, after falls or even minimal trauma.

   b. **The cauda equina syndrome** with buttock or leg pain, bladder or bowel dysfunction, and variable sensory loss is sometimes seen in long-standing AS. The cause is unknown but may involve arachnoiditis or stretching of the spinal cord or its roots by progressive spinal deformity. Myelography usually reveals lumbar arachnoid diverticulae.

   c. **Temporomandibular joints** may be affected, leading to local pain and dental malocclusion.

B. **Physical findings**

1. **Sacroiliac (SI) findings.** Early signs include local tenderness over the sacroiliac joints and tenderness with paraspinal muscle spasm at lumbosacral vertebral levels. Occult sacroiliac involvement can sometimes be elicited by special maneuvers to stress the joint.

   a. **Lateral compression of pelvis** with both the examiner's hands will elicit pain in involved joint(s).

   b. **Gaenslen's sign.** Instruct patient to lie supine on edge of examining table with knees flexed and with one buttock over the edge. Allow patient to drop the unsupported leg off the table. This maneuver will elicit pain in the contralateral sacroiliac joint by stretching it.

2. **Spine findings.** Loss of spinal motion (lateral and in flexion and extension) can be detected quite early in most cases, and several maneuvers can be reliably employed to detect and then follow such changes. With progression of disease, there is typically loss of the normal lordosis, progressive kyphosis of the thoracic spine, fixed flexion of the neck, and, ultimately, a stooped posture with fixed flexion contractures of the hips and knees. An important distinguishing finding involves **lateral flexion,** which is usually abnormal in AS but normal in lumbar disc disease. In addition, because the neurologic exam is usually normal in early AS, an abnormality supports the diagnosis of lumbosacral disc disease. Maneuvers used to detect and follow spinal involvement include:

   a. **Occiput to wall.** Patient stands erect with heels, buttocks, and back against wall and attempts to touch wall with back of head. Occiput to wall distance is measured.

   b. **Fingers to floor.** Patient bends forward with knees straight and attempts to touch fingers to floor. Distance from fingertips to floor is measured.

   c. **Spinal forward flexion.** Marks are made at three points along the spine (the lumbosacral junction and points 5 cm below and 10 cm above), and the distance between highest and lowest marks is measured in maximum forward flexion. Less than 5 cm of distraction is abnormal.

   d. **Lateral spinal flexion.** Two marks are made on the lateral trunk at the level of the xiphisternum and the iliac crest, and the distance between them is measured. The patient bends sideways, sliding the hand down the ipsilateral thigh, and the new distance between marks is measured. A difference of less than 3 cm is abnormal.

3. **Costovertebral involvement** is reflected in decreased chest expansion, which can be measured at the fourth intercostal space in men or under the breast in women. Less than 5 cm of chest expansion in the adult is considered reduced.

4. **Extraaxial joint involvement** is usually proximal (hips, knees, and shoulders) and often asymmetric and tends to cause early contractures. Passive and active range of motion of affected joints is correspondingly decreased. Occasionally, the enthesopathy of AS may be associated with palpable bony spurs, often on the heel.

5. **Other signs.** The signs associated with aortic regurgitation and acute iritis and upper lobe fibrosis are not specific. Rheumatoid nodules are notably absent. Fever is seldom present, although it can occur transiently during acute flares of arthritis.

C. **Laboratory findings**

1. **HLA-B27** is present in 95% of Caucasian spondylitics.

2. **Erythrocyte sedimentation rate (ESR)** is elevated in most cases but does not correlate well with disease activity.

3. **Hematologic tests.** A mild normocytic anemia is seen in severe cases. The peripheral white count is normal.

4. **Synovial fluid** contains a moderate number of mononuclear leukocytes in contrast to the increased polymorphonuclear leukocyte counts of RA fluid.

5. **Pulmonary function tests** in patients with thoracic involvement usually show diminished vital capacity (VC) and total lung capacity (TLC) and increased residual volume (RV) and functional residual volume (FRV). Flow measurements are usually normal.

6. **Immunologic tests.** A variety of nonspecific abnormalities are reported:

   a. Hypergammaglobulinemia.

   b. 7S IgG antiglobulins in serum.

   c. Variable reduction in serum complement activity.

   d. Conflicting data on presence of immune complexes in serum.

   e. Impaired mixed lymphocyte response (MLR) in B27 positive individuals.

7. **Other tests.** The alkaline phosphatase is often elevated, reflecting osteitis. Calcium and phosphorus are normal. IgM rheumatoid factors are notably absent.

D. **Radiographic findings.** The radiographic appearance of advanced AS is characteristic.

1. **SI joints.** The earliest radiographic changes often occur here and consist of punched-out **erosions, "pseudowidening"** of the joint, and adjacent **sclerosis.** Eventually bony bridging of the joint appears with complete loss of joint space.

2. **Spine.** Vertebral chondritis and adjacent subchondral osteitis followed by fibrosis and ossification lead to bony bridging of adjacent vertebrae (syndesmophytes). Earliest changes usually occur at the thoracolumbar junction. The

aptly named **bamboo spine** of AS represents the advanced radiographic appearance of this ossification process.

The **Romanus sign** is an erosion surrounded by sclerosis at a vertebral body margin. Occasionally, aggressive disc inflammation may erode the disc and adjacent vertebral bodies, mimicking septic discitis. Periostitis of the periphery of the vertebral body leads to early "squaring" of vertebral bodies.

Apophyseal and costovertebral joint capsules may become ossified and fused. Rigidity and instability may lead to **atlantoaxial subluxation.** The initial osteitis and erosions of the manubriosternal joint and the symphysis pubis appear as widening of the joint, followed by sclerotic new bone formation and fusion.

3. **Peripheral joints.** Initially, the x-ray appearance of proximal joints in AS may resemble RA. However, there is a greater tendency in AS to central articular erosion and often proliferative new bone formation in periarticular tissues with bony ankylosis. Concentric joint space narrowing and lateral femoral osteophytes are distinctive x-ray signs of hip disease in AS.

4. **Ligamentous-bony junctions.** Inflammation and secondary ossification at these junctions in areas such as the pelvis (sacrotuberous and sacrospinal ligament insertions), the greater trochanter of the femur, plantar fascia, and the Achilles tendon lead to proliferative bone margins and whiskery spicules.

E. **Nuclear scans.** Technetium stannous pyrophosphate bone scans can often detect areas of active inflammation in AS before standard radiographic changes are present. However, the bone scan is not of great clinical utility because it cannot distinguish among other causes of high uptake.

IV. **Differential diagnosis.** Distinguishing AS from the multitude of other causes of low back pain (LBP) represents a major diagnostic challenge. Testing for HLA-B27 is impractical and expensive to perform in all patients complaining of back pain. The **clinical history,** however, may be a sensitive and specific tool in the differential diagnosis. If four or more of the following five features are present, the diagnosis of AS should be strongly entertained:

1. Age of onset less than 40 years.
2. Insidious onset.
3. Duration of LBP more than three months.
4. Association with morning stiffness.
5. Improvement with exercise.

A. **Lumbosacral disc disease** and "lumbar strain" may be difficult to distinguish from AS; however, the clinical story of pain intensifying with rest and improving upon exercise in spondylitics may be useful. Although sciaticalike pain may occur in AS, accompanying neurologic signs of lumbar root compression are unusual.

B. **Pelvic inflammatory disease** in women or premenstrual tension syndromes with referred pain can usually be excluded by careful history and exam.

C. **Other SSA.** Any of the other SSA may develop skeletal inflammation essentially identical to classic AS. Usually the extraarticular manifestations of these diseases allow clinical distinction among the group, but there is probably an overlapping spectrum of features. The rheumatic syndrome usually follows the onset of other clinical manifestations but occasionally may precede it. For example, the spondylitis of **inflammatory bowel disease** may precede bowel symptoms by months or years. The spondylitis of **Reiter syndrome** and **psoriatic arthropathy** is usually less severe than that of typical AS, and syndesmophytes tend to appear on only one lateral margin of the vertebral body. Typical extraarticular features will eventually clinch the diagnosis in most cases.

D. **Degenerative joint disease (DJD)** of lumbosacral apophyseal and intervertebral joints is very common but the older age of the patient and typical osteophytes on x-ray usually facilitate differentiation. The SI joints can be affected by osteoarthritis but radiographic involvement is limited to the lower part of the joints, whereas complete involvement is the rule in AS.

E. **Ankylosing hyperostosis (Forrestier disease)** is a proliferative form of osteoarthritis seen in elderly subjects which can mimic AS but lacks apophyseal and sacroiliac involvement.

F. Occasionally, peripheral arthritis and minimal spine involvement may resemble **rheumatoid arthritis** or **lupus erythematosus** until the passage of time, acquisition of laboratory data, and radiographic evolution clarify the diagnosis. One should keep in mind that RA and AS can rarely coexist.

G. **Osteitis condensans ilii** is an asymptomatic sclerosis of iliac subchondral bone in parous women which may cause radiographic confusion with AS. Sclerosis is only on the iliac side of the joint in this condition.

H. **Osteitis pubis** is an erosive sclerosing disorder of the symphysis pubis seen in women who have undergone pelvic or urologic surgery. There is no skeletal disease elsewhere.

I. **Fractures** of the vertebral endplate might bear radiographic resemblance to some features of AS.

J. The vertebral discitis and osteitis of AS are sometimes intense enough to mimic **septic discitis** and **spinal osteomyelitis** and may even require needle aspiration to exclude infection.

K. **Septic sacroiliitis** is an acute process but can leave confusing radiographic signs that might later resemble AS.

L. **Paget disease** can involve bone adjacent to the sacroiliac joints, thus mimicing AS. Characteristic radiographic changes elsewhere and elevations of serum alkaline phosphatase and urinary hydroxyproline excretion are usually diagnostic.

M. **Metastatic cancer** to the pelvis or vertebral bodies always belongs in the differential diagnosis of back or pelvic pain.

N. **Fluorosis** can cause sclerosis of bone and radiographic changes indistinguishable from the sacroiliitis of AS.

O. **Others. Whipple disease, familial Mediterranean fever,** and **Behcet disease** rarely have associated sacroiliitis and arthritis.

P. The chest pain of AS can mimic **angina pectoris** or pleurisy; its association with LBP, nocturnal onset, and lack of "oppressiveness" can help separate it from ischemic cardiac pain.

V. **Therapy.** The **aims of management** in AS are to control pain, maintain maximum skeletal mobility, and prevent deformities. There is no specific therapy or cure for AS. Management requires patient education and cooperation and consists of lifelong dedication to a program of posture control, exercises, and judicious use of medications and surgical intervention when appropriate.

A. **Physical therapy.** All patients should be enrolled in a physiotherapy program. Maintenance of erect posture is critical in all activities including sitting, standing, and walking. Sleeping should occur in a prone position or supine on a firm mattress with one small or no pillow. Breathing and chest expansion exercises are important. Exercises to extend all parts of the spine and to move all peripheral joints fully should be taught and diligently followed. Walking, swimming, and jogging are excellent sports which maintain joint mobility. The following spine exercises are useful.

1. Lying flat on back, bring both knees to chest, hold to count of 5, and relax to full extension. Repeat three times.

2. Lying flat on back, squeeze shoulder blades together, keeping chin tucked in, and count to 5. Relax. Repeat three times.

3. Lying prone, lift head off surface, count to 5, relax. Repeat three times.

   a. Then, arching back, lift head and shoulders off surface, count to 5, relax. Repeat three times.

   b. Then lift head and shoulders off surface; grasp hands behind back, hold and count to 5, relax. Repeat three times.

B. **Drugs.** Today's drug therapy does not interrupt the progression of disease. The role of drugs is to relieve pain and inflammation in order to maintain posture and permit performance of an exercise program.

   1. At the Hospital for Special Surgery, the two most commonly employed agents are indomethacin and phenylbutazone.

      a. **Indomethacin** 25 to 50 mg TID or QID is the preferred drug because it is well-tolerated and has fewer side effects than phenylbutazone.

      b. **Phenylbutazone** 50 to 100 mg QID affords good relief of acute symptoms but has unpredictable bone marrow toxicity. It is best used in acute settings for one or two weeks, then tapered and replaced by other medication. In the occasional patient refractory to indomethacin and other modalities, longer-term phenylbutazone may be cautiously used, in the lowest dose possible. In such settings, frequent blood counts and careful examinations are mandatory to prevent serious marrow aplasia.

   2. **Naproxen** 250 mg BID or TID and **sulindac** 100 to 200 mg BID are reported to offer pain relief comparable to that of indomethacin in some series and, with time, may gain wider use.

   3. **Salicylates,** for unknown reasons, seldom provide an adequate therapeutic response in AS and are not often used at the Hospital for Special Surgery.

   4. **Gold, systemic corticosteroids, chloroquine, and cytotoxic agents** are not beneficial in this disease.

   5. **Intraarticular corticosteroids** may occasionally be useful for acutely inflamed joints. Indications and dosage are discussed in Chapter 3.

C. **Radiotherapy.** In the 1940s, radiotherapy to involved spine dramatically relieved symptoms in many patients but was followed by leukemia in some; thus such therapy was discontinued. There have been no controlled trials of low-dose radiation therapy.

D. **Surgery.** Surgical procedures are usually reserved for patients with far advanced disease causing painful deformities or loss of function. Total hip replacement is the most commonly performed procedure. However, total knee replacements, cervical and lumbar osteotomies to relieve severe spinal kyphosis, condylar resections of ankylosed temperomandibular joints (TMJs), and stabilization of atlantoaxial subluxation have also been performed. Unfortunately, the threat of spinal cord damage is increased in these patients, and the long convalescence and periods of postoperative bed rest exacerbate the natural tendency to reankylose. Indeed, all reported series of total hip replacements in AS include a percentage of patients with reankylosis.

VI. **Prognosis.** The course of AS varies. Symptoms may be persistent or intermittent over the years. In some patients, the disease progresses relentlessly (often in spite of therapy) with fusion of axial and peripheral joints. In others, bony ankylosis may develop gradually with little pain or discomfort. In still others, skeletal involvement may be limited to only mild sacroiliitis and never progress to serious spondylitis or ankylosing disease.

Although not curable, AS is an eminently rehabilitative disease. Most patients who maintain disciplined exercise and posture programs and take antiinflammatory medication judiciously are able to lead relatively normal and active lives with minor adjustments in lifestyle. Less than 10% develop relentlessly crippling disease. Most

longitudinal studies of AS show survival curves approximating that of the general population.
Well-defined causes of death resulting from the disease itself are few but include aortic insufficiency, uremia secondary to amyloidosis, and atlantoaxial subluxation and cord compression.

Bibliography

Calin, A., and Fries, J. F. Striking prevalence of ankylosing spondylitis in "healthy" W27 positive males and females. *N. Engl. J. Med.* 293:835, 1975.

Calin, A., Porta, J., Fries, J. F., and Schurman, D. J. Clinical history as a screening test for ankylosing spondylitis. *J.A.M.A.* 237:2613, 1977.

Hill, H. R. H., Hill, A. G. S., and Bodmer, J. F. Clinical diagnosis of AS in women and relation to presence of HLA-B27. *Ann. Rheum. Dis.* 35:267, 1976.

Moll, J. M. H., Hoslock, I., MacRae, I. F., and Wright, V. Associations between AS, psoriatic arthritis, Reiter's disease, the intestinal arthropathies, and Behcet's syndrome. *Medicine* 53:343, 1974.

Schlosstein, L., Terasaki, P., Bluestone, R., and Pearson, C. High association of an HL-A antigen, W27, with ankylosing spondylitis. *N. Engl. J. Med.* 288:704, 1973.

21. Bursitis and Tendinitis

Paul M. Pellicci and
Richard R. McCormack

Bursitis

I. Anatomic Considerations. A bursa is a closed sac containing a small amount of synovial fluid and lined with a cellular membrane similar to synovium. Bursae are present in areas where tendons and muscles move over bony prominences; they facilitate such motion. Approximately 160 formed bursae are present in the body, and others may form in response to irritative stimuli. The clinically important bursae follow.

A. Shoulder

1. **Subacromial** bursa lies between the acromion and the rotator cuff.

2. **Subdeltoid** bursa lies between the deltoid muscle and the rotator cuff.

3. **Subcoracoid** bursa lies at attachment of the biceps, coracobrachialis, and pectoralis minor tendons to the coracoid process.

B. Elbow

1. **Olecranon** bursa lies over the olecranon process.

2. **Radiohumeral** bursa lies between the common wrist extensor tendon and the lateral epicondyle.

C. Hip

1. **Iliopsoas** bursa may communicate with the hip joint and lies between the hip capsule and the psoas musculotendinous unit.

2. **Trochanteric** bursa surrounds the gluteal insertions into the greater trochanter.

3. **Ischiogluteal** bursa separates the gluteus maximus from the ischial tuberosity.

D. Knee

1. **Prepatellar** bursa lies between skin and the patellar tendon.

2. **Infrapatellar** bursa lies deep to the insertion of the patellar ligament.

3. **Popliteal** bursae are numerous. The largest lies between the semimembranosus muscle and the medial head of the gastrocnemius muscle.

E. Foot

1. **Achilles** bursa separates the Achilles tendon insertion from the posterior aspect of the calcaneus.

2. **Subcalcaneal** bursa is located at the insertion of the plantar fascia into the medial tuberosity of the calcaneus.

II. Etiology

A. Direct trauma to a bursal area may lead to the inflammatory response in the bursa of hyperemia, the exudation of fluid and leukocytes into the bursal sac.

B. Chronic overuse or irritation of a bursal area.

C. Manifestation of a **systemic disorder** such as rheumatoid arthritis or gout.

D. Septic bursitis may occur secondary to **puncture wounds,** surrounding **cellulitis,**

or after a **local therapeutic injection.** The organisms most frequently responsible are staphylococci (aureus, epidermidis) and streptococci.

III. Diagnosis

A. Localized pain is the presenting complaint, with radiation into the involved limb as an occasional feature.

B. Swelling is common in olecranon bursitis but is usually not seen in subdeltoid bursitis.

C. Erythema may be present and does not necessarily indicate sepsis.

D. Tenderness is always present.

E. Pain is usually elicited when the patient is asked to execute a maneuver that stresses the involved motor unit; for example, abduction of the hip against gravity will cause pain in trochanteric bursitis.

F. Radiographs may, on occasion, demonstrate deposits of calcium in the region of the bursae. Calcific bursitis and calcific tendinitis may be indistinguishable, both clinically and radiographically.

IV. Therapy

A. Rest

1. The region should be immobilized for seven to ten days.

2. The patient should be told to discontinue activities that aggravate the symptoms for one to two weeks.

B. Ice compresses to the acutely inflamed area reduce swelling and provide relief from pain.

C. Antiinflammatory medications

1. For **mild** symptoms, aspirin 650 mg PO QID, either buffered or with food.

2. For **moderate** symptoms, ibuprofen 400 mg PO QID with food.

3. For **severe** symptoms, indomethacin 25 mg PO QID with food or phenylbutazone 100 mg PO QID after eating; neither drug should be used for more than 5 to 7 days.

D. Aspiration of swollen subcutaneous bursae such as the olecranon bursa should be performed. Reaccumulation is common, and it is not unusual to perform two or three aspirations in order to resolve the problem. The fluid should be cultured and crystalline evaluation made. Incision of the bursa may lead to prolonged drainage or infection and is rarely indicated.

E. Injection of the offending bursa with 1% lidocaine 3 cc mixed with methylprednisolone acetate (Depo-Medrol) 40 mg is usually successful in relieving symptoms.

F. Surgery to excise a bursa is rarely necessary. However, if the procedures outlined in **IV.A.** through **IV.E.** have been repeatedly unsuccessful and the disability is significant, surgery may provide relief.

G. If **infection** is suspected, the bursa must be aspirated and the fluid smeared for direct Gram stain as well as sent for microbiologic culture. Pending results, patients with mild symptoms may be treated as outpatients with dicloxacillin 500 mg PO QID. Patients who have more severe infections or who are markedly symptomatic should be hospitalized and treated with nafcillin 1.5 gm IV every 4 hours. In chronic cases refractory to antibiotics, bursectomy may be indicated.

Tendinitis

Tendinitis is a general term used to describe any inflammation associated with a tendon. The inflammation may occur within the substance of the tendon (intratendinous lesion) or be associated with the tenosynovial sheath (tenosynovitis). Since bursae are often located near tendons, *tendinitis* and *bursitis* are often used interchangeably to represent the same affliction (see discussion of bursitis). Together these entities are the most common causes of soft tissue pain.

I. Pathology

A. **Intratendinous lesions** occur primarily later in life as the vascularity of the tendon diminishes. They are usually associated with repetitive motion and are felt to represent microtrauma or limited macrotrauma short of rupture within the substance of the tendon. Local signs and symptoms of inflammation are caused by the reparative process of vascular infiltration with acute and chronic cellular responses. During the reparative process, calcium salts, which are visible on radiographs, may be deposited in degenerated portions of the tendon, hence the term *calcific tendinitis.* Tennis elbow, calcific tendinitis in the supraspinatus, and trochanteric tendinitis are examples of intratendinous lesions.

B. **Acute or chronic paratendinous inflammation or tenosynovitis** may have several etiologies.

   1. **Repetitive motion with injury** is by far the most common etiology. Synovial tendon sheaths are located in areas where tendons pass over bony surfaces and where large tendon excursions are found, most commonly about the wrist and ankle. Repetitive motion causes inflammation with edema, and a decrease in the fine tolerances already present in these gliding areas. The result is decreased excursion and painful motion of the affected tendon, often with signs of mechanical blocking, such as may be seen with DeQuervain disease and trigger finger.

   2. These paratendinous inflammations may also be triggered by **direct or microtraumatic intratendinous injuries** and result from the reparative process initiated in the tenosynovium.

   3. Acute tenosynovitis may also be of **septic origin.** Most commonly, this disorder involves a direct wound contaminating the sheath. Alternatively, it may result from a generalized sepsis, especially in a compromised host, and may be multifocal. Because vascular supply is poor, infection is not well controlled with antibiotics alone and surgical drainage is usually necessary.

   4. Acute and chronic paratendinous inflammations are also commonly seen in the **inflammatory arthritides** and **collagen vascular diseases.**

II. Physical examination

A. The classic sign of inflammation within the tendon or tendon sheath is **pain on motion,** especially with passive stretch or contraction of the affected motor tendon unit against resistance.

B. Local **swelling, warmth, and tenderness** are usually present. Tenderness may be palpated along the course of the tendon. On deep structures, such as the supraspinatus or gluteus medius tendons, deep point tenderness in a specific and reproducible location may be elicited.

C. **Erythema** may or may not be present depending on the depth of the structure and the acuteness of the process. Since most tendons cross joints, tendinitis must be distinguished from acute **inflammatory** or **septic arthritis.** In the latter case, range of motion will be more severely restricted. Systemic signs may be present, and capsular tenderness should be distinguished from tenderness directly over the tendon. When in doubt, diagnostic arthrocentesis will resolve the matter.

III. Therapy. The therapy of tendinitis is similar to that of bursitis.

A. **Immobilization** is the most important modality. Methods are:

   1. A **splint** or **cast** for the affected region in the distal upper and lower extremity.

   2. A **sling** for lesions of the proximal upper extremity.

3. **Crutches** for lesions of the proximal lower extremity.
Gentle physical therapy within the limits of pain should be started as the inflammation resolves to avoid permanent stiffness.

B. **Local heat** is helpful in relieving symptoms and in alleviating painful muscle spasm associated with tendinitis. Hot packs, warm soaks, skin counterirritants (such as balms, ultrasound), or hot wax treatments are equally effective and should be utilized.

C. **Antiinflammatories**

1. **Aspirin** may be given in doses up to 0.6 gm every 4 hours as tolerated.

2. **Phenylbutazone** in doses of 100 to 200 mg TID with food or **indomethacin** 25 to 50 mg TID with food may be used for acute inflammation. These drugs should not be continued for more than five to seven days.

3. **Corticosteroids,** given systemically or locally as injections with a local anesthetic, can also be beneficial in certain cases. The injected area should be cooled with ice for 24 hours after injection, and adequate analgesics should be prescribed to counteract the pain experienced when the local anesthetic wears off. Methylprednisolone acetate suspension 20 to 40 mg is the most frequently used preparation. No more than three weekly injections should be used. Steroid preparations are contraindicated in the presence of infection.

D. **Surgery** is the treatment of choice when nonoperative therapy has failed. It involves repair of degenerative tendon such as in tennis elbow, release of fibroosseous tunnels such as in DeQuervain disease, and tenosynovectomy for chronic wrist tenosynovitis, a common manifestation of rheumatoid arthritis.

22. Fibromyalgia (Fibrositis) and Psychologic Aspects of Rheumatology

John F. Beary III

I. **Fibromyalgia.** This syndrome is characterized by symptoms of diffuse aching, sleep disturbance, and localized sites of deep myofascial tenderness in tense, anxious patients. The term *fibrositis* is a misnomer because pathologic studies reveal no inflammation of fibrous tissue. The sites of tenderness in the neck, low back, and other areas are said to be reproducible; however, the same phenomenon can be found in controls.

Histologic and laboratory studies are normal. Treatment is reassurance and salicylates as required.

II. **Psychogenic musculoskeletal syndrome.** Musculoskeletal symptoms that are secondary to psychologic stress or neurosis characterize this syndrome. The patient complains of vague, nonspecific problems that are greatly out of proportion to objective findings. A careful history may reveal a stressful situation involving the patient's occupation or primary personal relationship.

On examination, a reported tender area may "disappear" if the patient is distracted. Neurologic exam may elicit a nonanatomic pattern on sensory testing (midline or base of limb boundaries). Laboratory studies are normal. The sedimentation rate is a good screening test; a normal result is reassuring. Of course, patients with psychogenic complaints may have or develop organic disease; thus the physician must remain wary.

A. **Therapy**

1. **Reassurance** and emotional support. The *aequanimitas* concept of Sir William Osler can be usefully applied to such patients. It involves conveying to the patient in a kind, authoritative manner that he or she has a minor illness which is expected to resolve, and that the physician has seen several similar cases which have done well.

    If the patient feels that the physician is concerned and speaks with authority about the problem, the patient can then often understand and tolerate the symptoms.

2. **Patient education** about mind-body interaction.

3. **Avoidance of psychoactive drugs** or analgesics for which the patient may develop a dependence.

III. **Chronic pain.** Anxiety or depression is often a component of chronic pain and can pose a difficult management problem in any chronic rheumatic disease. About 10% of rheumatoid arthritis patients, at some time in their course, fail to respond to anti-inflammatory medications and develop severe, chronic pain that is unresponsive to conventional analgesic regimens. Pain of this nature makes it impossible to function at home or in the workplace.

A. **Therapy**

1. **Pain clinic referral.** In such a clinic, a team of specialists including psychiatrists, neurologists, neurosurgeons, and social workers evaluate the patient and develop a comprehensive therapeutic approach.

2. **Drugs** which may be of benefit, but which are withheld because of side effects or addiction potential until conventional analgesic therapy has failed, include the following.

   a. Tricyclic antidepressants give a synergistic effect with narcotic analgesics. The initial regimen is imipramine 75 mg at bedtime. The maintenance dose may be increased by 25 mg per week as necessary until a maximum maintenance dosage of 150 mg per week is reached. Sedation and anticholinergic effects are the most common adverse reactions.

   b. Methadone is a strong narcotic with a long duration of action. Dosage is 2.5 to 10 mg every 6 to 8 hours. Side effects may include nausea, dizziness, and constipation. The need to relieve severe pain and dysfunction must outweigh the addiction potential.

IV. Quackery. Because several of the rheumatic diseases as yet have no cure, patients may become very discouraged by pain and disability and turn to unconventional methods for relief. One can understand the motivation of these desperate people. Unfortunately, unethical promoters exploit that aspect of human nature which will believe the most improbable claim if it coincides with a desperate hope for relief. The Arthritis Foundation estimates that $400,000,000 every year is spent in the United States on such worthless so-called cures as trips to uranium mines, electrical devices, "immune milk," and filtered sea water.

The physician should be open-minded about proposed cures presented by the patient. If one gently reminds the patient to ask the following questions, most quack methods will be shown for what they are: (1) How much personal financial gain is the seller of the treatment receiving?, (2) What is the evidence for effectiveness?, and (3) What is the potential harm to the patient from participating in the treatment? The Arthritis Foundation sends a useful newsletter to all patients who ask to be put on their mailing list.* It discusses advances in arthritis treatment and debunks quack cures. An informed patient is less likely to fall prey to quack promoters who enrich themselves by exploiting desperate patients.

National Arthritis News, Arthritis Foundation, 3400 Peachtree Rd, Atlanta, GA   30326.

23. Gout

John F. Beary III

Gout is a complex disorder with primary and secondary forms characterized by hyperuricemia and urate crystal-induced arthritis. It is one of the first diseases known to ancient man. In the fifth century B.C., Hippocrates wrote a clinical description of gout, using the term *podagra*. The word *gout* was introduced in the thirteenth century; it is derived from the Latin word for drop, *gutta,* thus reflecting an early concept that gout was caused by a poison entering a joint drop by drop.

I. **Epidemiology.** The **prevalence** of all types of gout is 275 cases per 100,000 members of the United States population. Primary gout is thought to be a polygenic disease. In the United States, about 12% of family members of gout patients are affected. Ninety percent of primary gout patients are male. The peak age for the first attack of gouty arthritis is during the fifth decade.

II. **Disease classification**

A. **Primary gout.** In primary gout, hyperuricemia is thought to result from a disorder of purine metabolism or from abnormal excretion of uric acid. Most primary gout patients fall into an idiopathic category because no precise genetic or metabolic defect has been identified. In about 1% of the primary gout group, specific enzyme defects have been found. Deficiency of hypoxanthineguanine phosphoribosyltransferase (HGPRT) and increased activity of phosphoribosylpyrophosphate (PRPP) synthetase are the best studied examples.

B. **Secondary gout.** Secondary gout comprises about 10% of all gout cases. It can result from a variety of disorders that cause hyperuricemia as a result of **overproduction** or **impaired excretion** of uric acid (Table 23-1).

Asymptomatic Hyperuricemia

Asymptomatic hyperuricemia (AH) is arbitrarily defined as serum uric acid values that exceed the mean plus two standard deviations in an asymptomatic population. Therefore, by definition, 2.5% of the population will be affected. The uric acid levels of the normal population and the population with gout overlap. It should be stressed that most patients with hyperuricemia are asymptomatic and do not develop articular or renal disease.

I. **Diagnosis.** Most clinical laboratories use an autoanalyzer colorimetric technique based on the ability of urate to reduce phosphotungstic acid. For men, the upper limit of a normal uric acid is 8.0 mg/dl and for women, 6.5 mg/dl. Several common substances such as caffeine, vitamin C, and acetaminophen produce spurious uric acid elevations with the colorimetric technique. The true serum uric acid as measured by the uricase method is 1 mg/dl lower than the value measured by the automated technique. Evaluation of the AH patient includes exclusion of drug effects or other conditions listed in Table 23-1. Diuretic therapy is a particularly common cause of uric acid elevation and usually does not require treatment.

II. **Therapy.** Treatment of asymptomatic hyperuricemia is a subject of controversy. No strong evidence has been offered that AH results in chronic renal disease or joint deformity. Factors in the evaluation of the patient that might lead one to consider individualized therapy to lower serum uric acid include a family history of renal stones and the degree of hyperuricemia. Patients with repeated uric acid elevations greater than 10 mg/dl have an increased chance of suffering an acute gout attack or urolithiasis, and probenecid or allopurinol therapy (see Chronic Gout, **VI.B.3.**) to lower serum uric acid should be considered. There is no established treatment protocol for lesser degrees of hyperuricemia, but the cost and possible toxicity of long-term al-

Table 23-1. Classification of Hyperuricemia

Overproduction of Uric Acid
  Primary gout
  Myeloproliferative disorders
  Lymphoma
  Hemoglobinopathies
  Hemolytic anemia
  Psoriasis
  Cancer chemotherapy
Underexcretion of Uric Acid
  Chronic renal failure
  Lead nephropathy (saturnine gout)
  Drugs (diuretics except spironolactone and ticrynafen; ethambutol; low-dose aspirin)
  Lactic acidosis (alcoholism, preeclampsia)
  Ketosis (diabetic, starvation)
  Hyperparathyroidism
  Hypertension
Overproduction and Underexcretion
  Glycogen storage disease, Type I
Mechanism Unknown
  Sarcoidosis
  Obesity
  Hypoparathyroidism
  Paget disease
  Down syndrome

---

lopurinol or uricosuric therapy argue against their routine use in AH patients with uric acid levels less than 10 mg/dl.

Acute Gout

I. **Clinical presentation.** Acute gouty arthritis classically presents as acute monarthritis (72% of patients), but polyarticular inflammation is also seen in patients with acute gout. The onset is sudden and the patient complains of severe pain in the affected joint. Even the weight of bedsheets can be intolerable. An untreated attack usually lasts three to five days. The history may implicate diuretic use, recent surgery, chronic renal disease, or alcohol abuse as initiating or precipitating factors. A positive family history supports the diagnosis of primary gout.
The metatarsophalangeal joint of the big toe is most commonly involved (podagra), followed in frequency by other joints of the foot and the knee. Erythema is often observed over the affected joints and can mimic the appearance of cellulitis. Chills and fever (as high as 39°C) may occur, suggesting the presence of sepsis, which is an important consideration in the differential diagnosis.

II. **Laboratory findings**

A. **Synovial fluid examination.** The most important procedure in establishing the diagnosis of acute gouty arthritis is the examination of synovial fluid by compensated polarized microscopy.

1. **Principles of polarizing microscopy.** The polarizing microscope consists of normal microscope optics to which polarizer and analyzer lenses that orient white light into a single plane are added. When a birefringent crystal is examined and rotated into the proper position, it will appear as a bright object against a dark field. When a first-order red compensator is added to the system, the specimen background appears as rose (first-order red). Crystals examined

with a compensator have characteristic colors which change when they are rotated 90 degrees as a result of the optical properties of the crystals and the compensator's deceleration of a characteristic frequency of light. The complex physics underlying this phenomenon are clearly described elsewhere (*Clin. Rheum. Dis.* 3:91, 1977).

   2. **Crystal identification.** If carefully sought, **urate crystals** can be found in the synovial fluids of 85% of acute gout patients. Urate crystals are slender, needle shaped and have a strong **negative birefringence** under polarized light. (**Calcium pyrophosphate crystals** are pleomorphic, predominantly rhomboid shaped, and have weak positive birefringence.) In most joint fluids the urate crystals can be found inside neutrophils; however, in chronic gout, crystals are also found free in the synovial fluid. Under polarized light, urate crystals appear yellow when parallel to the axis of the red compensator and blue when perpendicular to the axis. An axis reference line is etched on the housing of the compensator. The calcium pyrophosphate crystals of pseudogout have the *opposite* orientation. Identification can be aided by the mnemonic "U Pay Peb": *U*rate crystals = *Pa*rallel *Y*ellow, *P*erpendicular *B*lue.

B. **Biochemical findings.** The serum uric acid is usually elevated but is normal in about 10% of patients with acute gout. The creatinine and urea nitrogen will be elevated if secondary gout attributable to renal failure is responsible for the acute attack. Lead poisoning, which can also cause nephropathy, can be detected by measuring an elevated level of coproporphyrin III or lead in the urine. If one of the genetic enzyme deficiencies of primary gout is suspected, erythrocyte enzymes can be assessed in a few specialized laboratories.

C. **Radiographic findings.** Radiographs usually show only soft tissue swelling in the first attack of acute gout. With recurrent or chronic disease, tophi and destructive joint changes may be seen.

III. **Differential diagnosis.** In addition to primary and secondary gout, the differential diagnosis of acute monarthritis includes septic arthritis, pseudogout, trauma, and atypical rheumatoid arthritis (RA). Infection can be ruled out *only* by a Gram stain and culture of the synovial fluid. Identification of calcium pyrophosphate crystals under compensated polarized light will support the diagnosis of pseudogout. However, it should be emphasized that gout and pseudogout can coexist. Trauma is suggested by the history. Atypical RA can, infrequently, present as an acute monarthritis, and months of observation may be required before a clinical pattern of disease consistent with classic RA emerges.

IV. **Therapy.** Acute gout is treated with one of the following drug regimens (listed in order of preference). Detailed information on individual drugs appears in Appendix G.

A. **Indomethacin** is better tolerated than oral colchicine and is thought to have somewhat less hematologic toxicity than phenylbutazone. The dose of indomethacin is 50 mg every 6 hours for 24 hours, then 50 mg TID for 2 days, 50 mg BID for 1 day, and 50 mg daily for 1 day. A therapeutic effect is seen in about 8 hours.

B. **Other nonsteroidal antiinflammatory drugs.** Alternative regimens for patients unable to tolerate indomethacin include:

   1. **Naproxen** 500 mg initially. Then 250 mg every 8 hours with gradual tapering over 5 days as inflammation subsides.

   2. **Ibuprofen** 800 mg initially. Then 400 mg every 6 hours with gradual dosage tapering over 5 days.

C. **Colchicine.** A therapeutic response to colchicine in acute gout was formerly claimed to be diagnostic but is now recognized to be nonspecific.

   1. **Oral colchicine** may cause major vomiting and diarrhea at the doses needed for control of an acute attack and is not recommended.

2. **Intravenous colchicine.** In patients with congestive heart failure or hypertension, for whom the salt-retaining effect of the nonsteroidal antiinflammatory drugs is undesirable, IV colchicine is optimal treatment. It is also the treatment of choice in patients with concurrent peptic ulcer disease because the IV form has no gastrointestinal toxicity. The dose is 2 mg IV diluted in 15 ml of saline and administered slowly over 15 minutes. The drug is diluted to avoid the inflammation which occurs if the intravenous line infiltrates the subcutaneous tissue. Relief of symptoms occurs in 6 to 8 hours.

D. **Allopurinol or probenecid** should *not* be started during an acute gout episode because fluctuation of the serum uric acid level may prolong the attack.

Interval Gout

Interval gout refers to the asymptomatic period between acute attacks. Some patients may never have another attack. The asymptomatic period is unpredictable and may range from several months to many years.

A conservative approach should guide therapeutic decisions in the patient with interval gout. Many will not need treatment. Factors that influence a decision to treat with uric acid-lowering agents include a history of renal calculi or uric acid excretion greater than 1,000 mg daily. See Chronic Gout for a complete discussion.

Chronic Gout

Chronic gout is characterized by recurrent episodes of acute polyarticular arthritis, chronic synovitis, joint deformity, tophi, or renal stones.

I. **Physical examination.** Tophi are found in about 15% of patents, particularly in the olecranon bursae, finger joints, and occasionally in the helix of the ear; they may ulcerate. Joint examination may reveal an asymmetric polyarthritis which can be very deforming and sometimes difficult to distinguish from RA (see **IV.**).

II. **Laboratory findings**

A. **Serum studies**

1. **Uric acid.** Elevated uric acid values occur in about 90% of patients.

2. **Creatinine.** Elevated levels may reflect gout-related nephropathy or primary renal disease.

B. **Urine studies.** Primary gout patients can be subdivided into **overexcretors** of uric acid (15% of patients) and **normal excretors** based on quantitative urinary excretion of urate. On a regular diet, a normal person will excrete 300 to 800 mg of uric acid every 24 hours. The patient should be instructed to avoid alcohol or aspirin ingestion and to eat only one moderate serving of meat daily during the three days preceding the urine collection. Foods with very high purine content such as organ meats (liver and kidney) and anchovies should also be avoided before the collection. A uric acid collection obtained during an acute gout attack is unreliable as a result of fluctuating serum acid levels not usually seen in the basal state.

III. **Radiographic findings.** Punched-out areas of bone destruction or soft tissue tophi may be seen radiographically. Pure urate stones are radiolucent and cannot be seen on the standard supine abdominal film; intravenous pyelography, therefore, is required to demonstrate urate urolithiasis.

IV. **Differential diagnosis.** The differential diagnosis includes RA, osteoarthritis, and pseudogout. Rheumatoid nodules cannot always be clinically distinguished from tophi and, in some cases, biopsy of a nodule may be necessary. The absence of synovial fluid urate crystals in osteoarthritis and the demonstration of calcium pyrophosphate crystals in pseudogout serve to distinguish these disorders.

V. Complications. Nephrolithiasis occurs in 20% of all gout patients with normal uric acid excretion and in 40% of those patients with elevated values. Uric acid stones, which are radiolucent, represent 10% of all renal calculi, but in gout patients 85% of renal stones are pure uric acid. Fifty percent of patients with all forms of nephrolithiasis have a recurrence within nine years.

Diagnostic evaluation of a renal stone includes chemical analysis of the calculus, if possible, and analysis of a 24-hour urine specimen for uric acid, calcium, and phosphate. An intravenous pyelogram should be performed to exclude ureteral obstruction. If the etiology of the stone is still unclear, serum and urine studies should be ordered to exclude hyperparathyroidism, cystinuria, or renal tubular acidosis. Uric acid is less soluble at acidic pH; therefore alkalinization of the urine may be helpful in some patients.

VI. Therapy

   A. Patient education. It is important that the patient realize that gout is a chronic disease and that certain lifestyle modifications, such as maintenance of an ideal weight and moderation of alcohol intake, are important. A purine-restricted diet has not been found to be of value in gout therapy. Other factors worth emphasizing are ingestion of at least 2 liters of fluids per day to help prevent renal stones, and avoidance of alcohol and aspirin, which aggravate hyperuricemia. Women should be counseled to avoid extremes in shoe fashion in order to prevent hallux valgus deformity, which can predispose the patient to gouty involvement of the metatarsophalangeal joint.

   B. Drug therapy. The goals of therapy are to prevent renal parenchymal damage and nephrolithiasis and to suppress articular flares. Drug strategy in chronic gout is determined by the pattern of 24-hour urate excretion and the severity of disease.

   1. Gout prophylaxis. Colchicine 0.6 mg daily or BID is effective in diminishing the frequency and severity of spontaneous gout flares and flares induced by initial allopurinol and probenecid therapy. Colchicine may be discontinued after a 6-month symptomfree interval.

   2. Recurrent gout attacks. Gout attacks are treated as described earlier (Acute Gout, **IV.**). The patient may be given a supply of indomethacin (the drug of choice for acute attacks) with instructions to take 50 mg every 6 hours at the first sign of a gout prodrome and to call the physician. When self-administered in this manner, a gout attack may be aborted with only two or three doses of indomethacin.

   3. Hyperuricemia. Patients are classified as overexcretors or normal urate excretors based on quantitative urinary studies as described in **II.B.**

   a. Uricosuric therapy

      (1) Indications (all must be present)

         (a) Normal urate excretor (less than 1,000 mg/24 hr)

         (b) Normal renal function

         (c) Absence of tophi

         (d) No history of renal calculi

      (2) Drug administration. Prophylactic colchicine 0.6 mg BID should be begun 3 days before therapy.

         (a) Probenecid is the uricosuric drug of choice. The initial dose is 250 mg BID for 1 week. The dose is increased to 500 mg BID or TID depending on serum uric acid response. Adequate hydration must be maintained to prevent uric acid precipitation in renal tubules.

         (b) Sulfinpyrazone is an alternative uricosuric agent for patients intolerant of probenecid. Initial dosage is 50 mg BID for 1 week. Maintenance dosage is 100 mg TID or QID.

b. Allopurinol therapy

(1) Indications (only one need be present)

(a) Hyperexcretion of urate (greater than 1,000 mg/24 hr)

(b) History of renal calculi

(c) Tophi

(d) Renal insufficiency and gout

(e) Uricosurics ineffective or allergenic

(f) Before cytotoxic therapy of neoplasia

(2) Drug administration. Prophylactic colchicine 0.6 mg BID should be started 3 days before initiating allopurinol therapy. Initial allopurinol dose is 100 mg daily, which is increased weekly until the maintenance dose of 300 mg daily is reached. Doses as high as 600 to 800 mg per day may be needed in a few patients to achieve clinical control. If the creatinine clearance is less than 20 ml per minute, the toxicity (skin rash, vasculitis, agranulocytosis) of allopurinol increases.

c. Combined uricosuric and allopurinol therapy. Occasional patients will require combination therapy to control gout and to reduce the serum uric acid level to 7.0 or less (autoanalyzer measurement). The drugs are used together at their usual dosages: allopurinol 300 mg per day and probenecid 500 mg BID.

4. Chronic synovitis. Joint aspiration and intraarticular injection of corticosteroid are often of value. The technique and dosage regimen are described in Chapter 3.

5. Prevention of nephrolithiasis. In patients with renal stones, the following measures are useful.

a. Urine alkalinization. A urine pH greater than 6.0 can be achieved with:

(1) Sodium or potassium citrate (Polycitra) 20 ml QID.

(2) Acetazolamide 500 mg at bedtime.

b. Large urine volume. The patient should be instructed to drink adequate fluids to produce at least 2 liters of urine daily.

C. Surgical therapy. Surgical removal of large tophi is indicated if they become infected or interfere with joint function.

VII. Prognosis. The prognosis of properly managed gout is good, and most patients have a normal life span. However, a few patients with severe tophaceous renal disease develop chronic renal failure.

Bibliography

Boss, G. R., and Seegmiller, J. E. Hyperuricemia and gout: Classification, complications, and management. *N. Engl. J. Med.* 300:1459, 1979.

Liang, M. H., and Fries, J. F. Asymptomatic hyperuricemia: The case for conservative management. *Ann. Intern. Med.* 88:666, 1978.

Smyth, C. J. Disorders associated with hyperuricemia. *Arthritis Rheum.* 18:713, 1975.

Wyngaarden, J. B., and Kelley, W. N. *Gout and Hyperuricemia.* New York: Grune & Stratton, 1976.

24. Infectious Arthritis

Robert D. Inman

The consequences of an untreated septic joint are devastating. Ankylosis, septic destruction of the joint, osteomyelitis, disseminated infection, and death often followed joint infections before the antibiotic era. With specific antimicrobial therapy now available, the clinician must maintain a high degree of suspicion of infection in evaluating any patient with arthritis.

I. Introduction

A. Sources of infection. Although contiguous sites of infection such as skin abrasions or lacerations can lead to infection in an adjacent joint, most joint infections arise from hematogenous dissemination of the organism. Some organisms appear to be more arthrotropic than others, as demonstrated by the higher incidence of joint infections caused by *Staphylococcus aureus* than by gram-negative bacilli, despite the higher frequency of gram-negative bacteremia.

B. Common organisms. The relative incidence of organisms in acute pyogenic arthritis is listed in Table 24-1. Some recent series report a higher incidence of gram-negative bacillary arthritis. Within this group, the most common organisms are *Pseudomonas aeruginosa, Escherichia coli, Proteus mirabilis, Serratia marcescens, Klebsiella pneumoniae,* and *Salmonella* species. Gram-negative cocci other than *Neisseria gonorrhoeae* include *N. meningitidis, Hemophilus influenzae* and *Streptobacillus moniliformis,* all of which can produce the pustulovesicular skin lesions characteristic of disseminated gonococcal infection. In older children, the gram-positive cocci predominate; in infants, however, *H. influenzae* (from six months to two years of age) and other gram-negative organisms (from birth to 6 months of age) are more common. Gonococcal arthritis has been reported in all age groups, but it is the most common cause of septic arthritis in the age group of 15 to 40 years.

C. Predisposing factors, in order of frequency, follow (the percentage of infectious arthritis cases associated with each factor appears in parentheses). Compromised host defences particularly facilitate onset of gram-negative bacillary arthritis.

1. Extraarticular infection (49%).

2. Previous damage to joint resulting from rheumatoid arthritis (RA), crystal-induced arthritis, trauma, or surgery (27%).

3. Serious underlying illness including malignancy, cirrhosis, diabetes, and heroin addiction (19%).

4. Previous antibiotic therapy (20%).

5. Immunosuppressive or corticosteroid therapy (50%).

II. Initial evaluation

A. Clinical presentation. History may reveal predisposing factors or portal of infection, such as skin, sinuses, middle ear, lungs, oropharynx, rectum, urethra, or pelvis. On examination systemic signs of infection are often present, including malaise, chills, and fever (90% of patients have temperature greater than 100°F). While knee or hip monarthritis is the most common joint finding, polyarthritis also occurs. Vesicular skin lesions with necrotic centers are particularly common in gonococcal infection.

B. General diagnostic measures

1. **Peripheral blood white blood cell count (WBC) and differential.** 30% of patients have WBC less than 10,000 cells.

Table 24-1. Incidence of Organisms in Acute Infectious Arthritis

Organism	Incidence (%)	
	Adults	Children
Neisseria gonorrhoeae	50	5
Staphylococcus aureus	35	45
Streptococcus pyogenes, S. pneumoniae, S. viridans	10	25
Gram-negative bacilli (*Escherichia coli, Salmonella, Pseudomonas*)	5	15
Hemophilus influenzae	1	10

2. **Culture** all possible foci of infection (sputum, urine, skin lesions, oropharynx, urethra, rectum) and obtain at least two blood cultures on both aerobic and anerobic media. In 49% of cases the same organism is cultured from an extraarticular site as well as from the joint.

3. **Radiographs** of the joint should be obtained to document extent of previous damage, to check for evidence of osteomyelitis, and to provide a baseline for follow-up studies.

4. **Radioisotope bone scan** may be of value in diagnostic problems involving deep-seated joints such as hip, shoulder, or spine. However, the findings are not specific, and the scan usually has little role in the initial evaluation of acute infectious arthritis.

C. **Arthrocentesis.** The physician must prove beyond a reasonable doubt that no infection is contributing to the arthritis. **Aspiration of synovial fluid** is mandatory for any joint inflammation in which infection is a possibility. Using sterile technique, arthrocentesis is safe (14 cases of introduced infection were found in reviewing 100,000 joint aspirations in 4,000 patients) and requires only familiarity with the anatomic landmarks of the joints. Initial aspiration is by closed needle technique, with a needle large enough (16- or 18-gauge) to permit aspiration of thick purulent material. The exception to this rule is the hip joint, where initial assessment should include the orthopedic surgeon since open surgical drainage may be required. (See Chap. 3 for details of joint aspiration.)
Synovial fluid analysis is the key to determining both preliminary and definitive treatment. The following studies are ranked in order of importance; if quantity of synovial fluid sample is small, culture and Gram stain receive priority.

1. **Culture.** Fluid must be inoculated onto media promptly at the bedside, or the sample must be hand-delivered by the physician to the laboratory. Media should be selected for gram-positive and gram-negative bacteria (blood agar, MacConkey agar), *N. gonorrhoeae* (chocolate or Thayer-Martin culture medium), *H. influenzae* (peptic digest of blood), anerobes (thioglycollate broth), and if indicated, fungi and mycobacteria.

2. **Gram stain.** Pending the results of cultures, the Gram stain is the cornerstone of initial antibiotic therapy (see sec. **III.A.**).

3. **Synovial fluid glucose.** In septic joints, this value is usually less than 50% of simultaneous serum levels; however, this relationship holds only for fasting specimens, since postprandial blood glucose may not equilibrate promptly with synovial fluid. Low synovial fluid glucose levels can be seen in noninfectious inflammatory arthritis such as RA. Gonococcal arthritis often does not have lowered synovial fluid glucose.

4. **Cell count and differential.** Synovial fluid leukocytosis with predominance of neutrophils is common, but the WBC range is wide (6,800 to 250,000 cells). Probability of infection increases with higher white cell counts: 40% of patients with infectious arthritis have synovial fluid WBC greater than 100,000, while RA or crystal-induced arthritis rarely produces these counts. Although there is a large overlap zone of infectious and noninfectious inflammatory arthritis, one series reported no instance of infection with a synovial fluid WBC less than 2,500 cells.

5. **Additional studies**

   a. **Countercurrent immunoelectrophoresis (CIE).** In some cases of arthritis caused by pneumococci, meningococci, and *H. influenzae*, the joint fluid is sterile, and a sample of synovial fluid for CIE detection of bacterial antigens may be of diagnostic value.

   b. **Lactic acid.** Synovial fluid lactic acid is elevated in nongonococcal infectious arthritis; however, since the levels in gonococcal arthritis are not significantly different from those in RA, SLE, or gout, this test remains of limited diagnostic value.

III. **Initial therapy**

A. **Antibiotic therapy,** based on Gram stain results, is summarized in Table 24-2. Antibiotic therapy should be initiated within 2 hours of patient presentation and should be administered parenterally to ensure prompt, reliable serum antibiotic levels. Intraarticular administration is not indicated since there is rapid equilibration of synovial fluid and serum antibiotic levels.
   It should be noted in Table 24-2 that, because *H. influenzae* occurs frequently in children, ampicillin should be included for either gram-negative organisms or a negative smear. *H. influenzae* arthritis also occurs in adults, and is often misdiagnosed as overdecolorized gram-positive cocci. It should also be emphasized that the recommendation of penicillin treatment in a healthy patient with a negative smear may result in undertreatment of the occasional *S. aureus* infection presenting with a negative smear. Present consensus does not recommend nafcillin as being optimal treatment for gonorrhea, so the clinician must decide which disease is most likely from the clinical evidence.

B. **Analgesics** that do not affect fever are used. Codeine 30 mg every 4 hours as needed.

C. **Joint splinting.** Immobilization of the joint by splinting may also produce pain relief.

D. **Antiinflammatory drugs** (e.g., aspirin, indomethacin) should not be used initially in order that the response to antibiotic therapy can be assessed.

IV. **Subsequent therapy**

A. **General measures.** Daily assessment of patient status includes temperature, strength and appetite, change in range of motion in the joint, blood WBC and differential, and resolution of the primary focus of infection. As joint symptoms improve, passive range of motion **exercises** should be started on a graduated schedule to avoid development of contractures in the recuperative period.

B. **Serial joint aspiration.** As long as an effusion persists in the joint, arthrocentesis should be performed once or twice a day. A flow sheet should be constructed in the chart so that the following data on the joint aspirates can be recorded: date and time, volume, cell count and differential, culture results, and minimum bactericidal concentration of the synovial fluid. When the organism is identified, therapy is adjusted according to Table 24-3.

C. **Duration of antibiotic therapy.** For nongonococcal septic arthritis, parenteral antibiotic therapy is usually continued at least seven days after the disappearance

Table 24-2. Initial Antibiotic Therapy Based on Patient Age and Gram Stain Results*

Age (yrs)	Gram-Positive Cocci	Gram-Negative Cocci	Gram-Negative Bacilli	Septic Clinical Picture but No Organism Present
< ½	Nafcillin	Penicillin G	Gentamicin	Nafcillin and gentamicin
½–2	Nafcillin	Penicillin G	Ampicillin	Ampicillin
2–15	Nafcillin	Penicillin G	Gentamicin	Nafcillin
15–40	Nafcillin	Penicillin G	Gentamicin	Penicillin G
> 40	Nafcillin	Penicillin G	Gentamicin	Nafcillin

*Gentamicin should be added where applicable if patient is a compromised host (cirrhosis, diabetes, intravenous drug abuse, or neoplasm).

Table 24-3. Intravenous Antibiotic Therapy Based on Culture Identification of Organism

Organism	Antibiotic	Alternate Drug
Staphylococcus	Nafcillin 100–150 mg/kg/24 hr in 4 doses	Cephalothin 100 mg/kg/24 hr
Streptococcus	Penicillin G 15–20 million units/24 hr in 4 doses	Cephalothin 100 mg/kg/24 hr
Neisseria gonorrhoeae	Penicillin G 6–10 million units/24 hr in 4 doses	Erythromycin 2 gm/24 hr
Hemophilus influenzae	Ampicillin 50 mg/kg/24 hr in 4 doses	Chloramphenicol 50 mg/kg/24 hr
Gram-negative organisms including *Escherichia coli, Enterobacter* spp., *Klebsiella, Proteus,* and *Salmonella*	Gentamicin 5 mg/kg/24 hr in 3 doses	Amikacin 15 mg/kg/24 hr
Pseudomonas	Tobramycin 5 mg/kg/24 hr in 3 doses	Amikacin 15 mg/kg/24 hr

of signs of joint inflammation. For *S. aureus* and gram-negative bacilli, three to four weeks of parenteral and two to four weeks of oral therapy are recommended.

    D. Open surgical drainage. In most instances, closed needle drainage is adequate, but infection in the hip demands consideration of prompt surgical drainage, and the orthopedic surgeon should be involved in the *initial* evaluation of any possible hip infections. Adequate drainage of purulent exudate is critical since the efficacy of antibiotics is limited in this situation. Large collections of pus result in low intraarticular pH, increased hydrolytic enzymes, and bacteria in a relatively dormant phase. Cartilage destruction is accelerated by the intraarticular pressure and the enzymes in the exudate. **Indications** for open surgical drainage are:

        1. Hip infection.

        2. Failure of needle aspiration to drain the joint adequately because adhesions and loculations of pus are present. (Widely varying WBC values in repeated aspirates suggest loculated pockets of pus.)

        3. Lack of local or systemic response to therapy (e.g., joint fluid cultures remain positive, patient remains febrile after 72 to 96 hours of antibiotic therapy). A low threshold for early exploratory arthrotomy should be maintained in the compromised host with gram-negative bacillary arthritis.

V. Specific entities and problems

    A. Gonococcal arthritis

        1. Diagnostic features

            a. Polyarthritis and monarthritis occur in roughly equal proportions at presentation.

            b. Pustulovesicular lesions that develop a necrotic central eschar occur in 44% of cases.

            c. Tenosynovitis occurs in 68% of cases.

            d. Positive culture results are: synovial fluid 60%, urethra 81%, blood 24%, rectum 13%, and pharynx 17%.

        2. Therapy. The current Center for Disease Control (CDC) recommendations for the therapy of the arthritis-dermatitis syndrome (equivalent regimens) follow in order of preference.

   a. **Ampicillin** 3.5 gm or **amoxicillin** 3.0 gm orally, each with probenecid 1.0 gm, followed by ampicillin 0.5 gm or amoxicillin 0.5 gm orally 4 times daily for 7 days; or

   b. **Tetracycline** 0.5 gm orally 4 times daily for 7 days. Tetracycline should not be used for complicated gonococcal infection in pregnant women; or

   c. **Spectinomycin** 2.0 gm intramuscularly twice daily for 3 days (treatment of choice for disseminated infections caused by penicillinase-producing *N. gonorrhoeae*); or

   d. **Erythromycin** 0.5 gm orally 4 times daily for 7 days; or

   e. **Aqueous crystalline penicillin G** 10 million units intravenously daily until improvement occurs, followed by ampicillin 0.5 gm 4 times daily to complete 7 days of antibiotic treatment.

   Indications for **hospitalization** are (1) inability of patient to follow or tolerate outpatient regimen, (2) uncertain diagnosis, or (3) presence of a purulent joint effusion.

B. Tuberculous arthritis

1. **Diagnostic features.** Presentation is typically a chronic monarthritis or spondylitis. The chest x-ray is often normal and constitutional symptoms may not be present. Skin test with purified protein derivative (PPD) is almost always positive. Synovial fluid cultures are positive in 80% of cases, and synovial tissue cultures obtained by biopsy are positive in 90% of cases.

2. **Therapy** consists of isoniazid 300 mg daily and ethambutol 15 to 20 mg/kg daily for a minimum of 24 months.

C. Fungal arthritis

1. **Diagnostic features.** Fungal arthritis usually presents as a chronic monoarticular disease, but an acute polyarthritis with or without erythema nodosum can be seen. Diagnosis usually requires culture of synovial fluid or synovial tissue on appropriate media, but serologic tests can also be of value. Key features of the common fungal organisms follow.

   a. **Blastomycosis** usually exhibits pulmonary and cutaneous foci; osteomyelitis. Large joint monarthritis.

   b. **Candidiasis** may be late manifestation of transient candidemia. Immunosuppressed host.

   c. **Coccidioidomycosis and histoplasmosis** both exhibit an acute transient polyarthritis with erythema nodosum. A chronic granulomatous synovitis may occur.

   d. **Cryptococcosis** rare; secondary to adjacent bone infection. Spondylitis.

   e. **Sporotrichosis.** Two forms include a chronic oligoarticular pattern and a disseminated systemic form with bone, joint, and skin involvement.

2. **Therapy** for fungal arthritis usually consists of amphotericin B (1.0 mg kg daily IV for a total dose of 2 to 3 mg/24 hr for 10 weeks) and sometimes 5-fluorocytosine (150 mg/kg daily PO for 6 weeks). Surgical debridement is sometimes required to clear the infection.

D. Viral arthritis.

Rubella and hepatitis B viruses are the most common pathogens, although arthritis can be a manifestation of mumps, infectious mononucleosis, and arbovirus infections. Polyarthritis develops in approximately 30% of women after rubella vaccination or rubella infection. The arthritis, which follows the onset of the rash, lasts from a few days to two weeks.

Hepatitis B infection may be preceded by a polyarthritis associated with urticaria. The arthritis lasts from a few days to a few weeks and is usually gone by the time jaundice develops. A chronic synovitis can be seen also in association with chronic active hepatitis.

No specific therapy is available for viral arthritis. Symptoms can be controlled with aspirin 600 mg PO every 6 hours.

E. Infarction versus infection can be a difficult diagnostic problem in the patient with sickle cell disease and in the lupus patient on corticosteroid therapy, which predisposes to osteonecrosis. In either circumstance, evidence for infection should be sought aggressively. Both represent compromised host situations and gram-negative bacilli (*Salmonella*) as well as gram-positive cocci may cause acute arthritis.

F. Prosthetic joints. Both loosening and infection can result in pain in the area of the joint prosthesis. Ancillary studies (radiologic changes, WBC, erythrocyte sedimentation rate, fever) are often of diagnostic help. Joint aspiration is mandatory if infection remains a possibility. Infection in a joint prosthesis usually necessitates removal of the prosthesis for complete eradication of the infection.

Antibiotic prophylaxis should be administered to all patients with joint prostheses who are undergoing any procedure that might result in bacteremia (dental work, gastrointestinal [GI] or genitourinary [GU] surgery). Recommendations for choice of antibiotics are the same as those for prophylaxis of bacterial endocarditis.

1. **Oropharyngeal procedures.** Procaine penicillin G 1.2 million units IM 30 minutes before procedure, then penicillin V 500 mg PO every 6 hours for 2 days. If allergic to penicillin, give erythromycin 1 gm PO 1½ hours before procedure, then 500 mg every 6 hours for 2 days.

2. **GI or GU procedures.** 30 minutes before procedure, give procaine penicillin G 2.4 million units IM every 8 hours for 1 day (or ampicillin 1.0 gm IM every 8 hours for 1 day) *plus* gentamicin 1.0 mg/kg IM or IV (not to exceed 80 mg) every 8 hours for 1 day. If allergic to penicillin, give vancomycin 1.0 gm IV *plus* gentamicin in dose listed above *or* streptomycin 1.0 gm IM.

G. Causes of culture-negative infectious arthritis

1. Inappropriate media (e.g., Thayer-Martin needed for gonococcus).

2. Inappropriate specimen handling (e.g., anerobes).

3. Previous antibiotic therapy.

4. Immune complex–mediated arthritis (pneumococcal, meningococcal).

5. "Reactive arthritis." Both postvenereal and postdysenteric arthritis are sterile and likely represent an immune complex–mediated phenomenon in a genetically susceptible host.

6. Viral arthritis.

Bibliography

Bayer, A. S., et al.   Gram-negative bacillary septic arthritis. Clinical, radiographic, therapeutic and prognostic features. *Semin. Arthritis Rheum.* 7:123, 1977.

Goldenberg, D. L., Brandt, K. D., Cohen, A. S., and Cathcart, E. S.   Treatment of septic arthritis. A comparison of needle aspiration and surgery as initial modes of joint drainage. *Arthritis Rheum.* 18:83, 1975.

Goldenberg, D. L., and Cohen, A. S.   Acute infectious arthritis. A review of patients with nongonococcal joint infections. *Am. J. Med.* 60:369, 1976.

Newman, J. H.   Review of septic arthritis throughout the antibiotic era. *Ann. Rheum. Dis.* 35:198, 1976.

Schmid, F. R.   Bacterial Arthritis. In D. J. McCarty (Ed.), *Arthritis and Allied Conditions.* Philadelphia: Lea & Febiger, 1979. Pp. 1363–1379.

25. Juvenile Rheumatoid Arthritis

Stephanie Korn

Juvenile rheumatoid arthritis (JRA) is the currently accepted term for a group of disease patterns having in common chronic idiopathic synovitis in children. Arthritis beginning after age 16 is arbitrarily labeled *adult rheumatoid arthritis* (RA). Whether JRA includes several distinct entities and whether it is a different disease from adult RA cannot be known until etiology and pathogenesis are clear. Infectious, immunologic, and genetic factors are suspected but not established as playing causal roles.

  I. Prevalence. The Arthritis Foundation estimates that 250,000 children in the United States have JRA. The onset of JRA ranges from the first year of life to the late teens.

 II. Classification. The American Rheumatism Association (ARA) definition of JRA is persistent arthritis of one or more joints for at least six weeks if other conditions causing or simulating arthritis are excluded (Table 25-1). Subjective symptoms without objective joint findings are insufficient for diagnosis. Manifestations during the first six months of disease determine onset subtype. Joints are counted individually; exceptions are the cervical spine, counted as one joint; the carpal joints of each hand, counted as one joint each; and the tarsal joints of each foot, counted as one joint each. Small joints of the hands and feet are counted individually.

  A. Systemic onset JRA (Still disease) includes 20% of total JRA patients.

   1. Clinical features. Girls and boys are affected equally, and onset may be at any age. High spiking fever, lymphadenopathy, hepatosplenomegaly, polyserositis, and typical rash are commonly seen. (The unique features of this pattern of disease have been recognized with increasing frequency in adults.) The rash consists of pale pink macules of variable size, appearing mostly on the trunk and proximal extremities, less commonly on the face and distal extremities. The rash is evanescent, appears commonly with fever, local heat, or scratching of the skin (Koebner phenomenon), and is rarely pruritic. Arthritis may not be apparent in the first weeks or months of disease. It can be a minor aspect of the illness, occurring only during febrile flares, or it can progress to severe chronic polyarthritis in about 20% of patients. The diagnosis of systemic JRA should not be considered definite unless arthritis is evident. Myalgias and myocarditis may also be seen.

   2. Laboratory findings. Granulocytosis (white blood cell [WBC] count up to 90,000/mm^3), thrombocytosis (WBC up to 1 million/mm^3), anemia, and elevation of sedimentation rate are frequent. Antinuclear antibody (ANA) and rheumatoid factor are rarely positive.

  B. Polyarticular onset JRA is defined as involvement of five or more joints at onset and is seen in 30% to 40% of JRA patients.

   1. Clinical features

    a. Rheumatoid factor–positive patients in this subset tend to be adolescents, often girls, and frequently have severe erosive arthritis similar to adult RA. Large and small joints are involved symmetrically. Joint stiffness is a feature. The cervical spine is often involved. Systemic symptoms, if present, are less severe than those of the systemic subset. Subcutaneous nodules may occur.

    b. Rheumatoid factor–negative patients with polyarticular arthritis may present at any age in childhood, may be male or female, and have less destructive arthritis.

Table 25-1. Disease Exclusions Required for Diagnosis of JRA

Other Rheumatic Diseases
  Rheumatic fever
  Systemic lupus erythematosus
  Ankylosing spondylitis
  Polymyositis and dermatomyositis
  Vasculitis
    Anaphylactoid purpura (Henoch-Schönlein)
    Polyarteritis
    Serum sickness and other allergic reactions
    Mucocutaneous lymph node syndrome and infantile polyarteritis
  Scleroderma
  Psoriatic arthritis
  Reiter syndrome
  Sicca syndrome
  Mixed connective tissue disease
  Behcet syndrome

Infectious Arthritis
  Bacterial arthritis (including tuberculosis)
  Viral, fungal, and mycoplasmal arthritides
  Nonbacterial arthritis associated with bacterial infections

Inflammatory Bowel Disease

Neoplastic Diseases Including Leukemia and Lymphoma

Nonrheumatic Conditions of Bone and Joints
  Osteochondritis
  Toxic synovitis of the hip
  Slipped capital femoral epiphysis
  Trauma
    Battered child syndrome
    Fractures
    Joint, ligament, and muscle injuries
    Congenital indifference to pain
  Chondromalacia of the patella
  Congenital anomalies and genetically determined abnormalities of musculoskeletal system (including inborn errors of metabolism)
  Idiopathic tenosynovitis

Hematologic Diseases
  Sickle cell anemia
  Hemophilia

Functional Limb Pains

Miscellaneous Diseases
  Immunologic abnormalities
  Sarcoidosis
  Hypertrophic osteoarthropathy
  Villonodular synovitis
  Chronic active hepatitis
  Familial Mediterranean fever

Source: Adapted from J. G. Schaller and V. Hanson, Proceedings of the conference on the rheumatic diseases of childhood. *Arthritis Rheum.* 20: Suppl., 1977.

2. **Laboratory findings.** Mild to moderate leukocytosis, anemia, and elevation of sedimentation rate may be seen. Nonspecific pattern of ANA without either anti-DNA antibodies or complement abnormalities may occur, especially in patients with positive rheumatoid factor.

3. **Radiographic findings.** Early x-ray changes are soft tissue swelling and juxtaarticular osteoporosis. Elevation of the periosteum, growth arrest lines, zones of metaphyseal rarefaction, epiphyseal overgrowth, and premature closure of epiphyses may also be seen. Destructive changes occur later in the disease course.

C. **Oligoarticular (pauciarticular) onset JRA** indicates that four or fewer joints are involved. About 50% of patients present with this pattern.

1. **Chronic uveitis subset features.** These patients often have a positive ANA and a high incidence of chronic uveitis. Young age at onset (average 3 years), positive ANA, and female sex are strong risk factors for development of uveitis, which usually occurs around the same time as arthritis, although its onset can range from months before to ten years after. The knee is more commonly involved than the ankle, hip, elbow, wrist, and single small joints of the hands or foot. Arthritis is often asymmetric and mild. The greatest long-term morbidity is associated with eye involvement, which is insidious with occasional symptoms of pain, tearing, redness, and photophobia which may progress to loss of vision (see sec. **IV.B.**). Systemic symptoms are not prominent.

2. **Sacroiliitis subset.** Adolescent boys with involvement primarily of hips and knees often demonstrate sacroiliitis clinically or on x-ray. More than 50% are positive for HLA-B27 antigen, and a high proportion develop ankylosing spondylitis. They are ANA negative. Acute iritis may occur.

D. **Differential diagnosis** (See also Table 25-1.)

1. **Infection of bone or joints** occurs frequently in childhood and should be carefully ruled out. Joint aspiration, blood culture, bone scan, counterimmunoelectrophoresis of joint fluid or urine and, in difficult cases, synovial biopsy, are techniques that may be employed to identify the infectious agent.

2. **Malignancies,** particularly leukemia, lymphoma, and neuroblastoma, can present as arthritis of one or more joints or as fever of unknown origin. Radiographic findings and bone marrow aspiration may lead to the correct diagnosis.

3. **Other rheumatic diseases,** especially acute rheumatic fever (ARF) and systemic lupus erythematosus (SLE), should be carefully excluded by clinical and laboratory criteria. As the arthritis of ARF, compared to JRA, tends to respond dramatically to aspirin, it is helpful to observe the pattern of joint involvement before instituting antiinflammatory therapy. Acetaminophen can be used for symptomatic relief until the diagnosis is clear. SLE is suggested by nephritis, leukopenia, thrombocytopenia, anti-DNA antibodies, and hypocomplementemia.

4. **Serum sickness–like illness** caused by drug hypersensitivity may be recognized by a history of an allergic diathesis, exposure to a drug during the two weeks preceding the illness, and the appearance of urticaria.

5. **Inflammatory bowel disease** may present before, with, or after related arthritis. Symptoms of abdominal pain, diarrhea, and erythema nodosum suggest the diagnosis.

6. **Traumatic synovitis** is common in childhood.

7. **Hemophilia** may present as acute arthritis. A chronic synovitis may result from the irritating effect of repeated bleeding into a joint. A child with a coagulopathy may not have been previously diagnosed before presenting with joint problems.

III. Therapy

A. General measures

1. **Adequate rest** and avoidance of excessive stress and fatigue are needed along with a proper balance of exercise and activity.

2. **Eating** is often a problem in ill children. Diets high in protein and calories with plenty of fluid should be prescribed. Obesity, however, will stress joints.

3. **Psychosocial problems** in patients with chronic illness and their families often compound physical limitations and require careful long-term attention in a team approach.

4. **School** progress is a high priority. Assignment to a special class may be necessary when the school cannot accommodate an arthritic child's needs.

B. Drug therapy

1. **Aspirin** is the initial drug of choice once the diagnosis of JRA is established. The starting dose is 70 to 80 mg/kg per day, divided in 4 to 6 doses daily. Giving the drug with milk or meals helps avoid gastric irritation; otherwise, antacids may be used, but the dose required for therapeutic effect will tend to be higher because absorption will be decreased. Therapeutic effect without toxicity is generally reached at a serum level between 20 and 30 mg/dl. Several days should be allowed for stabilization of the serum level following a dose change. When therapeutic effect is not achieved by the initial dose, the dose may be gradually increased to 100 mg/kg daily. For unknown reasons, some children, especially those with systemic JRA subset, do not readily achieve therapeutic levels, even at high dose. Once the level is adequate, four daily doses may be given at breakfast, lunch, dinner, and bedtime, thus avoiding awakening the child at night. Liver enzymes should be checked periodically to monitor for aspirin hepatotoxicity.

   As a result of the pharmacokinetics of aspirin, increasing the dose as tissue saturation is approached produces a large rise in the serum level of aspirin. Pushing the dose to toxicity is a dangerous approach in young children since early symptoms may not be expressed or accurately interpreted by parents. Fluid, electrolyte, and pH disturbances develop rapidly in small children, and salicylism, usually resulting from accidental ingestion, is still too frequently a cause of death.

   Used properly, aspirin is well tolerated and effective in most arthritic children. After several months without evidence of active disease, aspirin may be gradually withdrawn.

   a. **Preparations.** Chewable, flavored **baby aspirins** are preferred by young children and are available in tablets of 75 mg. When the number of baby aspirins required per dose is inconvenient to take, regular adult tablets (325 mg each, equaling 4 baby aspirins) may be given. They are better accepted when crushed in a teaspoon of applesauce. **Ascriptin** is useful when an aspirin and antacid combination is needed.

2. **Nonsteroidal antiinflammatory drugs (NSAIDs)** other than aspirin have not yet been widely tested in children, with the exception of tolmetin. Started at 15 mg/kg daily and gradually increased to 30 mg/kg daily in JRA patients, tolmetin was found to be safe and comparable to aspirin in efficacy (*J. Pediatr.* 90:799, 1977). Response to tolmetin occurs in a few days to a week. A more detailed discussion of clinical experience with nonsteroidal agents in JRA may be found in J. J. Miller's *Juvenile Rheumatoid Arthritis*.

3. **Gold** therapy is used in JRA when therapeutic doses of aspirin and other nonsteroidal agents have been inadequate in controlling disease for a period of months. Gold salts are given intramuscularly, 1 mg/kg per week (maximum 50 injections), following 3 test doses of 0.25, 0.5, and 0.75 mg/kg per week. The patient should be carefully monitored for toxicity, including observations of

skin and mucous membranes, urinalysis, complete blood count (CBC), platelet count, and periodic liver function tests. Toxic reactions are usually reversible by stopping the drug. About 40% of patients are said to respond well to gold treatment after several months. After 20 weekly injections, gold may be discontinued if no improvement has occurred. When disease activity responds to gold, injections may be extended to every two weeks and later to every three or four weeks. Gold may be discontinued when one year of full remission has been achieved. If disease activity flares when gold is withdrawn, gold may have to be continued indefinitely.

4. **Corticosteroids** should be used with great caution. They are indicated for systemic manifestations that are uncontrollable after an adequate trial of aspirin and NSAIDs, and for potentially life-threatening problems such as myocarditis or severe pericarditis. When local treatment of uveitis is ineffective, a course of oral corticosteroid is indicated to help prevent serious eye complications including blindness. Steroids are rarely used for joint manifestations alone. The severity and certainty of steroid complications increase with dose and duration of treatment and may include infection, adrenal suppression, hypertension, osteoporosis, growth retardation, and cataracts. For control of serious disease manifestation, prednisone up to 1 to 2 mg/kg daily (or equivalent doses for intravenous treatment) in 3 doses may be given for as short a period as possible. When improvement occurs, prednisone is consolidated in steps to a single morning dose and gradually tapered. Use of aspirin or other agents concurrently may help to decrease steroid requirement. To reduce long-term side effects, daily steroid treatment should not extend beyond four months and, whenever possible, an alternate day regimen should be used.

5. **Antimalarials,** penicillamine, and cytotoxic drugs are rarely used to treat JRA.

C. Physical therapy

1. **Exercise** is important to maintain joint function and muscle strength and mass. Joints should be rested when acutely inflamed, but prolonged immobilization is harmful. As the pain of inflammation improves, gentle passive and active range of motion exercises should be begun, then advanced as tolerated. Swimming is an ideal exercise since muscles are worked and joints moved freely without the stress of weight bearing. An exercise program beginning three times weekly with a physical therapist and continued by the family at home is valuable.

2. **Heat** helps to relieve stiffness and swelling and increase range of motion.

   a. Warm tub bath upon arising improves morning stiffness. During acute phases, baths may be prescribed two or three times a day.

   b. Ambulation in a heated pool in a physical therapy department is of great benefit in promoting the exercise program.

   c. Paraffin baths to the hands and wrists are beneficial when care is taken to control the temperature and create an enjoyable atmosphere for the child.

3. **Splints** applied to the wrist or knee at night are often used to maintain gains in range of movement obtained with daily exercise.

4. **Occupational therapy** helps promote independence in activities of daily living.

D. Surgical treatment

1. **Synovectomy** is controversial but may have a role in selected cases of medically resistant synovitis of one or two joints if done before destructive radiographic changes occur.

2. **Jaw reconstructive surgery** for micrognathia caused by temperomandibular joint involvement has recently been developed and gives good results; it is performed once adolescence is reached and most facial growth is complete.

3. **Total joint replacements** are being performed with increasing frequency in patients with significant disability once skeletal growth is complete.

IV. Complications

   A. **Growth.** Disease and corticosteroid therapy are major impediments to growth. Compensatory growth occurs following discontinuation of steroids but may not be complete.
   Localized growth problems may result in bony overgrowth caused by hyperemia. Premature closure of epiphyses may result in ultimate undergrowth and leg length discrepancy. Underdevelopment of the mandible is a particularly common problem.

   B. **Chronic uveitis** in JRA is an insidious inflammation of the anterior uveal tract (iridocyclitis). It occurs predominantly in the subset of ANA-positive girls with oligoarticular arthritis beginning in the first five years of life; however, it occurs in the other JRA subsets as well. Patients are often asymptomatic. Without periodic slit lamp examination, severe complications of scarring from prolonged inflammation may occur, including band keratopathy, cataract, glaucoma, and blindness. Findings on ophthalmoscopic exam may include injection around the limbus, excessive tearing, decreased pupil reactivity, or scalloped pupil edges caused by synechiae, cloudiness, or opacities in the anterior chamber. Slit lamp examination will reveal signs of inflammation which cannot be seen with the ophthalmoscope. It should be routinely performed every six months in JRA patients and every three to four months in the high-risk subset. Uveitis is treated with topical mydriatics and corticosteroids under the supervision of an ophthalmologist. Subconjunctival injections of steroid are used in resistant cases. When these measures fail, a course of oral prednisone 1 to 2 mg/kg daily is indicated. Prompt diagnosis and treatment of uveitis are of high priority in JRA management.
   Acute uveitis in HLA-B27 positive boys with sacroiliitis is more easily recognized than the chronic form of uveitis because symptoms (pain, photophobia) and signs noted above are prominent. It also responds better to treatment and poses less of a long-term problem.

   C. **Hepatic dysfunction** in JRA seems to result primarily from a toxic effect of aspirin and occurs most frequently in the systemic subset. Mild to moderate elevation of hepatic enzymes without hyperbilirubinemia is common and generally responds to temporary withdrawal of aspirin. Reinstitution of aspirin is usually well tolerated. Symptoms of hepatic dysfunction are less prominent than laboratory abnormalities, but cases of hepatic failure have been reported.

   D. **Infection** is increased in JRA patients. Systemic infection is largely responsible for the 1.4% mortality rate in JRA in the United States and is concentrated in the group with systemic disease onset at a young age. These patients are also most likely to receive corticosteroid treatment.

   E. **Renal failure from amyloidosis** is rare in the United States, although regularly seen, for unknown reasons, in Europe. It is the major factor in the 4% mortality rate of European JRA series. Presentation is always with proteinuria and, less commonly, with gastrointestinal symptoms, edema, hypertension, or hepatosplenomegaly, as well. Reports from England indicate that chlorambucil may be beneficial for this serious complication.

V. Prognosis.
Thirty to fifty percent of children have active disease at any given point 5 to 15 years after onset, and 70% to 90% are in functional class I or II. The 10% to 30% with marked disability divide almost equally between the systemic and polyarticular subsets. Prognosis may be difficult to predict as the disease course may be unicyclic, polycyclic, or continuous. However, with prompt and long-term attention to maintenance of joint mobility and avoidance or control of complications, the long-term outlook is generally optimistic. Many, but not all, children will have remission of disease, and most will not be significantly disabled.

Bibliography

Ansell, B. M. (Ed.).   Rheumatic disorders in childhood. *Clin. Rheum. Dis.* 2:2, 1976.

Arden, E. B., and Ansell, B. M. (Eds.).   *Surgical Management of Juvenile Chronic Polyarthritis.* New York: Academic, 1978.

Levinson, J. E., and Brewer, E. J.   *Juvenile Rheumatoid Arthritis: Diagnosis and Management.* Fort Washington, Pa.: McNeil Laboratories, 1978. This two-part film may be borrowed and monograph obtained free of charge from: Professional Services, McNeil Laboratories, 500 Office Center Dr., Fort Washington, PA   19034.

Miller, J. J. (Ed.).   *Juvenile Rheumatoid Arthritis.* Littleton, Mass.: PSG Publishing, 1979.

Schaller, J. G., and Hanson, V.   Proceedings of the conference on the rheumatic diseases of childhood. *Arthritis Rheum.* 20:Suppl., 1977.

26. Lupus Erythematosus

Robert P. Kimberly

Systemic Lupus Erythematosus

Systemic lupus erythematosus (SLE) is a multisystem disease with a spectrum of clinical manifestations and a variable course characterized by exacerbations and remissions. Lupus is marked by both humoral and cellular immunologic abnormalities, including multiple autoantibodies which may participate in tissue injury. Antinuclear antibodies (ANAs), especially those to native DNA, are common immunologic abnormalities found in the disease.

During the 19th century, lupus was considered to be a skin disease. The erosive nature of some of the skin lesions seemed to resemble the damage inflicted by the bite of a wolf, thus leading to the name *lupus*. In 1872, Moritz Kaposi described systemic symptoms in association with cutaneous disease. At the turn of the century, Sir William Osler described arthritis and visceral manifestations in conjunction with polymorphic skin lesions. The presence of circulating immunologic factors became apparent about 50 years later with the discovery of the LE-cell phenomenon by Hargraves in 1948, the recognition of the LE-factor as an antinuclear antibody in 1953, and the identification of antibodies to native DNA in 1956. Identification and characterization of abnormal autoantibodies continue to be major areas of clinical and immunochemical interest.

The development of sensitive laboratory tests for autoantibodies has enabled the recognition of milder forms of systemic lupus, with a consequent change in both reported prevalence and prognosis. The broad clinical spectrum of SLE challenges the diagnostic and therapeutic acumen of the physician.

I. Epidemiology

A. Sex. A female-male ratio of 9 : 1 is seen in most series of adult patients. The female predominance is less striking in childhood lupus (disease onset preceding puberty) and in elderly SLE patients.

B. Age. First symptoms usually occur between the second and fourth decades of life but may be seen in any age group. The presentation of SLE in the elderly (as much as 10% of the total lupus population in some series) may differ from that in younger patients.

C. Ethnic distribution. While lupus occurs in all races, its prevalence is not equally distributed among all groups. SLE occurs more commonly in the United States than in England and more in blacks than in whites. The average annual incidence in the United States is approximately 27.5 per million population for white females and 75.4 per million for black females. The reported prevalence figures for women vary widely from 1 per 1,000 to 1 per 10,000.

II. Genetics. The presence of a genetic component in SLE is supported by family studies.

A. Clinical disease. Family members of SLE patients are more likely to have lupus or another connective tissue disease. Concordance of disease among monozygotic twin pairs is high but not complete. Fraternal twins do not have a higher frequency of lupus than other first-degree relatives.

B. Immunologic abnormalities. Family members are more likely to have a false positive test for syphilis, antinuclear antibodies, antilymphocyte antibodies, and hypergammaglobulinemia. Lupus and lupuslike syndromes are associated with hereditary complement component deficiencies, most commonly C2 deficiency but also C1r, C1s, C1INH, C4, C5, and C8 deficiencies.

C. Histocompatibility studies. Lupus is associated with the B-cell alloantigen alleles HLA-DR2 and HLA-DR3.

III. Pathogenesis

A. Pathology. While no histologic feature is pathognomonic for SLE, several features are very suggestive: (1) fibrinoid necrosis and degeneration of blood vessels and connective tissue, (2) the hematoxylin body (the in vivo LE-cell phenomenon), and (3) "onion skin" thickening of the arterioles of the spleen.

1. Histopathology. Routine histologic examination of tissue specimens reveals a broad range of findings.

a. Skin. Skin biopsy may demonstrate a leukocytoclastic angiitis, especially in palpable purpuric lesions. The typical lupus rash usually shows epidermal thinning, liquefaction degeneration of the basal layer with dermal-epidermal junction disruption, and lymphocytic infiltration of the dermis. Rheumatoidlike nodules with palisading giant cells are uncommon, and panniculitis is rare.

b. Synovium. Synovial biopsies may show fibrinous villous synovitis. The presence of pannus formation or bone and cartilage erosions is rare.

c. Muscle. Muscle biopsies usually show a nonspecific perivascular mononuclear infiltrate, but true muscle necrosis, as seen in polymyositis, can occur. Muscle biopsy may be helpful in evaluating the possibility of steroid-induced myopathy or chloroquine-induced myopathy, a rare entity in patients taking antimalarials.

d. Kidney. The kidney has been the most intensively studied organ. The entire range of glomerulonephritis (membranous, mesangial, proliferative, and membranoproliferative) is seen (see Table 26-1). Crescentric and necrotizing vasculitic lesions may be found. Interstitial abnormalities are being increasingly recognized. There is no single renal lesion diagnostic of SLE. Tubuloreticular structures are not restricted to SLE.

In general, renal biopsy provides one indicator of prognosis, characterizing patients with diffuse membranoproliferative lesions as having the poorest five-year survival (40% to 85% depending on the series). However, the more recent recognition that the histologic class of the biopsy may not be static and may either deteriorate or improve has emphasized the need for defining renal disease activity sequentially.

Table 26-1. International Pediatric Classification of Lupus Nephritis

Classification	Findings
IA.	Normal
IB.	Minimal change
IIA.	Focal mesangial disease
IIB.	Diffuse mesangial disease
IIIA.	Focal lesions; <20% of glomeruli with proliferative or sclerotic lesions
IIIB.	Focal lesions, 20–50% of glomeruli with proliferative or sclerotic lesions
IV.	Severe focal; >50% of glomeruli with proliferative or sclerotic lesions
VA.	Diffuse proliferative or sclerotic lesions
VB.	Diffuse membranoproliferative lesions
VI.	Membranous
Arteritis	
End-stage	

e. **Central nervous system (CNS)** lesions vary and reflect a spectrum of neurologic involvement ranging from vasculitis with a concomitant stroke to microhemorrhages and focal perivascular infiltrates. Normal brain tissue is often present despite clinical abnormalities. Cytoid bodies, seen as white fluffy exudates on fundoscopic examination, represent superficial retinal ischemia.

f. **Other viscera.** Other visceral pathologic findings include nonbacterial verrucous endocarditis (Libman-Sachs endocarditis), redundant mitral valvular leaflets with lengthened chordae tendineae (mitral valve prolapse syndrome), pulmonary fibrosis, and nonspecific pleural thickening. Necrotizing vasculitis may be present in the viscera and lead to secondary events including bowel infarction, myocardial infarction, pancreatitis, and possible accelerated atherosclerosis. In the spleen, the concentric periarterial fibrosis of small arteries (onion skin lesions) may be an end-stage consequence of earlier vasculitis.

2. **Immunopathology**

a. **Skin.** Immunofluorescence shows deposits of immunoglobulins and complement at the dermal-epidermal junction (lupus band test) in 80% to 100% of lesional skin and 36% to 100% of nonlesional skin. Attempts to correlate a positive lupus band test with active SLE or the presence of lupus nephritis have given inconsistent results. Positive lupus band tests are not specific for lupus; they are commonly associated with bullous pemphigoid and dermatitis herpetiformis (IgA). Dermal-epidermal immunofluorescence may also be seen in rheumatoid arthritis, scleroderma, dermatomyositis, lepromatous leprosy, multiple sclerosis, cystic fibrosis, chronic active hepatitis, primary biliary cirrhosis, amyloidosis, and, according to some reports, normals.

b. **Kidney.** Glomerular immunofluorescence to determine the distribution, pattern, and density of immunoglobulin, immunoglobulin class, and complement components does not appear to have prognostic or therapeutic significance. The presence of immunofluorescence for immunoglobulin or complement is not restricted to SLE; it is, however, compatible with immune complex–mediated diseases.

B. **Immunology**

1. **Humoral immunity.** Overactivity of the humoral component of immunologic responsiveness is manifested by hypergammaglobulinemia, autoantibodies, and circulating immune complexes.

a. **Various autoantibodies** may contribute to tissue injury. Anti-DNA antibodies have been found in renal glomerular lesions. Attempts to correlate specific clinical patterns of disease with specific types of autoantibodies have been partially successful; for example, sicca syndrome with SLE has been associated with SS-B (Ha) antibodies. While the titer of antinuclear antibodies does not necessarily correlate with disease activity, the levels of anti-DNA antibodies may vary with clinical disease. Because results vary, this test alone cannot be used to guide therapy.

b. **Circulating immune complexes** are commonly found in active SLE and are often associated with **hypocomplementemia.** Immune complex deposits are found in many tissues. Isolated determinations of circulating complexes do not consistently correlate with disease activity. Sequential patterns of change may be of value, especially when used in conjunction with determinations of reticuloendothelial system clearance of complexes.

2. **Cellular immunity.** Lupus is characterized by lymphopenia and often by monocytosis. The normal complex immunoregulatory balance among cells is lost. Anergy, diminished delayed hypersensitivity skin testing reactions, is

common. Immunoglobulin-producing B-cells are hyperactive. Suppressor T-cells are deficient, and monocyte-macrophages elaborate increased amounts of suppressor substances inhibitory to T-cells. The primary defect has not been identified.

C. Provocative agents. Although the etiologic agents in lupus have not been identified, several factors that may exacerbate the disease are known.

   1. Ultraviolet light. Sun exposure may precipitate either the onset or a flare of clinical disease, causing both dermatologic and systemic manifestations in about one-third of patients. Since complete avoidance of the sun is impractical, patients should wear long-sleeved shirts, trousers rather than shorts, wide-brimmed hats, and use sunscreens. Many effective sunscreens are available commercially; however, none can completely obviate the potential for large sun exposure to exacerbate SLE (see Appendix G).

   2. Situational stresses. Some patients may experience increased disease activity during periods of fatigue or emotional stress (e.g., when encountering school examinations or interpersonal conflict). The significance of such factors should not be overlooked, and such stress should be reduced as much as possible.

   3. Infection. Viral infection has been suggested as an etiologic event in lupus. Although unproven as such, viral infection may provoke a flare of disease by an unknown mechanism. Concern that exposure to foreign antigen might be harmful has led to some reluctance to immunize patients with lupus. However, current studies with influenza and pneumococcal vaccines suggest that such vaccination confers protection without causing increased lupus disease activity. Specific antibody response may be lower than that in normals.

   4. Drugs. Many drugs have been associated with the development of antinuclear antibodies and, in some cases, of a clinical lupuslike syndrome (Table 26-2); procainamide and hydralazine are the most commonly implicated. However, the potential to induce these serologic changes in nonlupus patients does not preclude the use of these drugs in lupus patients. Although most physicians prefer to avoid them if an alternative drug is available, the use of these drugs in lupus has not been associated with documented exacerbation of disease activity.

IV. Clinical presentation. Lupus is a multisystem disease whose diagnosis rests on the recognition of a *constellation* of clinical and laboratory findings. No single finding makes the diagnosis although some findings, such as antibodies to double-stranded DNA or a characteristic malar rash, are more suggestive than others. As a result of the wide spectrum of manifestations and severity of disease, criteria for diagnosis have been devised to ensure at least a minimum uniformity for disease classification in clinical studies (Table 26-3). The presence of four criteria (not necessarily simultaneous) is required to classify a patient as presenting with SLE. The fluorescent antinuclear antibody test has replaced the LE-cell phenomenon in most centers.

A. Fever. Fever is a common manifestation of active SLE. Although often above 103°F at times, sustained fever of such magnitude is not common. Acute severe disease ("lupus crisis") may be accompanied by fever up to 106°F.

B. Skin. Facial erythema is more common than the classical "butterfly" eruption, but almost every type of skin lesion has been described in lupus. Chronic discoid lesions with central atrophy, depigmentation, and scarring or nonscarring alopecia are common occurrences in 20% to 30% of patients. Mucous membrane lesions with hard palate ulcers and nasal septal perforations may be present. Raynaud phenomenon may be associated with acrosclerosis and, uncommonly, digital ulceration. Purpura and ecchymosis may occur as a result of either disease or corticosteroid treatment.

C. Musculoskeletal system

   1. Arthritis is common and affects both small and large joints in a symmetric pattern. The axial spine is not involved. Even in the face of long-standing

Table 26-2. Drugs Implicated in Drug-Induced LE-like Syndrome

Anticonvulsants
  Phenytoin
  Carbamazepine
  Primidone
  Mephenytoin
  Trimethadione
  Ethosuximide

Antihypertensives
  Hydralazine
  Methyldopa
  Reserpine

Antibiotics
  Isoniazid
  Aminosalicylate (PAS)
  Penicillin
  Tetracycline
  Streptomycin
  Sulfonamides
  Griseofulvin

Antiarrhythmics
  Procainamide
  Practolol

Antithyroidals
  Propylthiouracil
  Methylthiouracil

Other Drugs
  Penicillamine
  Oral contraceptive pills
  Chlorpromazine
  Phenylbutazone
  Thiazides

arthritis, bony erosions are uncommon. Reducible joint deformity is caused by capsular laxity and both tendinous and ligamentous involvement which lead to partial subluxation. Tendon ruptures may occur. Articular symptoms may also derive from osteonecrosis, most often in large weight-bearing joints.

2. **Inflammatory myositis** may occur in 2% to 3% of patients. Muscle weakness may also reflect corticosteroid-induced myopathy or, rarely, chloroquine-induced myopathy, or a myasthenia gravis–like syndrome associated with SLE.

D. **Cardiovascular system.** The major cardiovascular morbidity associated with lupus appears to be accelerated coronary atherosclerosis and ischemic coronary disease.

1. **Pericarditis** is the most common cardiovascular manifestation. Pericardial effusions demonstrable by echocardiogram may be present in up to 60% of patients. Symptomatic pericarditis occurs in about 25% of patients. Tamponade is rare.

2. **Myocardial disease,** evidenced by signs ranging from persistent tachycardia to frank myocardial infarction, may also occur. The basis is often unknown but may include coronary vasculitis or antiheart antibodies.

3. **Verrucous endocarditis** (Libman-Sachs endocarditis) is a pathologic diagnosis since it rarely causes clinically significant valvular lesions or embolic complications.

Table 26-3. Preliminary ARA Criteria for Classification of SLE

Manifestations	Frequency (%)
Facial erythema (butterfly rash)	40–64
Discoid lupus	17–31
Raynaud phenomenon	19–44
Alopecia	40–71
Photosensitivity	17–41
Oral or nasopharyngeal ulcerations	15–36
Nondeforming arthritis	86–100
LE-cells	48–92
Positive ANA	~100
Chronic false positive serologic test for syphilis	8–26
Proteinuria >3.5 gm/24 hr	16–25
Urinary casts (cellular or granular)	17–48
Pleuritis or pericarditis	30–60
Pericarditis alone	17–23
Psychosis, convulsions	16–20
Hematologic abnormality	
Hemolytic anemia	14–54
Leukopenia <4,000/mm^3	40–47
Thrombocytopenia <100,000/mm^3	11–14

4. **Peripheral vascular manifestations** include vasculitis that usually affects small arteries, arterioles, and capillaries, especially those of the skin. Thrombophlebitis may occur and recur in some patients as a sign of disease activity. Gangrene is rare. Raynaud phenomenon may be a feature in up to 25% of patients.

5. **Other manifestations** include the rare occurrence of aortic insufficiency and the occasional presence of pulmonary hypertension.

E. **Pulmonary system**

1. **Pleuritis** is the most common pulmonary symptom. Pleural effusions may occur in up to 50% of patients and pleuritic pain in 60% to 70% of patients. While it is impractical to analyze the pleural fluid of each patient during each occurrence, effusions may be secondary to processes other than active lupus, and infection should always be considered in the differential diagnosis.

2. **Pneumonitis** as evidenced by rales on physical examination and patchy infiltrates or platelike atelectasis on chest x-ray is a diagnostic problem. Since SLE patients are often compromised hosts, infection by either common or uncommon agents must be considered. "Lupus pneumonitis" does occur, but this diagnosis requires rigorous exclusion of other processes. Progressive lupus pneumonitis ending in acute pulmonary insufficiency is uncommon. Lung biopsy may be required to establish a diagnosis, especially in the setting of persistent or progressive findings. Abnormal pulmonary function tests with moderate restrictive and obstructive deficits are common, but patients usually have mild or no associated symptoms.

F. **Gastrointestinal system.** Abdominal pain is a common complaint and may reflect gastrointestinal distress associated with medications or intrinsic pathology. Sterile peritonitis (serositis) and mesenteric vasculitis are difficult to document. Intestinal perforation, especially in patients on corticosteroids that can mask

Table 26-4. Autoantibodies in SLE

Antigen Source	Antibody Nomenclature	Incidence in SLE(%)	Specificity for SLE
Nuclear			
All determinants	ANA	100	—
ds DNA	Anti-DNA (double-stranded or native)	80–90	High
ss DNA	Anti-DNA (single-stranded)	80–90	—
Deoxyribonucleoprotein histones	LE-cell antibody	50–90	—
Acidic nucleoproteins	SM	30	High
	RNP	30–40	—
	SS-A	25	—
	SS-B (Ha)	15–20	—
Cytoplasmic			
RNA	rRNA, rRNP, Ro, La	Uncertain	—
Cell Surface Determinants			
RBC	Direct Coombs	30	—
WBC	Antilymphocyte antibodies	Common	—
	Antineutrophil antibodies	Uncommon	—
Platelets		Common	—
Others			
Clotting factor phospholipids	Lupus anticoagulant	10	—
Cardiolipin	False positive serologic test for syphilis	10–25	—

symptoms, must be considered as well as spontaneous bacterial peritonitis. Pancreatitis may also occur. Hepatomegaly may occur in one quarter of patients, but abnormal liver function tests are usually drug-related rather than indicative of intrinsic lupus-associated liver damage. Chronic active hepatitis with positive tests for LE-cells or antinuclear antibodies (lupoid hepatitis) is not part of the spectrum of SLE.

G. Other systems. Lymphadenopathy is common but obviously not specific. Conjunctivitis, keratoconjunctivitis sicca, episcleritis, and retinal exudates (cytoid bodies) may be present. Parotid enlargement with or without a dry mouth (xerostomia) is reported in up to 8% of patients.

V. Laboratory abnormalities

A. Autoantibodies to nuclear and cytoplasmic antigens occur in lupus. Their detection is diagnostically significant although the sensitivity and specificity for lupus vary with each specific autoantibody (Table 26-4). Since these autoantibodies may participate in immunologically mediated tissue damage, correlation between disease activity and antibody titer has been sought with the hope that antibody level (especially anti-DNA antibody level) might provide an index of disease activity and a guide to therapeutics. The utility of this approach, however, is controversial since some patients with persistently abnormal values do not develop severe disease despite conservative treatment. Indeed, there are some patients who have had only laboratory abnormalities with no symptoms for many years. Different techniques are available for measuring any given autoantibody, but they do not necessarily provide comparable results. Although both IgM and IgG rheumatoid factors may occur in up to one-third of patients, their presence does not correlate with the presence of articular disease.

B. Serum complement is often abnormally low in conjunction with elevated autoantibody titers. Hypocomplementemia per se is not specific for lupus and may reflect any immunologically mediated disease accompanied by complement consumption, a hereditary complement component deficiency, impaired synthesis, or an improperly handled serum sample. In the context of lupus, hypocomplementemia is often, but not invariably, associated with nephritis. As with anti-DNA antibody levels, complement titers are valuable as a therapeutic guide in some but not all patients.

C. Routine laboratory examination may reveal many abnormalities.

1. Hematology

    a. Anemia occurs in more than 50% of patients, especially during active disease. Most anemias in SLE are of the chronic disease type (normochromic, normocytic with low serum iron and total iron binding capacity [TIBC]). The direct Coombs test may be positive in approximately 25% of patients; true hemolytic anemia occurs in 10% of patients. The Coombs test may represent cell surface immunoglobulin (IgG), complement (C3, C4), or both.

    b. Leukopenia. Lupus patients are often leukopenic, especially during periods of disease activity. Lymphopenia caused by antilymphocyte antibodies is the most common type, but antibody-mediated neutropenia can occur. Anti-stem cell antibodies are rare.

    c. Thrombocytopenia. Antiplatelet antibodies have been demonstrated by a direct Coombslike test.

    d. Prolongation of the partial thromboplastin time. Antibodies to both individual components of the clotting cascade (VIII, IX, XII) and to the prothrombin converting complex have been described. The lupus anticoagulant is not corrected by addition of normal plasma to the patient's plasma. In the presence of normal platelets, the lupus anticoagulant does not appear to cause clinically significant bleeding.

    e. False positive serologic test for syphilis. A small percentage of biologic false positive reactions give a "positive" fluorescent treponemal antibody (FTA) which can be distinguished from a true positive because of its beaded appearance. Circulating anticoagulants are associated with a false positive serologic test for syphilis.

    f. The sedimentation rate is frequently elevated but is an inconsistent index of disease activity. It is not useful in differentiating active lupus from an intercurrent process.

2. Biochemistry. Apart from hypergammaglobulinemia, routine biochemical screening reflects the pattern and degree of organ involvement. Mild hyperkalemia in the absence of renal insufficiency reflects a lupus-related renal tubular defect.

VI. Differential diagnosis. The diagnostic strategy for lupus involves recognition of a multisystem disease, the presence of certain serologic findings, and the absence of any other recognized disease process to explain the findings. Not all clinical and laboratory findings are of equal specificity: acute pericarditis and psychosis, as well as proteinuria and leukopenia, have many causes other than SLE. Conversely, discoid lupus rash and high-titer antinative DNA antibodies or Sm antibodies strongly support the diagnosis. The art of diagnosis rests in the recognition of a constellation of findings, each of which is given the appropriate clinical weight. Since there are many and varied presentations of lupus, the full differential diagnosis includes most of internal medicine.

A. **The most common presentation** is a young female with polyarthritis; however, lupus is not the most likely cause of her symptoms. Infectious arthritis, especially gonococcal arthritis, must be considered first since specific, curative therapy is available. Early in the course of uncomplicated lupus polyarthritis, radiographs of the joints are usually not helpful. However, radiographs are important in evaluating and following infectious arthritis. The single most useful laboratory test is the antinuclear antibody determination. While not completely specific (Table 26-5), it is highly sensitive. A positive test is a signal to consider the diagnosis further, and a negative test in a patient not receiving corticosteroid therapy makes the diagnosis unlikely.

B. **Organ systems that may be affected** by SLE include skin and mucous membranes (rash, ulceration, alopecia); joints (nondeforming, often symmetric polyarthritis and periarthritis); kidney (glomerulonephritis); serosal membranes (pleuritis, pericarditis, abdominal serositis); blood (hemolytic anemia, leukopenia, thrombocytopenia); lungs (transient infiltrates, rarely progressive hemorrhagic pneumonitis); and nervous system (seizures, psychosis, peripheral neuropathies).

C. **Other rheumatic diseases.** Patients with multisystem disease and antinuclear antibodies may have a condition other than SLE. Ten to twenty percent of patients with rheumatoid arthritis may have LE-cells; up to 40% may have positive antinuclear antibodies. Systemic sclerosis (scleroderma), especially in the early phase of disease, and mixed connective tissue disease must be considered as well as systemic necrotizing vasculitis, Wegener granulomatosis, and chronic active hepatitis with persistent synovitis.

D. **Drug-induced SLE-like syndrome.** See Table 26-2.

VII. **Therapy.** The diagnosis of SLE does not mandate the use of corticosteroids. The poor prognosis reported in earlier series has been altered because the capability to diagnose milder forms of the disease now exists. This expansion of the mild end of the disease spectrum affects not only the overall prognosis but also the therapeutic approach to patients with the diagnosis of SLE.

The pleomorphic manifestations of lupus, even within a single organ system, have hampered the design and evaluation of both controlled and uncontrolled therapeutic studies. Treatment must be individualized. The therapeutic strategy must consider both the pattern and the severity of organ system involvement.

General measures include adequate rest and avoidance of stress. Specific measures follow.

A. **Fever.** Aspirin 600 to 900 mg QID. Indomethacin 25 to 50 mg TID, acetaminophen, or other nonsteroidal antiinflammatory drugs are also effective antipyretics which can be used in aspirin-intolerant patients. Corticosteroids are not indicated for fever alone.

B. **Skin rash.** Avoidance of ultraviolet exposure in order to prevent exacerbation of both cutaneous and systemic disease is paramount. Sunscreens, wide-brimmed hats, long sleeves, and long pants should be used by all patients. Highly protective sunscreens (Total Eclipse, SuperShade, Block Out) should be applied liberally 1 to 2 hours before exposure and reapplied after any swimming or sweating.

  1. **Topical therapy.** Active skin disease should be treated initially with topical corticosteroid preparations (triamcinolone, fluocinonide) two to three times daily. Occlusive dressings with cellophane wrap may be used at night, particularly on the upper extremities.

  2. **Systemic therapy.** The antimalarial hydroxychloroquine, 200 mg PO BID is used to supplement topical treatment of extensive lesions. Regular ophthalmologic examination at 3- to 6-month intervals should include slit lamp examination and measures of light and color perception. The drug should be tapered as soon as disease control permits. Systemic corticosteroids are not indicated for skin disease alone.

Table 26-5. Differential Diagnosis of Common Serologic Tests

	Antinuclear Antibodies	Anti-DNA Antibodies	Low CH_{50}	Rheumatoid Factor
SLE Incidence	~100%	80%	80%	20–40%
Diseases with high incidence	Discoid lupus Drug-induced LE Sicca syndrome Scleroderma	Discoid lupus Drug-induced LE (single-stranded)	Hereditary complement deficiency Hereditary angioedema Membranoproliferative glomerulonephritis Cryoglobulinemia	Rheumatoid arthritis Sicca syndrome
Diseases with occasional incidence	Rheumatoid arthritis Dermatomyositis Idiopathic pulmonary fibrosis Chronic active hepatitis Aging	Chronic active hepatitis Sicca syndrome Rheumatoid arthritis Scleroderma Dermatomyositis	Rheumatoid arthritis Serum sickness Serious infection: gram-negative sepsis, pneumococcal sepsis	Dermatomyositis Juvenile rheumatoid arthritis Scleroderma Sarcoidosis Subacute bacterial endocarditis Idiopathic pulmonary fibrosis Aging
Diseases with rare incidence	Necrotizing vasculitis	Necrotizing vasculitis	Necrotizing vasculitis	Insulin-dependent diabetes Normals

C. Arthritis

1. **Nonsteroidal antiinflammatory drugs.** Aspirin 600 to 900 mg QID or indomethacin 25 to 50 mg PO TID. Gastrointestinal intolerance may limit therapy with nonsteroidal antiinflammatory drugs (NSAIDs) in some patients. Occasionally, large elevations of liver enzymes may occur and require either reduction or termination of therapy. Transient changes in renal function with any NSAID may occur. The increasing experience with NSAID other than aspirin includes several apparently idiosyncratic reactions in lupus patients manifested by fever and aseptic meningitis.

2. **Systemic corticosteroid.** Oral prednisone, 10 to 20 mg daily, is reserved for patients with accompanying constitutional symptoms unresponsive to NSAID.

D. Serositis.
NSAID as outlined for arthritis. Rarely, pericarditis presents with a large pericardial effusion necessitating immediate high-dose prednisone (20 mg TID) therapy. Adverse effects of chronic high-dose corticosteroid therapy are discussed in **VII.I.1.**

E. Pneumonitis.
Transient pulmonary infiltrates that clear spontaneously without therapy may occur. The major significance of the radiologic findings lies in differential diagnosis rather than therapeutics. Infection with routine or opportunistic pathogens must be considered. Infiltrates secondary to lupus require no specific therapy.

Fulminant pneumonitis with hemorrhage, which is rare, requires aggressive therapy with high-dose corticosteroids (prednisone 20 mg TID) and often cytotoxics (azathioprine 2 to 3 mg/kg/24 hr or cyclophosphamide 2 to 3 mg/kg/24 hr).

F. Hematologic abnormalities

1. **Hemolytic anemia** is uncommon but may be severe and require corticosteroid therapy if the anemia is symptomatic. Young patients can tolerate hemoglobin levels of 7 to 8 gm/dl. When required, prednisone 40 to 60 mg per day is given in two or three divided doses and tapered as quickly as possible using the hemoglobin and reticulocyte count as guides.

2. **Immune thrombocytopenia** secondary to lupus usually responds to corticosteroid therapy. Platelet counts of 80,000 to 100,000 are considered adequate. Life-threatening thrombocytopenia unresponsive to several weeks of prednisone 60 mg daily may improve with splenectomy. The role of azathioprine or vincristine has not been established; administration of vinca alkaloid–loaded platelets for steroid-resistant thrombocytopenia is a promising experimental therapy.

3. **Leukopenia** in lupus usually represents lymphopenia rather than neutropenia and is not associated with the serious risk of infection that accompanies the leukopenia of cancer chemotherapy. Leukopenia does not warrant specific treatment per se.

G. Vasculitis.
Small vessel cutaneous vasculitis, usually found on the digits and palm of the hand, may be managed with low-dose prednisone, 20 mg per day. Medium vessel and large vessel vasculitis, although uncommon, require 60 mg per day in divided doses.

H. Neurologic disease

1. **Seizures** require the use of anticonvulsants. Initial therapy is phenytoin 300 to 400 mg daily with monitoring of serum drug level. Phenobarbital 20 to 60 mg TID is added if needed to achieve seizure control.

2. **Psychosis** may be secondary to either steroid therapy or SLE.

   a. **Steroid-induced psychosis** will improve with tapering of systemic corticosteroids. Major tranquilizers such as haloperidol 1 mg BID initially will assist in control of psychotic manifestations.

b. SLE-related psychosis. The occurrence of SLE-related psychosis does not necessarily require an increase in steroid therapy. If adequate behavioral control is achieved with major tranquilizers and no organic signs are present on either physical examination or CSF analysis, corticosteroids are not initiated or increased.

3. Parenchymal central nervous system disease. In the presence of new focal neurologic findings, prednisone 20 mg TID is given until either improvement or toxicity is observed. Some neurologic lesions are not steroid-responsive. If no improvement is evident after about three to four weeks of high-dose therapy, prednisone is tapered to avoid complications. Use of doses greater than 60 to 80 mg daily of prednisone rarely produces additional therapeutic benefit but markedly increases the risk of serious drug side effects. Any trial of very high-dose prednisone in severe disease should last for a predetermined, limited period of time. The value of cytotoxic agents in CNS disease has not been determined, and their role is limited to steroid-unresponsive, desperately ill patients.

4. Peripheral nerve disease. Peripheral neuropathy is common. Mononeuritis multiplex usually represents small vessel vasculitis. If unresponsive to prednisone 60 mg daily in three divided doses, azathioprine 2 to 3 mg/kg or cyclophosphamide 2 to 3 mg/kg may be initiated.

I. Renal disease. The management of renal disease is controversial. Evaluation of therapeutic outcomes has been hampered by the pleomorphic nature of lupus nephritis. Renal biopsy in general shows some correlation between morphologic severity and outcome. Patients with diffuse proliferative or membranoproliferative glomerulonephritis have the worst prognosis, but the natural history of clinically silent, diffuse proliferative disease with normal renal function has not been determined. Any therapeutic regimen must consider both short-term and long-term side effects encountered during the management of chronic nephritis.

1. Corticosteroid therapy. The initial management of active renal disease (celluria, cylindruria, proteinuria, or declining clearance function) is prednisone 60 mg per day. Serum hemolytic complement and anti-DNA binding activity are used to assist in guiding therapy in the subgroup of patients who show close correlation between serologic and clinical activity. Resolution of signs of active disease may permit tapering of prednisone, while return of an active sediment, increased proteinuria, or decreased function may prompt an increase in prednisone dosage.

While prednisone clearly helps ameliorate acute exacerbations of disease, there are many **serious side effects** of chronic corticosteroid therapy.

a. Physical appearance is altered by weight gain producing truncal fat deposition (moon facies, buffalo hump), hirsutism, acne, easy bruisability, and purple striae. Although individual patients differ in their susceptibility to these changes, reduction of the steroid dose will eventually reduce the severity of these manifestations.

b. Infection occurs with greater frequency in corticosteroid-treated patients. Corticosteroids may mask both local and systemic signs of infection. Minor infections have a greater potential to become systemic.

Latent infections, especially mycobacterial varieties, may become activated, and opportunistic agents such as fungi, *Nocardia*, and *Pneumocystis carinii* may cause serious clinical problems. Skin testing for delayed hypersensitivity to *Mycobacterium tuberculosis* should be performed before the initiation of corticosteroid therapy. However, a negative reaction may reflect the altered immunity of active SLE rather than lack of previous exposure to *M. tuberculosis*.

c. Mental function may be altered. Minor reactions include irritability, insomnia, euphoria, and inability to concentrate. Major reactions may include severe depression, mania, and paranoid psychoses.

d. Glucose intolerance may be induced or exacerbated by corticosteroids. Insulin may be required to control hyperglycemia and should be adjusted as the corticosteroid dosage is changed.

e. Hypokalemia may be caused by preparations with mineralocorticoid activity. Serum potassium should be checked frequently, especially if congestive heart failure, nephrosis, or peripheral edema producing secondary hyperaldosteronism is present.

f. Sodium retention, edema, and hypertension may be induced by all corticosteroid drugs. When these effects become clinically significant, agents with less salt-retaining properties can be used. Alternative steroid preparations are listed in Appendix G. Since steroids should be given only for major SLE manifestations, it is usually not feasible to control hypertension by a reduction in dose; therefore, blood pressure must be controlled by standard antihypertensive therapy.

g. Myopathy may occur in patients receiving long-term high-dose steroids. The muscles are not tender and, unlike inflammatory myositis, steroid-induced myopathy is usually not characterized by elevated serum muscle enzymes. Proximal weakness is the most common symptom. Pelvic girdle weakness is more common than shoulder girdle symptoms. Biopsy may be useful in distinguishing inflammatory SLE-related myositis from non-inflammatory corticosteroid-induced myopathy. Drug-induced myopathy will gradually improve with a reduction of corticosteroid dose.

h. Skeletal abnormalities include osteopenia and osteonecrosis. Corticosteroids may reduce gastrointestinal calcium absorption, induce secondary hyperparathyroidism, and also reduce collagen matrix synthesis by osteoblasts. Compression fractures in the vertebral spine represent a major secondary complication. They occur in about 15% of steroid-treated patients. Prophylactic vitamin D (50,000 units twice per week) and calcium (1,500 mg daily) are being evaluated, but are not used routinely (see Chap. 30).
Osteonecrosis occurs most frequently in weight-bearing joints, especially the femoral heads. The mechanism is unknown (therapy is discussed in Chap. 29). Reduction in corticosteroid dose whenever possible is desirable, although it is unlikely to affect established osteonecrosis.

i. Hypoadrenalism may occur during periods of physiologic stress in patients with suppression of the hypothalamic-pituitary-adrenal axis resulting from exogenous steroid administration. During episodes of surgery or major intercurrent illness, it is advisable to provide supplemental steroid therapy to patients who are receiving corticosteroid therapy or who have discontinued such therapy within the previous year.
Hydrocortisone 300 mg, or equivalent dosage, per day in three divided doses may be given intravenously or intramuscularly during the period of maximum stress, and subsequently tapered over 5 days. The stress of major nonsurgical illness may be managed with an increase in daily steroid dosage to at least a 30-mg prednisone equivalent.

j. Other side effects of corticosteroids include increased intraocular pressure, which may precipitate glaucoma, and the occurrence of posterior subcapsular cataracts. Although dyspepsia may accompany the use of steroids, it usually responds to antacids and administration of medication with meals. Enhancement of peptic ulcer disease probably does not occur. Routine treatment of corticosteroid-treated patients with antacids is not necessary. Menstrual irregularities, night sweats, and pancreatitis have been associated with corticosteroid therapy. Pseudotumor cerebri, associated with rapid steroid dose reduction, is a rare complication.

2. Cytotoxic drugs. Controlled trials of azathioprine and cyclophosphamide in lupus nephritis have shown conflicting results. They are used in either severe corticosteroid-resistant disease or the context of unacceptable steroid side effects. Azathioprine 2 to 3 mg/kg/24 hr, avoids the potential complications of alopecia, sterility, and hemorrhagic cystitis associated with cyclophosphamide. Both agents require careful monitoring of complete blood cell counts. Allopurinol should not be used with azathioprine because it inhibits azathioprine catabolism.

Evidence is mounting that long-term toxicity with cytotoxic agents may include both hematopoetic malignancy and solid tumors (reticulum cell sarcoma with azathioprine; bladder carcinoma with cyclophosphamide).

3. **Other regimens.** Plasmapheresis and high-dose intravenous "pulse" methylprednisolone are experimental therapies. Guidelines for their use have not been established.

J. Special management considerations

1. **Idiopathic drug reactions.** The possibility of an increase in allergic drug reactions in lupus patients is controversial. However, some observations suggest that sulfonamide drugs may exacerbate lupus. Fever and meningeal irritation have been reported in SLE patients taking ibuprofen.

2. **Drug-induced lupus.** Medications associated with drug-induced lupus (Table 26-2) have been used extensively and effectively in idiopathic lupus patients. Although the risk of exacerbating the underlying disease is often discussed, such risk has not been established and does not contraindicate the use of an otherwise indicated medication.

3. **Pregnancy.** The effects of pregnancy on SLE and SLE on pregnancy are variable. The incidence of spontaneous abortions and premature deliveries is higher than normal in patients with SLE. While perinatal mortality does not appear to be higher in infants born to mothers with lupus, there is a small incidence of congenital heart block in such infants. The mother is most likely to have flares of disease activity during the third trimester and the first two postpartum months. Disease activity may be relatively quiescent during early pregnancy. Patients with renal disease or active lupus during the six months immediately preceding pregnancy seem more likely to experience a difficult pregnancy and postpartum period. The differential diagnosis of preeclampsia and active SLE may be very difficult; patients should be managed optimally for both conditions unless the diagnosis is clear.

Since lupus is a disease of women in the childbearing age, contraception is an important issue. Because hormonal manipulation may exacerbate SLE, many physicians prefer to avoid the use of oral contraceptives. The condom and diaphragm are preferable because they have no adverse effects, but the patient's willingness to use these methods effectively must be considered.

4. **Hemodialysis.** SLE patients appear to tolerate chronic hemodialysis as well as any chronic renal failure population. Clinical impressions suggest that SLE patients may be more quiescent once on dialysis but still occasionally experience lupus disease activity.

5. **Transplantation.** Lupus patients may undergo renal transplantation without any apparent increase in morbidity compared to other transplantation populations.

VIII. **Prognosis.** The prognosis of SLE has improved, largely because milder forms of disease have been recognized, but also through the availability of potent antibiotics, the development of intensive care units, and probably the use of corticosteroids in the more severely ill patients. Prognosis depends on the pattern of organ involvement; renal and central nervous system disease have the worst five-year survival. Infection continues as a major cause of death. Recent series show five-year survivals of about 90%.

Drug-Induced Lupus

Many drugs (Table 26-2) have been implicated in the induction of a lupuslike syndrome with manifestations ranging from an isolated positive ANA test to a full clinical lupus syndrome. Procainamide and hydralazine are the most common drugs reported to produce a lupuslike syndrome.

I. Clinical features. Skin rash, arthritis, pleural and pericardial effusions, lymphadenopathy, splenomegaly, anemia, leukopenia, elevated sedimentation rate, and transient false positive serologic test for syphilis may all be included. Renal disease is characteristically absent. Most manifestations resolve after discontinuation of the drug.

II. Laboratory findings. The laboratory profile of a patient with drug-induced lupus may help distinguish the syndrome from SLE. Serum complement is rarely reduced in the drug-induced syndrome and antibodies to native (or double-stranded) DNA are usually absent. However, antibodies to single-stranded DNA may be present.

III. Therapy of drug-induced lupus involves discontinuation of the offending agent and symptomatic management of the clinical manifestations. Since most manifestations are reversible, therapy is usually of short duration. The occurrence of a positive ANA test alone should prompt review of the indications for use of the inciting agent but does not per se require the addition of therapeutic agents.

Discoid Lupus Erythematosus

Disease may be limited to the skin and assume the chronic discoid form with scaling red plaques and follicular plugging. Healing of these lesions is associated with central scarring and atrophy. While chronic discoid disease remains primarily cutaneous in the majority of patients, a small percentage (about 5%) will develop systemic disease. Conversely, patients with systemic disease may have discoid lesions among the cutaneous manifestations of their disease. Certain types of skin lesions such as subacute cutaneous lupus erythematosus may reflect a specific immunogenetic predisposition.

Therapy of discoid lupus follows the same principles as those outlined for skin disease in systemic lupus: avoidance of sun and ultraviolet exposure, and use of topical steroids and hydroxychloroquine.

See Chapter 10 for more information regarding discoid lupus.

Bibliography

Decker, J. L. (Moderator).   Systemic lupus erythematosus. Evolving concepts. *Ann. Intern. Med.* 91:587, 1979.

Dubois, E. L. (Ed.).   *Lupus Erythematosus* (2nd ed.). Los Angeles: University of Southern California Press, 1976.

Estes, D., and Christian, C. L.   The natural history of systemic lupus erythematosus by prospective analysis. *Medicine* 50:85, 1971.

Fries, J. F., and Holman, H. R.   *Systemic Lupus Erythematosus. A Clinical Analysis.* Philadelphia: Saunders, 1975.

Ginzler, E. M., Bollet, A. J., and Friedman, E. A.   The natural history and response to therapy of lupus nephritis. *Annu. Rev. Med.* 31:463, 1980.

Ropes, M. W.   *Systemic Lupus Erythematosus.* Cambridge, Mass.: Harvard University Press, 1976.

Rothfield, N. F. (Ed.).   Systemic Lupus Erythematosus. *Clinics in Rheumatic Disease,* vol. 1(3). Philadelphia: Saunders, 1975.

27. Osteoarthrosis (Osteoarthritis, Degenerative Joint Disease)

Steven K. Magid

Osteoarthrosis (OA) is a common, progressive joint disease which is classified into primary and secondary forms depending on whether a pathogenetic factor has been identified. It is primarily noninflammatory in nature, but secondary inflammation may occur. It is characterized by joint cartilage destruction with formation of osteophytes. Weight-bearing joints are particularly involved. Over 50 names exist for this disease of which *osteoarthrosis, osteoarthritis,* and *degenerative joint disease* (DJD) are the most common. *Osteoarthrosis* will be used in this chapter because it denotes that inflammation is usually a secondary phenomenon.

The disease has been described in the skeleton of Neanderthal man and in dinosaur fossils.

I. Epidemiologic and genetic factors

A. Epidemiology. The incidence and prevalence of OA depend on the means used to detect the disease. Autopsy studies show that OA may begin by age 20, and by 40 years of age, 90% of the population will be affected. X-ray changes are often seen by age 30, and the prevalence increases progressively with age. Under age 45, men are more affected, and over age 55, women predominate. Older women tend to have proximal interphalangeal (PIP), distal interphalangeal (DIP), and first carpometacarpal (CMC) joint involvement. Men tend to have more hip involvement (perhaps related to occupational factors) than women. Racial and ethnic differences in prevalence and pattern of disease exist, which may be accounted for by differences in occupation and lifestyle, as well as by possible differences in predisposing factors such as rheumatoid arthritis (RA), congenital dysplasia of the hip, and slipped capital femoral epiphysis.

B. Genetics. The genetics of OA have been described for two groups.

1. Heberden nodes present. In generalized OA with Heberden nodes, the inheritance is probably through a single autosomal gene which is dominant in females and recessive in males.

2. Heberden nodes absent. Generalized OA in this setting is more common in men than women, and is statistically associated with seronegative arthritis, hyperuricemia, and hypertension.

II. Pathogenesis

A. Primary OA. OA probably results from an imbalance between cartilage synthesis and degradation. The forces exerted on a joint by motion and weight bearing are dissipated by joint cartilage, subchondral bone, and surrounding structures (joint capsule and muscles). Joint cartilage has unique properties of compressibility and elasticity, attributable to the presence of an intertwined mesh of both collagen and proteoglycan. Cartilage collagen is type II. Proteoglycans (PGs) are large molecules that individually consist of a protein core with negatively charged glycose-amino-glycan (GAG) side chains composed of keratan and chondroitin sulfate. Proteoglycans exist mostly as aggregates and are attached as side chains by a link protein to a core of hyaluronic acid. The PGs bind a large amount of water molecules which are released when the cartilage is compressed, and recaptured when compression is removed. Various mechanisms have been proposed for the development of OA:

1. Aging results in a decrease in the total amount of PGs and is a common feature of OA. With normal aging, an increase in the keratan-chondroitin sulfate ratio occurs. The opposite is found in OA, suggesting that OA is a pathologic process, not simply an extension of the natural process.

2. **Mechanical factors** may allow PGs to escape into the synovial fluid, thus causing synovial inflammation and enzyme production.

3. **Proteolytic enzymes** may gain entry into the cartilage matrix and cause damage.

4. **Chondrocytes** may play a role in the destructive process by releasing various enzymes. They may also be unable to compensate for cartilage destruction effectively with increased synthetic activity.

5. **Abnormal nutrient diffusion.** Nutrients must diffuse from the synovial fluid since cartilage does not have a blood supply. It is postulated that this process is abnormal in OA.

6. **Abnormal joint stress** may lead to microfractures in the subchondral bone. Subsequent repair may lead to stiffening and inability of the bone to act as a shock absorber.

B. **Secondary OA.** Known disorders that can cause the above changes follow.

1. **Trauma**

   a. **Acute.** An immediate inflammatory reaction often occurs after the traumatic event. After several months, the inflammation subsides and is followed by a bony, often painless, enlargement of the involved joint.

   b. **Chronic.** Repetitive, minor occupational trauma produces disease patterns such as (1) bus driver; shoulders, (2) coal miners; spine and knees, and (3) pneumatic drill operators; shoulder, elbows, and hands.

2. **Bleeding dyscrasias.** Hemarthrosis occurs in 90% of patients with hemophilia, most commonly in the knee, ankle, and elbow. With recurrent hemarthrosis a proliferative synovitis occurs, which promotes development of secondary OA. Large cystic areas and evidence of osteonecrosis may be seen on radiographs.

3. **Neuropathic joint disease.** Loss of pain or proprioception leads to decreased joint protection and subsequent secondary OA. Examples of diseases responsible for the development of neuropathic arthropathy include diabetes, syphilis, syringomyelia, pernicious anemia, spinal cord trauma, and peripheral nerve injury. X-ray findings reveal severe OA changes with loss of cartilage, exuberant osteophyte formation, bizarre bony overgrowth, fragmentation of subchondral bone with pathologic fractures, and, eventually, disintegration of the joint structure.

4. **Intraarticular steroid injections** may be associated with OA. Two mechanisms are postulated: (1) intraarticular injection affords pain relief and allows overuse of an already damaged joint, and (2) cartilage may be directly damaged by injected steroids.

5. **Alkaptonuria.** These patients lack homogentisic acid (HGA) oxidase, which results in increased urinary excretion of HGA as well as increased HGA binding to connective tissue. The latter result presumably is responsible for the secondary OA seen in this disorder. The pigment is deposited in cartilage, skin, and sclera. Degenerative disease of the spine with calcification of the intervertebral discs is characteristic.

6. **Wilson disease.** Premature OA, pseudogout, and chondromalacia patellae are articular manifestations of this disorder of copper metabolism.

7. **Chondrocalcinosis.** Generalized OA is often seen in these patients and some authors feel the two diseases may share a common pathogenesis. OA and chondrocalcinosis are also associated with joint hypermobility disorders.

8. **Kaschin-Beck disease** is a growth disturbance seen in Northeast Asian children that produces abnormal enchondral bone growth leading to epiphyseal and metaphyseal abnormalities. The disease may be related to fungus-contaminated grain.

9. **Miscellaneous disorders.** Noninflammatory disorders, such as aseptic necrosis, as well as inflammatory conditions such as rheumatoid arthritis, septic arthritis, and seronegative spondyloarthritis may alter joint dynamics and lead to secondary OA.

III. **Pathology.** The earliest change is a softening of articular cartilage. The following features are seen as the disease progresses.

A. **Structural breakdown** of cartilage. In order of progression, this process consists of:

1. Fibrillation and fissuring.

2. Focal and diffuse erosions of the cartilage surface.

3. Thinning and complete denudation of cartilage.

B. **Changes in subchondral bone**

1. Sclerosis.

2. Cyst formation.

3. Bone thickening with eburnation.

4. Reactive proliferation of new bone and cartilage at joint periphery, producing osteophytes.

C. **Synovitis** (occasional)

IV. **General clinical presentation**

A. **Symptoms.** Symptomatic patients are usually over age 40. They complain of pain of insidious onset in one or a few joints. The pain is aching and poorly localized. It first occurs after normal joint use and can be relieved by rest. As the disease progresses, pain during rest develops. Morning stiffness and stiffness after inactivity are common, although usually not as severe as in rheumatoid arthritis. The most common sites of involvement are the DIP and first CMC joints of the hand and the first metatarsal phalangeal (1st MTP) joint in the foot; the hips; the knees; and the lumbar and cervical spine. OA almost never involves the metacarpophalangeal joints, wrists, elbows, and shoulders, unless secondary to trauma. In general, there is little correlation between joint symptoms and x-ray or pathologic changes. Only 30% of patients who have x-ray changes in a specific joint will actually have symptoms referrable to that joint. However, if more severe radiographic findings are required for diagnosis, a better correlation exists. The cause of pain in OA is multifactoral and includes:

1. Elevated periosteum.

2. Pressure on exposed subchondral bone.

3. Trabecular microfracture.

4. Intraarticular ligament disease.

5. Capsule distention.

6. Synovitis and entrapment of inflamed synovial villi between opposing joint surfaces.

7. Periarticular tendon and fascia inflammation.

8. Muscle spasm.

B. **Physical examination.** Joints may be tender, especially if swelling, warmth, and erythema (synovitis) are present. However, tenderness may be present without signs of inflammation. Pain on weight bearing may be present without pain on passive range of motion.

Joint enlargement may result from the presence of fluid accumulation, synovial hyperplasia, or osteophytes.

In later disease stages, there may be crepitus, gross deformity and subluxation caused by cartilage loss, collapse of subchondral bone, or bone cysts and gross bony overgrowth. Limitation of motion increases as disease progresses, perhaps caused by joint surface incongruity, muscle spasm and contracture, capsule contracture, or mechanical blockage resulting from osteophytes or loose bodies.

C. **Radiographic findings** may lag a stage behind the patient's symptoms. In addition, OA is so common that one should look carefully for coexisting RA or fracture. Special views are often required to evaluate the extent of involvement.

   1. **Characteristic radiographic findings** of OA are:

      a. **Joint space narrowing** secondary to degeneration and disappearance of articular cartilage.

      b. **Subchondral sclerosis (eburnation)** secondary to new bone formation.

      c. **Marginal osteophyte formation** secondary to proliferation of cartilage and bone.

      d. **Periarticular bone cysts**, which range from several millimeters to several centimeters.

      e. **Subluxation and deformity** in advanced disease.

      f. **Absence of ankylosis.**

   2. **Radiographic grading** has been described using the above criteria:

      a. **Grade 0:** no OA.

      b. **Grade 1:** doubtful OA.

      c. **Grade 2:** minimal OA.

      d. **Grade 3:** moderate OA.

      e. **Grade 4:** severe OA.

D. **Laboratory findings.** No specific or diagnostic abnormalities are seen in primary OA.

   1. **Blood and urine.** The sedimentation rate, complete blood count (CBC), antinuclear antibody (ANA), rheumatoid factor, calcium, phosphate, alkaline phosphatase, and urinalysis are generally normal. They are helpful in evaluating associated conditions and causes of secondary OA, as well as in excluding other causes of arthritis.

   2. **Synovial fluid,** when present, is usually noninflammatory (see Chap. 4).

   3. **Radionuclide scans.** Isotope uptake is normal in typical OA; however, if an inflammatory component is present, uptake may be increased.

   4. **Arthroscopy** may be of diagnostic value in patients with mechanical derangement associated with OA and is of therapeutic value in removing loose bodies.

V. **Specific joint disease patterns**

A. **Hands**

   1. **Symptoms.** DIP joints are the most frequent site of hand involvement in OA. PIP joints are also affected; however, MCP joints are rarely involved. The first CMC joint may be involved, especially in patients whose occupations require repetitive use of this joint. Joint involvement is usually symmetric.

   2. **Physical examination.** In patients with Heberden or Bouchard nodes, swellings over the joint are present, and there is decreased range of motion. The

nodes are usually nontender. In some patients, small gelatinous cysts occur on the dorsal aspect of the DIP joints; they seem to be attached to tendon sheaths, resemble ganglia, and usually precede the development of Heberden nodes. When the first CMC joint is affected, range of motion becomes limited, and a tender prominence develops at the base of the first metacarpal bone, which may lead to a squared-off appearance of the hand. When the trapezioscaphoid joint is involved, there may be pain and swelling on the volar aspect of the wrist.

3. **Radiographic findings.** Patients with mild radiographic changes usually have no symptoms. X-rays of Heberden nodes show joint space narrowing, subchondral sclerosis, cysts, and spurs. Although nodes may feel hard and bonelike, they may not be radiodense. When the first CMC joint is involved, subluxation of the base of the first metacarpal bone may be noted.

B. Hips

1. **Symptoms.** As a result of the hip's role in locomotion, patients with OA of the hip may be significantly disabled. Patients are usually older than those with hand involvement. Males are more often affected than females. Twenty percent of patients with unilateral disease will develop contralateral disease after eight years. Patients often complain of pain that increases with motion and weight bearing and decreases with rest. They may also complain of stiffness and a limp.

   True hip pain is felt on the outer aspect of the groin or inner thigh. Pain that originates in the hip may be perceived as originating in the medial knee or distal thigh (20% of patients), buttocks, or sciatic region. Patients may walk with an antalgic gait, which may cause pain in other lower extremity joints or the back. Sitting or rising may be especially difficult in these patients. It is important to distinguish true hip pain from pain caused by a lumbar radiculopathy, femoral hernia, or vascular insufficiency (see Chap. 16).

2. **Physical examination.** Decreased range of motion and pain on motion are the primary findings. Internal rotation is affected first. As deterioration progresses, there is further loss of rotation, and loss of extension, abduction, and flexion. Patients may develop joint contractures. In the early stages of OA, flexion may not cause pain; however, extension and rotation will. In cases where the radiation of the pain is atypical (to the thigh or knee), symptoms attributed to the hip can be reproduced by moving the hip through the extremes of motion while fixing all motion of the knee. Shortening of the limb caused by contracture or progressive lateral and upward subluxation of femoral head may be observed. Compensatory lordosis of spine may also be observed secondary to flexion contracture of the hip.

3. **Radiographic findings.** Less than 1.7% of patients under age 55, 3% of patients over age 55, and over 10% of patients over age 85 have radiographic evidence of OA. Compared to OA symptoms in other joints, hip symptoms correlate better with x-ray findings. Virtually all patients with severe x-ray findings will have complaints attributable to the hip. Anteroposterior (AP) views of the **pelvis** should be done routinely when OA of the hips is suspected to obtain information about both hips, sacroiliac (SI) joints, and pelvic bones. Advanced cases may show protrusio acetabuli.

4. **Associated and predisposing conditions.** Some authors feel that OA of the hip is usually secondary to a developmental abnormality.

   a. **Congenital dysplasia of the hip (CDH)** may account for 25% of OA in older white patients. The acetabulum does not develop properly and is shallow, which often results in femoral head subluxation and secondary degenerative changes. Patients may present with a limp in childhood or with premature OA in adulthood.

   b. **Slipped capital femoral epiphysis (SCFE).** Just before the femoral epiphysis closes (between ages 16 and 19), the femoral head may be displaced posteromedially. These patients may present with a painful limp in adolescence or early adulthood.

    c. Legg-Calvé-Perthes disease is idiopathic osteonecrosis of the proximal femoral capital epiphysis which occurs in young (3- to 8-year-old) males. The osteonecrosis often results in an abnormally large, flat femoral head with a wide short neck.

C. Knees

1. **Symptoms.** The knee is frequently affected by OA. Patients complain of trouble with kneeling, climbing stairs, and getting in and out of chairs. Locking of the knee may result from loose joint bodies.

2. **Physical examination.** Osteophytes may be palpated as irregular bony masses. Crepitus may be felt with the examiner's hand held over the patella during knee motion. Quadriceps atrophy may be present.

    a. Medial and lateral compartment disease. Genu varus commonly occurs with medial compartment disease. Genu valgus, although less common, may occur when there is involvement of the lateral compartment. The joint may be unstable as a result of cartilage loss and secondary lengthening of the collateral ligaments. It is important to compare the degree of varus-valgus deformity (of the extended knee) with and without weight bearing. If a change into varus alignment or an increase in the degree of deformity occurs with weight bearing, it is evidence of cartilage loss and compartment deformity rather than of ligamentous laxity alone.

    b. Patellofemoral disease. With patellofemoral OA, the patella loses side-to-side mobility, resulting in loss of about 10% of extension and flexion. Pain and tenderness are most marked anteriorly. Pain may be elicited if the patella is held firmly against the femur and the quadriceps are isometrically contracted. Patellofemoral disease may occur alone without medial or lateral compartment disease.

3. **Radiographic findings**

    a. Standard views are anteroposterior (AP) and lateral. It is important to obtain these films while weight bearing to assess amounts of varus-valgus deformity and joint space narrowing. **Standing** films show the femoral cartilage and tibial plateau cartilage in direct contact and demonstrate cartilage thinning and joint space narrowing more reliably than non–weight-bearing films.

    b. Tunnel view is taken with the knee in slight flexion to expose the intercondylar notch. This view allows evaluation of loose bodies, intraarticular spurs, and changes in the tibial intracondylar spines.

    c. Merchant view is taken tangential to the flexed knee and allows evaluation of the patellofemoral articulation.

4. **Associated and predisposing conditions**

    a. Fractures of tibial plateau or femoral condyles with mechanical incongruence.

    b. Ligamentous injuries causing instability.

    c. Chronic patellar dislocation.

    d. Severe varus and valgus deformities.

    e. Internal derangement; torn menisci predispose to OA, as do absent menisci after meniscectomy.

    f. Chondromalacia is a degeneration of the patellar cartilage most prominent in the age group of 15 to 30 years. There is pain on activity, especially descending stairs. Pain is elicited when the patella is pressed into the femoral groove as the patient tightens the quadriceps muscle.

D. Spine. Degenerative disease of the spine may be divided into OA and **spondylosis**. Because the posterior apophyseal joints are true diarthrodial joints, they may undergo the usual changes of OA, including joint space narrowing, sclerosis, and spur formation. The degenerative changes that affect the discs and vertebral bodies should properly be referred to as *spondylosis*. Discs may herniate and compress the spinal cord or nerve roots. Degenerative changes of the vertebral bodies result in osteophytes which may cause mechanical compression of vital structures (spinal cord, nerve root, and, rarely, vessels).

1. Symptoms

   a. Local pain and stiffness may be due to paraspinal ligament or joint capsule involvement or paraspinal muscle spasm.

   b. Radicular symptoms are common at all spinal levels.

   (1) Cervical spine involvement usually occurs at the neural foramen secondary to impingement by osteophytes. Radicular symptoms have a predilection for the cervical spine because neural foramina and the spinal canal are relatively small in this area. Symptoms include neck pain which often radiates to the shoulder and more distal aspects of the upper extremity. Weakness and paresthesias of the hand and arm may also occur.

   (2) Thoracic spine. Radicular pain often radiates around the chest wall. It should be differentiated from angina, herpes zoster, cholecystitis, and pleuritic pain. Degenerative disease is uncommon in the thoracic spine, and the diagnosis of a neoplastic process must be entertained.

   (3) Lumbar spine. Patients complain of low back pain which often radiates down the buttocks and may even extend into the legs and feet. The pain may increase with coughing and straining. With severe lesions, motor and sensory abnormalities may be present. A cauda equina syndrome with sphincter dysfunction may also occur.

   c. Cord compression from intervertebral ridges at cervical levels may result in progressive myelopathy with minimal or no radicular pain.

   d. Mechanical compression of vital structures also occurs mostly at the level of the cervical spine. Large anterior spurs may cause dysphagia, hoarseness, or cough. Compression of vertebral arteries may produce symptoms of vertebrobasilar insufficiency with vertigo, double vision, scotomata, headache, or ataxia. These symptoms often vary with head and neck position. Compression of the anterior spinal artery may produce a central cord syndrome.

2. Physical examination. The spinal examination may reveal decreased range of motion and local tenderness. A careful neurologic evaluation to determine absent reflexes, long tract signs, and a radicular pattern of weakness and sensory abnormalities is important.

3. Radiologic findings. Severe degenerative changes may be present on x-ray, with few symptoms. In contrast, a small spur that is critically placed may cause significant morbidity. **Oblique films** must be ordered in order to evaluate neural foramina. Standard AP and lateral views will not demonstrate impingement by a bone spur or subluxed apophyseal joint. Osteophytes usually arise from the anterior and anterolateral aspects of vertebral bodies and are best seen on lateral films. A decrease in the intervertebral disc space secondary to disc degeneration is seen most often in the lower cervical and lumbar spine. A **vacuum phenomenon** indicative of disintegration of the nucleus pulposus may also be present. Anterior vertebral wedging may be seen. Myelograms may be useful in determining the cause of neurologic symptoms.

E. Feet

1. **Symptoms.** The first MTP joint is one of the most common sites of OA involvement. Acute swelling and pain may be caused by bursal inflammation at the medial side of the metatarsal head (bunion). Patients often have a history of using improper footwear. In contrast, OA of the ankle or tarsal joints is rare and, when present, usually secondary to trauma.

2. **Physical examination** may reveal tenderness over the first MTP joint and hallux valgus deformity. The great toe is unable to bear weight normally, and added stress is placed upon the metatarsal heads. Metatarsalgia may ensue.

3. **Radiographic findings.** Typical changes of OA, such as sclerosis, joint space narrowing, and osteophyte formation, may be seen at the first MTP joint. Subluxation of the great toe with hallux valgus deformity may be noted. Radiographic changes in the midtarsal joints are common; however, they are infrequently associated with symptoms.

F. Shoulder.
OA of the glenohumeral joint is rare unless secondary to trauma or some other predisposing condition such as inflammatory arthropathy or osteonecrosis. In contrast, soft tissue degenerative diseases such as subacromial bursitis, supraspinatus tendinitis, and bicipital tendinitis are common over age 40. Radiographs may show changes of OA with spur formation, calcification of the bursa, or calcification in the tendons.

Acromioclavicular joint involvement may cause poorly localized shoulder pain, and shoulder range of motion is affected.

G. Manubriosternal
involvement is very rare.

H. Sacroiliac joint.
Sclerosis with osteophytes may occur at the lower end of the joint, especially when contralateral arthritis of the hip or knee is present.

I. Temporomandibular joint.
Crepitus, tenderness, and pain (often referred to the ear) are common problems which are sometimes related to dental malocclusion. Radiographic characterization of this joint is difficult; tomograms provide the best views.

J. Elbow.
OA is usually related to a malunited fracture or to repeated minor trauma (as with pneumatic drill operators). Both the radiohumeral and ulnohumeral articulations may be involved.

VI. Differential diagnosis.
OA can be confused with other forms of arthritis because it may occasionally present as an inflammatory polyarthritis of the hands or monoarticular arthritis. In addition, radiographic evidence of OA is so common that its presence may be unrelated to the true etiology of the patient's complaints (see Chaps. 12–18, which discuss diseases in specific anatomic areas).

A. Rheumatoid arthritis

1. **Monarticular.** When RA presents as a monarticular arthritis of a large joint, differentiation from OA may be difficult and is based on:

   a. **Synovial fluid analysis.** The fluid contains more white blood cells, a greater percentage of neutrophils, and poorer viscosity than OA fluid (see Chap. 4).

   b. **Radiographs** in patients with RA often show erosions and osteoporosis. Osteophytes, subchondral bone cysts, and sclerosis suggest OA. However, Heberden nodes and other degenerative abnormalities may coexist with RA.

   c. **Blood studies.** The ESR is usually elevated, and latex fixation is often positive in RA.

   d. **Follow-up observations.** These may eventually reveal a pattern of joint destruction typical of RA.

2. Polyarticular

a. Distribution of joint involvement is important when differentiating RA from inflammatory erosive OA.

(1) RA: MCP and DIP and wrist involvement.

(2) OA: DIP and PIP joints characteristically affected.

b. Radiographic features (see sec. **IV.A.1.**). General features of RA that help distinguish it from OA are:

(1) More inflammation with greater loss of joint function.

(2) Involvement of a greater number of joints.

(3) Quicker progression.

(4) Less knee involvement.

(5) More hand involvement.

(6) Morning stiffness, though present, lasts for less time.

(7) Frequent association with a positive test for rheumatoid factor.

B. Seronegative spondyloarthropathy. These diseases frequently involve the interphalangeal joints, single large joints, and the spine. Differentiating features are:

1. Psoriasis. Skin and nail lesions and typical patterns of psoriatic arthropathy affecting interphalangeal joints (see Chaps. 10 and 35).

2. Reiter syndrome. Presence of conjunctivitis, urethritis, and characteristic skin lesions (see Chap. 37).

3. Inflammatory bowel disease. Complaints referrable to the large or small intestine (see Chap. 9).

4. Ankylosing spondylitis. Sacroiliitis and fine, symmetric, marginal syndesmophytes (see Chap. 20).

C. Crystal-induced arthritis

1. Gout affects primarily the first MTP joint as well as other joints of the foot and lower extremity. Tophaceous deposits over the small joints of the hand may be confused with osteophytes. The diagnosis of gout is confirmed by identification of urate crystals in the joint fluid (see Chap. 23).

2. Pseudogout may coexist with OA. The wrist, shoulder, knee, and ankle joints are commonly involved. Radiographs reveal chondrocalcinosis in most pseudogout patients. Diagnosis is confirmed by identifying positively birefringent, rhomboidal calcium pyrophosphate dihydrate (CPPD) crystals in the joint fluid (see Chap. 34).

D. Other disorders that may coexist with OA but are important to identify include:

1. Chronic infection. Tuberculosis can be identified by culture.

2. Neoplastic synovitis. Lymphoma or leukemia may be identified by synovial fluid cytology.

3. Pigmented villonodular synovitis. The joint effusion is usually bloody. Diagnosis is confirmed by synovial biopsy.

4. Neoplastic metastasis to juxtaarticular bone. Bone scan is a useful diagnostic measure.

VII. Therapy

A. Correction of predisposing factors should optimally take place before anatomical changes occur.

B. **Joint rest.** Excessive use of an involved joint may increase symptoms and accelerate degenerative changes. It is important to protect joints. Weight-bearing joints may be unloaded by use of a cane (held in the hand opposite to the involved extremity and extended in tandem with it), crutches, or a walker. A lumbar corset and cervical collar may be useful for lumbar or cervical OA.

1. **Obesity.** Weight reduction is important.

2. **Malalignment.** Valgus-varus knee deformity and eversion-inversion ankle deformity should be surgically corrected.

3. **Occupational changes** may be necessary.

C. **Physical therapy** helps to relieve pain and stiffness, maintain and recover joint mobility, and strengthen supporting muscles.

1. **Therapeutic exercise.** See Appendix B.

2. **Heat** generally relieves pain and muscle spasm. Many modalities are available, including diathermy and ultrasound (for deep pain), infrared, hot packs, warm pool, and paraffin bath (for hands). See Appendix A for regimens.

D. **Occupational therapy** helps patients to adapt to their disabilities and helps minimize the stress placed on involved joints during activities of daily living. See Appendix B.

E. **Drugs.** The following agents are used.

1. **Salicylates** are the first line of therapy since they have both analgesic and antiinflammatory properties. The major side effects involve gastrointestinal disturbances (10% to 30%), occult bleeding (70%), exacerbation of peptic ulcer disease, and inhibition of platelet function. Therapeutic salicylate levels are 20 to 30 mg/dl.

   a. **Aspirin** (acetylsalicylic acid) is the drug of choice. It is the oldest and least expensive of all the nonsteroidal antiinflammatory drugs (NSAIDs) and is usually as effective as the others. Its major drawback is gastrointestinal (GI) intolerance. Dosage is two or three 325-mg tablets QID. Less aspirin is required to treat OA than to treat RA.

   b. **Ascriptin** (aspirin 325 mg plug 150 mg magnesium-aluminum hydroxide [Maalox]) may produce less GI irritation than aspirin. Dosage is 2 to 3 tablets QID.

   c. **Ecotrin** (enteric-coated aspirin). Dosage is 325-mg pills, 2 to 3 pills PO QID. Absorption is not as reliable as with aspirin and ascriptin.

   d. **Choline salicylate and choline magnesium trisalicylate** do not inhibit platelet function and are indicated for use in OA secondary to a bleeding dyscrasia. See Appendix G for dosage.

2. **Nonsteroidal antiinflammatory drugs (NSAIDs).** If patients are unable to tolerate ASA, substitution of another NSAID is indicated. Moreover, some patients who do not respond to aspirin may respond to one of the newer NSAIDs. A NSAID can frequently be added to an existing aspirin regimen with good results. One of the major drawbacks of these drugs is their expense. Side effects common to most of the NSAIDs include dyspepsia, CNS dysfunction, fluid retention, platelet abnormalities, and hepatic or renal dysfunction. Each drug is discussed fully in Appendix G. The NSAIDs listed here are of approximately equal potency.

   a. **Ibuprofen.** Dosage is 400 mg QID. Maximum response occurs in two to six weeks. Supplied as 300-, 400-, and 600-mg tablets.

   b. **Indomethacin** may cause significant adverse effects and is usually reserved for severe OA of large joints (hips, knees), especially if a significant inflammatory component is present. GI symptoms occur in about 57% of patients.

CNS symptoms including headache, vertigo, and dizziness are common in the first few weeks of treatment, especially in the elderly. Dosage is 25 mg BID or TID. The dose may be increased by 25 to 50 mg weekly to a maximum of 200 mg daily. Response may occur between one week and one month after starting therapy. Supplied as 25- and 50-mg capsules.

c. Naproxen is a proprionic acid derivative. Patient compliance is enhanced because of its long duration of action. Dosage is 250 mg BID. Supplied as 250-mg tablets.

d. Fenoprofen is also a proprionic acid derivative. Initial dosage is 300 to 600 mg QID. The maximum daily dosage is 3,200 mg. Supplied as 300-mg capsules and 600-mg tablets.

e. Sulindac, an analogue of indomethacin, also has the advantage of BID dosage. The dose is 150 mg PO BID. Supplied as 150- and 200-mg tablets.

f. Tolmetin is a pyrrole alkanoic acid derivative which is chemically different from the other NSAIDs. Dosage is 400 mg TID initially. Maximum daily dosage is 1,800 mg. Supplied as 200-mg tablets that contain 18 mg of sodium.

3. Analgesics may be used to supplement antiinflammatory agents. Useful drugs are listed in order of potency.

    a. Acetaminophen. The dose is 325 to 650 mg TID or QID.

    b. Propoxyphene is a nonnarcotic but potentially addictive analgesic. It is more effective when taken with aspirin. The dose is 65 mg every 4 to 6 hours.

    c. Codeine 30 mg may be given with 325 to 650 mg of either ASA or acetominophen.

    d. Percocet contains 325 mg of acetominophen plus 5 mg of oxycodone. Dosage is one tablet every 6 hours.

    e. Percodan contains 325 mg of aspirin and nearly 5 mg of oxycodone. Dosage is one tablet every 6 hours. Percodan is considered to be more addicting than codeine.

    f. Narcotics more potent than those above are rarely indicated because addiction potential is increased.

4. Steroids

    a. Oral steroids are *not* indicated in OA since they are of equivocal benefit yet have serious side effects.

    b. Intraarticular steroids may help some patients with synovitis. Pain relief may last from days to months. Intraarticular injections should be performed no more than two to four times a year. Dosages and precautions are discussed in Chapter 4.

F. Surgery

1. Indications

    a. Relief of pain or severe disability after failure of conservative measures to reverse or alleviate the pathologic process.

    b. Correction of mechanical derangement that may lead to OA.

2. Contraindications

    a. Infection.

    b. Poor vascular supply.

   c. Emotional instability or occupational factors that make surgical rehabilitation unlikely to succeed.

   d. Obesity (relative contraindication).

   e. Serious medical illness (relative contraindication).

3. Knee procedures

   a. Osteotomy consists of removal of a single wedge of bone from the proximal tibia (single osteotomy) or from both the tibia and distal femur (double osteotomy). It realigns the joint by correcting angular deformity and provides relief of pain. Osteotomy is especially useful in unicompartmental disease when the patellofemoral compartment is not involved. It is a relatively conservative procedure since total knee replacement can be performed later, if required.

   b. Arthrodesis may transform a painful unstable leg into a painless stable leg. However, disadvantages include permanent loss of joint mobility and additional stress on other joints, particularly the ipsilateral hip. It is never indicated when knee disease is bilateral.

   c. Total knee prosthesis. This procedure is indicated for relief of severe pain and functional disability. There is reservation concerning its use in young patients since the long-term durability of the prosthesis is not known, and an increased failure rate exists in physically active patients; however, for the severely handicapped patient, there may be no alternative. Relative contraindications include osteoporosis, loss of bone (prosthesis cannot be properly anchored), and the presence of soft tissue contractures. The total condylar prosthesis is currently the type most widely used. Complications include sepsis, cement loosening, and phlebitis.

4. Hip

   a. Osteotomy. Sections of bone are excised in order to improve joint congruence and decrease the load on the joint. This approach may be indicated in young patients who have preservation of joint space and mild deformity. A total hip replacement (THR) may be reserved for the future if required.

   b. Excision arthroplasty. The femoral neck is excised to afford relief of pain, but the procedure results in limb shortening and joint instability. **Indications** are:

   (1) Salvage operation for a failed THR.

   (2) Relief of pain for patients who, for other reasons, have limited weight-bearing activities.

   c. Arthrodesis. Mobility is sacrificed for relief of pain and joint stability. All articular cartilage is removed, and bone surfaces are brought together. The procedure may be considered for active young patients who have only one hip involved and whose level of disability cannot be otherwise controlled. A THR can be performed later in life. The knees, contralateral hip, and spine are subjected to increased stress following the procedure.

   d. Total hip replacement attempts to reconstruct normal joint dynamics by insertion of a metal femoral head into a polyethylene pelvic socket. Both elements are held in place by methylmethacrylate cement. Ninety-six percent of patients achieve relief of pain, and 90% have increased range of motion. Indications and contraindications are noted above. **Surgical complications** include:

   (1) Intraoperative bone cement reaction, producing hypotension and cardiopulmonary arrest.

   (2) Femoral nerve, artery, or vein damage.

(3) Femoral hematoma.

(4) Infection. During the first 4 postoperative days, 75% of patients are febrile. Fever between the fourth and eighth days may represent either infection or hematoma. Fever occurring eight days or more following surgery is usually caused by infection.

The diagnosis is made by hip aspiration and culture. If infection is confirmed or strongly suspected, surgical exploration should be performed with excision of necrotic tissues and evacuation of hematomas. If no bone infection is present, conservative management with systemic antibiotics and possibly open joint irrigation should be attempted. (In 70% to 80% of such patients, the THR may be saved.)

If infected bone is found on reexploration, removal of the prosthetic joint and long-term antibiotic therapy are indicated. Attempts to treat late infection conservatively usually fail, since bone involvement by infection has invariably occurred by the third postoperative month.

(5) Thromboembolic disease is common following THR surgery. Controlled studies reveal no prophylactic effect with subcutaneous minidose heparin therapy. Aspirin, however, may be of benefit. Treatment of thromboembolic disease with therapeutic doses of anticoagulants increases the risk of hematoma and subsequent infection.

(6) Cement loosening may be caused by technical factors or, more commonly, infection. It may be radiographically detected as a lucent line at the cement-bone interface. A characteristic symptom is pain that abates after the first few steps.

VIII. Prognosis is highly variable. With DIP involvement of the hand, there is moderate pain and stiffness but little limitation of overall function. Weight-bearing joints are more likely to cause disability. The time between onset of hip pain and the development of high level of disability averages eight years. OA of the knee carries a worse prognosis than OA of the hip. Varus knee deformity and early onset of pain are poor prognostic signs.

Osteoarthrosis Variants

I. Ankylosing hyperostosis (diffuse idiopathic skeletal hyperostosis, Forestier disease). This disease is felt to be a disorder of bone formation and is more common in the elderly. Extensive spurs form along the anterior aspect of the vertebral bodies in a flowing pattern. Perispinal soft tissue ossification is also present.

Extraspinal manifestations are common and consist of large irregular bone spurs that form at the olecranon process and the calcaneus, as well as diffuse calcification of ligaments. Spinal stiffness is the primary complaint, and range of motion is well preserved. HLA-B27 antigen occurs in 30% of these patients.

II. Inflammatory osteoarthritis. Mild degrees of inflammation, whether primary or secondary, are common to all forms of OA. However, terms such as *primary generalized osteoarthritis* have been applied to those subjects who have more marked inflammatory manifestations and who lack features of RA or other inflammatory arthropathies. The PIP and DIP joints are most commonly involved, and the MCP joints may also be affected. Postmenopausal women are most frequently affected. Severe inflammation and proliferative synovitis may occur. **Bony erosion,** as well as cartilage loss, spur formation, and subchondral sclerosis occur. The picture may be clinically indistinguishable from RA, although rheumatoid factor is absent. Some authorities believe that inflammatory OA represents a variant of seronegative RA.

Bibliography

Coventry, M. B. (Ed).   Total joint arthroplasty symposium (Part I). *Mayo Clin. Proc.* 54:257, 1979.

Moskowitz, R. W. Management of osteoarthritis. *Hosp. Pract.* 14:75, 1979.

Peyson, J. G. Epidemiologic and etiologic approach to osteoarthritis. *Semin. Arthritis Rheum.* 8:288, 1979.

Tan, E. M., and Ziff, M. (Eds). Symposium on osteoarthritis. *Arthritis Rheum.* [Suppl] 20:S96, 1977.

Wright, V. (Ed). Osteoarthrosis. *Clin. Rheum. Dis.* 2:495, 1976.

28. Osteomyelitis

Robert D. Inman

Although the distinction made between acute and chronic (greater than 3-month duration) forms of osteomyelitis has some value in therapy and prognosis, no abrupt shift from one category to the other occurs in most cases. A more useful classification, based on pathogenesis, divides cases into three types: hematogenous osteomyelitis, osteomyelitis secondary to a contiguous focus of infection, and osteomyelitis associated with peripheral vascular disease. Relative frequencies in one large series were 19%, 47%, and 34% of patients, respectively.

I. Disease classification

A. Hematogenous osteomyelitis

1. **Epidemiology.** Age distribution in this type of osteomyelitis shows a predilection for children under age 16 and adults over 50 years of age.

2. **Anatomic foci.** The most common sites in children are the metaphyseal regions of the tibia and femur; for adults, the spine is the most common site.

3. **Causative organisms.** *Staphylococcus aureus* is the most common pathogen. Gram-negative bacillary infections are increasing in frequency. Tuberculous and fungal infection make up a small percentage of cases. Antecedent foci of infection vary with the organism: *S. aureus* derives from soft tissue infection or postsurgical wounds; gram-negative bacilli from a gastrointestinal (GI) source; tubercle bacilli or fungus from a pulmonary focus. Two special patient groups should be noted with regard to pathogenic organisms. Drug addicts are predisposed to gram-negative bone infection, particularly from *Pseudomonas aeruginosa*. In patients with sickle cell disease, *Salmonella* osteomyelitis is a common entity, with serotypes *S. choleraesuis, S. paratyphi,* and *S. typhimurium* predominating.

4. **Clinical presentation.** In the majority of patients, the clinical presentation is characterized by pain and swelling in the limb with fever (75%) and chills, usually of less than 3-week duration. Vertebral osteomyelitis often follows a more subacute course with continual dull back pain and few systemic symptoms.

5. **Radiographic changes** consist of lytic lesions and areas of increased density but are often not visible until weeks after the onset of infection. Although the lytic process occurs first, and proceeds at a faster rate than the blastic response, changes are not visible radiographically until 30% to 50% of bone mineral has been removed. Bone sclerosis suggests that the infection has been present more than one month. There is a 10-day period after matrix formation before mineralization is complete. Similarly, there is usually a delay in radiographic improvement during the healing phase. Thirty percent of patients show worsening on x-ray while improving clinically on therapy.

6. **Radionuclear scanning.** The bone scan can become positive as early as 24 hours after the onset of symptoms, that is, 10 to 14 days before radiographic changes. A negative bone scan is reasonably strong evidence against osteomyelitis, although isolated cases of acute osteomyelitis with negative scans have been reported. The bone scan may also be of value in differentiating bone infarction from bone infection in patients with sickle cell disease. If the scan is performed within two days of the onset of symptoms, a "cold" area of decreased radionuclide uptake is seen in the area of bone infarction, as distinguished from the increased uptake seen in acute osteomyelitis from the onset. If the timing of the scan is delayed, reactive periostitis will mask the avascular

nature of the infarction, and a "hot" area of increased uptake will be seen with both infection and infarction.

B. Osteomyelitis secondary to a contiguous focus of infection. Most cases of this type occur in adults over 50 years of age and arise from postoperative infections. Osteomyelitis of the hip after open reduction of a hip fracture is a common example. This infection can be insidious, with little local inflammatory reaction. This type of osteomyelitis also occurs after the spread of a soft tissue infection to bone, as in hands and toes. Less common instances are dental infections leading to osteomyelitis of the mandible and frontal bones. *S. aureus* is again the most common organism in this group, but a polymicrobial infection is common. An important entity recently described is osteomyelitis due to *P. aeruginosa* in children following a puncture wound in the foot. These patients characteristically have a period of one to two weeks of improvement after the initial posttraumatic inflammation, followed by worsening of the local signs.

C. Osteomyelitis associated with peripheral vascular disease. This group consists mainly of adults between 50 and 70 years of age who present with peripheral vascular insufficiency secondary to diabetes or artherosclerosis. Most commonly, toes and small bones of the foot are involved. Local pain, swelling, and erythema are usually present on admission with chronic cutaneous ulcers often serving as the portal of entry for the infection. The characteristic radiologic finding is the presence of mottled lytic lesions, occurring usually five to six weeks after the clinical appearance of the infection. Although staphylococci and streptococci predominate among the pathogens, anaerobic infection (bacteroides, fusobacteria, anaerobic cocci) plays a significant role in this group, and appropriate culture conditions should be obtained.

II. Therapy

A. Antibiotic therapy. While the pathogenic classification recorded in section I. is of diagnostic value, therapy is dictated usually by duration of infection. In acute osteomyelitis, a 90% cure rate is achieved with antibiotic therapy alone. Blood cultures are positive in up to 50% of hematogenous osteomyelitis and allow precise selection of antimicrobial therapy. If the bone infection is uncomplicated (e.g., metaphysis of tibia or femur in a normal host), some authors recommend empiric therapy for staphylococci (nafcillin 1.5 gm every 4 hours IV). Complicated problems (e.g., in drug addicts or other compromised hosts) require bone aspiration and bone biopsy. Choice of antibiotic is based on the culture and sensitivity, and parenteral therapy is maintained for four to six weeks (Table 28-1).

B. Surgical therapy. Surgery is indicated in the following circumstances:

1. For biopsy in atypical or unresponsive cases.

2. For debridement of necrotic tissue and drainage of loculated pus.

3. If neurologic abnormalities develop during cranial or vertebral osteomyelitis.

4. If infection spreads into the hip joint.

Table 28-1. Antibiotic Therapy of Potential Pathogens in Osteomyelitis

Organism	Antimicrobial Agent	Dosage
Staphylococcus aureus	Nafcillin	1.5 gm IV every 4 hours
Pseudomonas sp.	Gentamicin	1.5 mg/kg every 8 hours (serum level 5–7 kg/ml)
Salmonella sp.	Ampicillin	0.25–0.5 gm IV every 6 hours

5. If an ischemic toe or foot has failed to respond to parenteral antibiotics, amputation may be required.

III. Prognosis. In general, the cure rate for chronic osteomyelitis is far below that achieved for acute infections, largely because it is difficult to deliver adequate antibiotic levels into necrotic, chronically infected bone. Success has been achieved with prolonged (6-month to 1-year) monitored antibiotic therapy combined with surgical excision of necrotic tissue. Oral antibiotic therapy has a role in such prolonged treatment programs but should be monitored with serum antibiotic levels.

Bibliography

Brank, B. A., and Black, H. Pseudomonas osteomyelitis following puncture wounds in children. *J. Bone Joint Surg.* 56-A:1637, 1974.

Handmaker, H., and Leonards, R. The bone scan in inflammatory osseous disease. *Semin. Nucl. Med.* 6:95, 1976.

Kelly, P. J. Osteomyelitis in the adult. *Orthop. Clin. North Am.* 6:983, 1975.

Lewis, R. P., Sutter, V. L., and Finegold, S. M. Bone infections involving anerobic bacteria. *Medicine* 57:279, 1978.

Lutzker, L. G., and Alavi, A. Bone and marrow imaging in sickle cell disease: Diagnosis of infarction. *Semin. Nucl. Med.* 6:83, 1976.

Musher, D. M., Thorsteinsson, S. B., Minuth, J. N., and Luchi, R. J. Vertebral osteomyelitis: Still a diagnostic pitfall. *Arch. Intern. Med.* 136:105, 1976.

Waldvogel, F. A., Medoff, G., and Swartz, M. N. Osteomyelitis: A review of clinical features, therapeutic considerations and unusual aspects. *N. Engl. J. Med.* 282:198, 260, 316, 1970.

29. Osteonecrosis

Bernard N. Stulberg
and Joseph M. Lane

Osteonecrosis (formerly called *aseptic* or *avascular necrosis*) is a focal degeneration of bone, probably secondary to ischemia, which occurs most commonly in the femoral head and proximal humerus. Early diagnosis is important to allow therapeutic intervention before irreversible bone damage occurs.

I. Pathogenesis. The etiology of osteonecrosis (ON) is not known, although most investigators agree that the ultimate disease pathway involves the inadequacy of the blood supply to meet the metabolic needs of the involved bone segment. The initiating event in ON may occur at either a macroscopic level (usually secondary to trauma) or a microscopic level (possibly the result of repeated microvascular injury). ON secondary to traumatic events will not be discussed here as it is most commonly considered in operative orthopedics.

A. Disease association factors. A large proportion of findings formerly felt to reflect idiopathic ON have been shown to be associated with a number of clinical conditions. Table 29-1 contains a partial listing of the more common associations.

B. Lesion type. Osteonecrotic lesions may be diaphyseal or juxtaarticular. The former may result in bone infarction, which is usually asymptomatic and clinically unimportant. Juxtaarticular lesions are often symptomatic, may lead to subsequent joint incongruity, and thus may result in severe secondary osteoarthritis. This discussion considers only juxtaarticular lesions.

C. Stages of disease. A pattern of evolution based on clinical and radiographic criteria has been described for juxtaarticular lesions. However, the problem occurs in the absence of associated disease in older subjects and may result in severe hip and knee osteoarthritis.

1. Stage I. Normal radiographic findings; patient may be completely asymptomatic; diagnosis by bone scan.

2. Stage II. Minimal or no pain; radiographic appearance of irregular lucent areas; often with marginal sclerosis.

3. Stage III. Moderate to severe symptoms; radiographs show subchondral fracture with the "crescent" sign (implying osteochondral fracture with collapse); joint architecture minimally disturbed.

4. Stage IV. Severe symptoms with advanced subchondral collapse and joint destruction; advanced changes of osteoarthrosis.

II. Diagnosis

A. Clinical symptoms. The major presenting symptom of osteonecrosis is pain, often out of proportion to radiographic findings. It has a sudden onset and is often localized to the periarticular area. Most common areas of involvement are the proximal femur, distal femur, proximal tibia, and proximal humerus. Osteonecrotic lesions have been identified in all bones of the skeleton. Multiple bone involvement, particularly of the contralateral joint, necessitates careful evaluation of the opposite limb.

B. Physical findings

1. Localized bone tenderness

2. Normal joint mobility is the rule because lesions are periarticular. Early lesions are often associated with full, painless passive range of motion.

Table 29-1. Conditions Associated with Osteonecrosis

High Association
  Alcoholism
  Congenital malformations
  Corticosteroid therapy
  Cushing syndrome
  Decompression syndrome
  Gaucher disease
  Hematopoetic disorders (Hemophilia)
  Hemoglobinopathy (particularly SC disease)
  Hyperuricemia
  Irradiation
  Systemic lupus erythematosus
  Thermal injuries or frostbite
  Trauma
Moderate Association
  Diabetes mellitus
  Fat embolism
  Gout and hyperuricemia
  Rheumatoid arthritis
Reported but Uncertain Association
  Hypercholesterolemia
  Hypertriglyceridemia
  Lymphoma

C. **Laboratory data.** In the majority of patients with ON, there is antecedent recognition of an associated condition, such as systemic lupus erythematosus (or other illness requiring corticosteroid therapy), alcoholism, or hemoglobinopathy; thus extensive laboratory study is not required. In the absence of a recognized basis for ON, a general health evaluation should be obtained, which may include performance of the following tests:

  1. Complete blood count (CBC), urinalysis, erythrocyte sedimentation rate (ESR), serum chemical profile (including uric acid, glucose, serum glutamic-oxaloacetic transaminase [SGOT], alkaline phosphatase).

  2. Antinuclear antibody (ANA).

  3. Serum hemoglobin electrophoresis.

  4. Serum amylase and lipase.

  5. Prothrombin time and partial thromboplastin time.

  6. Serum lipoprotein electrophoresis and triglycerides.

  7. Glucose tolerance test.

D. **Radiographic evaluation**

  1. Routine anteroposterior (AP) and lateral x-rays of the involved bone and joint to determine the disease stage as described in **I.C.**

  2. Total body bone scan.

  3. AP and lateral x-rays of previously unstudied areas with bone scan positivity.

  4. Tomography of involved joint if diagnosis is still not established.

E. **Differential diagnosis**

  1. **Early osteoarthrosis (OA)** is difficult to distinguish from ON. The diagnosis of OA is suggested by old age, Heberden nodes, and the absence of ON-associated disorders.

2. Osteomyelitis is suggested by systemic signs and an extraskeletal focus of infection. Diagnosis is confirmed by bone biopsy and culture.

III. Therapy. Identification and treatment of associated diseases listed in Table 29-1 are the initial therapeutic measures.

Once an osteonecrotic lesion has reached the point of subchondral fracture and collapse (stage III), only surgical intervention will be helpful. The recommended therapy follows.

A. Stage I lesions

1. Hip and knee lesions

a. Rest (bedrest if necessary).

b. Crutches or cane to decrease joint forces for three months.

c. Limitation of vigorous activities.

d. Maintenance of full active and passive range of motion (pool therapy if necessary).

e. Radiographs or bone scan every three months.

f. Mild analgesics such as aspirin 650 mg QID.

2. Shoulder lesions

a. Sling until pain diminished.

b. Same as outlined above in **1.c.–f.**

B. Stage II lesions

1. Hip and knee lesions. Same as for stage I (sec. **III.A.1.**) *except* protected weight bearing for at least six months.

2. Shoulder lesions. Same as for stage I (sec. **III.A.2.**) *except* limitation of activities for six months.

C. Stage III lesions

1. Hip and knee lesions. Use conservative measures as outlined for stage I (sec. **III.A.1.**). If unsuccessful in relieving pain, osteotomy or prosthetic joint replacement is recommended.

2. Shoulder lesions. Use conservative measures as outlined for stage I (sec. **III.A.2.**), but consider hemiarthroplasty or total joint replacement if pain is unrelieved.

D. Stage IV lesions

1. Hip and knee lesions. Total joint replacement if level of symptoms and disability warrant it.

2. Shoulder lesions. Total joint replacement if warranted by level of symptoms and disability.

E. Experimental measures. Two important modalities aimed at reversing the disease process have been reported. The authors have limited experience with these methods and feel they should be limited to investigational use at the present.

1. Decompression. The method records venous pressure of bone in the periarticular area. The venous pressure is reported to be elevated in ON. Bone decompression with trephine may reverse stage I lesions.

2. Bone grafting with or without muscle-pedicle transfers has been recommended for stage II lesions. Best results are reported when grafting is done before subchondral collapse.

IV. Prognosis. Only early lesions (mostly stage I and some stage II lesions) respond well to conservative management. The early identification and treatment of associated disease entities (such as decreased use of corticosteroids) represent the only circumstances in which conservative management may successfully prevent the evolution of the osteonecrotic process.

Bibliography

Cruess, R. L.   Experience with steroid-induced avascular necrosis of the shoulder and etiologic considerations regarding osteonecrosis of the hip. *Clin. Orthop.* 130:86, 1978.

Hungerford, D. S., and Zizic, T. M.   Alcoholism-associated ischemic necrosis of the femoral head. *Clin. Orthop.* 130:144, 1978.

Jacobs, B.   Epidemiology of traumatic and nontraumatic osteonecrosis. *Clin. Orthop.* 130:51, 1978.

Jones, J. P., Jr.   Osteonecrosis. In D.J. McCarty (Ed.), *Arthritis and Allied Conditions* (9th ed.), Philadelphia: Lea & Febiger, 1979. P. 1121.

Park, W. M.   Spontaneous and Drug-Induced Aseptic Necrosis. In J.K. Davidson (Ed.), *Aseptic Necrosis of Bone.* Amsterdam: Amsterdam Excerpta Medica, 1976.

30. Osteoporosis

Bernard N. Stulberg
and Joseph M. Lane

Osteoporosis (OP) involves a state of bone loss characterized by a reduction in total bone mass to a level below normal for an individual's age, sex, and race. Osteoporosis is classified into primary and secondary forms. The term *osteopenia* refers to a radiographic finding of decreased bone density. In OP, the bone loss occurs in cancellous (spongy) bone more rapidly than in cortical bone.

Osteoporosis implies a decrease in bone mineralized and unmineralized matrices; *osteomalacia* refers to a decrease in mineralized matrix, thus causing the ratio of mineralized to unmineralized matrix to decrease. In osteomalacia, bone mass may be normal, low, or even increased. However, many patients have a mixture of OP and osteomalacia.

Osteoporosis is the most common metabolic bone disease and occurs in 25% of women and 17% of men over age 70.

I. **Pathogenesis.** The exact cause of OP is unknown, although net bone resorption is the final result. Bone volume diminishes as a function of age, and bone strength varies directly with bone volume; thus the susceptibility to fracture increases with age.

The following **continuing factors** have been identified.

A. **Immobilization**

B. **Endocrine**

   1. Postmenopausal.

   2. Corticosteroid excess.

   3. Congenital 17-hydroxylase deficiency (estrogen deformity).

   4. Hyperparathyroidism (secondary form much more common than primary form).

   5. Hyperthyroidism.

   6. Diabetes mellitus.

   7. Acromegaly.

C. **Age (greater than 65 years)**

D. **Iatrogenic**

   1. Chronic heparin therapy.

   2. Corticosteroid therapy.

E. **Nutritional abnormalities**

   1. Lactase deficiency.

   2. Inadequate calcium intake.

   3. Malabsorption.

   4. Metabolic acidosis.

   5. Alcoholism.

   6. High phosphate intake (milk-alkali syndrome).

   7. Vitamin D deficiency.

   8. Scurvy.

F. Genetic and sex factors

1. Females are born with less total bone mass than males.

2. Black populations have higher ratio of cortical to cancellous bone (61% to 35%) than white populations; therefore, OP is rare in blacks.

3. Ethnic populations of Northern European origin are most susceptible; Slavic populations and Mediterranean populations are most resistant.

II. Clinical presentation. Back pain and fractures are the most characteristic presenting symptoms. Vertebral compression fractures (often multiple and most commonly T12 to L2), proximal femur fractures (femoral neck and intertrochanteric), distal radius fractures, and pelvic fractures are the most common fracture types. The loss of height secondary to multiple vertebral fractures is quite characteristic of osteoporotic patients.

A. History may reveal early menopause, low dietary calcium, back pain, malabsorption symptoms, steroid therapy, or Northern European heritage.

B. Physical examination. Kyphosis, scoliosis, loss of height, and localized bone tenderness (particularly spinal) are common findings.

C. Laboratory studies. Serum calcium, phosphorus, and alkaline phosphatase are normal. Urinary calcium is high initially but is normal in chronic OP.

D. Radiographic findings. Early changes include osteopenia, particularly in the spine and pelvis, and loss of horizontal trabeculations in vertebral bodies.
Spinal compression fractures with biconcave ("codfish") deformities are common particularly at T12, L1, and L2. Schmorl nodes (disc protrusion through vertebral endplate) are seen. No focal lytic or blastic lesions occur.

E. Bone biopsy. Bone biopsy reveals decreased bone mass with a normal mineral-matrix ratio.

F. Bone densitometry. Densitometry reveals decreased bone mass.

III. Differential diagnosis. Diagnosis should emphasize the identification of treatable secondary causes of OP. Causes of OP follow.

A. Multiple myeloma. Decreased alkaline phosphatase, monoclonal gammopathy, lytic lesions on x-ray, and generalized bone tenderness suggest the diagnosis.

B. Metastatic malignancy may be manifested by increased alkaline phosphatase, hypercalcemia, cortical erosions on x-ray, x-ray evidence of vertebral pedicle destruction, and positive bone scan.

C. Genetic disorders. Ehlers-Danlos syndrome, Marfan syndrome, and osteogenesis imperfecta.

D. Hyperthyroidism is suggested by weight loss, heat tolerance, elevated serum thyroxine, and elevated urinary calcium and hydroxyproline.

E. Hyperparathyroidism (primary). Elevated calcium, decreased or normal PO_4, elevated parathormone. Radiographic evidence of endosteal and periosteal resorption. Biopsy reveals osteitis fibrosa cystica, increased number of osteoclasts, and bone resorption (dissecting resorption).

F. Osteomalacia. Low serum calcium and phosphorus levels. Elevated alkaline phosphatase. Radiographs reveal pseudofractures. Biopsy reveals osteoid seams and a decreased mineralized-unmineralized matrix ratio.

G. Renal osteodystrophy. Uremia, elevated PO_4, decreased calcium, and ectopic mineralization are diagnostic clues.

H. Scheuermann disease is seen in the adolescent age group and manifested by wedge fractures of T6, T7, and T8.

I. Gastrointestinal disease. Symptoms of malabsorption or a history of previous gastrointestinal surgery suggest a cause for OP.

IV. Therapy

  A. Fracture management. Therapy of **limb** fractures (e.g., femur and distal radius fractures) follows usual routine, since fracture healing is normal in OP patients. **Vertebral compression** fractures caused by OP may be treated by the following regimen.

    1. Analgesics and bedrest. The disease is self-limiting, and subjective response is a reasonable indication to resume graded physical activity.

    2. Pool exercise therapy, progressing to ambulation and ultimately to flexion and extension exercises.

    3. Lumbosacral support, Knight-Taylor brace, or other appropriate back support is prescribed for a 3-month trial.

  B. Medical therapy of OP. Follow-up bone biopsy at two years to monitor therapy and assess results is recommended.

    1. Calcium carbonate 1,300 mg TID (equivalent to daily dose of 1,500 mg elemental calcium).

    2. Sodium fluoride 1 mg/kg per day in 3 divided doses. Gastric discomfort, joint pain, and ankle edema may occur.

    3. Vitamin D 400 units per day (as part of a multivitamin). Periodic monitoring (3 times monthly) of 24-hour urine calcium. Levels below 250 mg per day will help to avoid renal calculi. Exercise and physical therapy programs are essential to maintain bone mass.

    4. Estrogen therapy is controversial. It prevents OP during early menopause (for three to six years), but the risk of endometrial cancer precludes recommending its routine use.

V. Prognosis. Preventive measures are most important because severe bone damage, once present, is irreversible. About 4% of elderly osteoporotic individuals will sustain a femoral fracture. Only 60% of these fracture patients will survive two years.

Bibliography

Avioli, L. V., and Krane, S. M. *Metabolic Bone Disease*, Vol. 1. New York: Academic, 1977.

Jaffe, H. L. *Metabolic Degenerative and Inflammatory Diseases of Bones and Joints.* Philadelphia: Lea & Febiger, 1972. P. 367.

Jowsey, J. *Metabolic Diseases of Bone.* Philadelphia: Saunders, 1977.

Lane, J. M. Metabolic Bone Disease and Fracture Healing. In R. B. Heppenstall (Ed.), *Fracture Treatment and Healing.* Philadelphia: Saunders, 1980.

Riggs, B. L., et al. Treatment of primary osteoporosis with fluoride and calcium. *J.A.M.A.* 243L:446, 1980.

Singh, M. M., Nagrath, A. R., and Maini, P. S. Changes in trabecular pattern of the upper end of the femur as an index of osteoporosis. *J. Bone Joint Surg.* 52-A:457, 1970.

31. Paget Disease of Bone

Bernard N. Stulberg
and Joseph M. Lane

In 1877, Sir James Paget described several cases of a condition he termed *osteitis deformans*, a disease of bone characterized by severe, extensive skeletal involvement and obvious deformity of individual long bones.

I. **Definition.** Paget disease of bone is characterized by increased bone resorption (osteoclastic activity) and subsequent reactive bone formation (osteoblastic activity). The etiology is unknown. The disease may involve only one bone (monostotic) or multiple bones (polyostotic). The polyostotic form is characteristically asymmetric.

II. **Epidemiology.** Although Paget disease was once considered to be quite rare, the recognition of its monostotic form, coupled with improvements in roentgenographic and scintiscanning technology, reveal the disease to be radiographically present in 3% to 4% of the population. Geographic and racial differences in occurrence of the disease have been cited; however, no genetic pattern has been identified.

There is a slight male predominance. Paget disease is usually not discovered until after age 40, and most patients are over 50.

III. **Pathogenesis.** Paget disease of bone is characterized by a marked stimulation of osteoclastic and osteoblastic activity and a significantly increased rate of bone turnover. Grossly, the newly formed bone is of poor structural integrity; resulting deformity and pathologic fracture are commonly seen in involved bones. Radiographically, the involved bone may demonstrate either a lytic or blastic picture or, more commonly, both. A characteristic V pattern of the advancing osteolytic front may be seen. Grossly, the involved bone appears spongy, of poor structural integrity, and somewhat pumicelike. Histologically, the pattern of irregular segments of mature (lamellar) bone with multiple cement lines is considered diagnostic. Cement lines imply reversal of osteoclastic resorption and subsequent new bone formation. The resultant "mosaic" or "jigsaw" pattern is classically associated with Paget disease.

IV. **Clinical presentations.** Most patients with Paget disease are asymptomatic, and the disease is usually recognized fortuitously when a roentgenogram is obtained for another purpose (e.g., intravenous pyelogram [IVP], trauma). Symptomatic patients most commonly present with pain, deformity, or pathologic fracture. However, other important clinical features may result from the alteration of joint architecture and function, compression of neural structures, change in temperature of overlying skin and subcutaneous tissues, and, rarely, bone sarcoma in an area of Paget disease ("Paget sarcoma"). (See Table 31-1.)

A. **Sites of involvement.** The most common sites of bone involvement in Paget disease are:

1. Sacrum, 56%

2. Spine (lumbar most frequent), 50%.

3. Right femur, 31%.

4. Cranium, 28%.

5. Sternum, 23%.

6. Pelvis, 21%.

7. Left femur, 15%.

8. Clavicle, 13%.

9. Tibia, 8%.

Table 31-1. Radiographic and Clinical Manifestations of Paget Disease of Bone

Location	Radiographic Findings	Clinical Symptoms
Skull	Osteoporosis circumscripta	None
	Cranial enlargement	Occasionally painful
	Basilar invagination	Occipital neuralgia; lower cranial nerve impingement; medullary compression; syringomyelia with ventricular obstruction and increased intracranial pressure; vertebral basilar artery insufficiency
	Temporal bone involvement	Hearing loss
	Auditory osicle involvement	Hearing loss
Facial, jaw-bones	Unilateral radiographic changes	Proptosis; trigeminal neuralgia; displacement of teeth
Spine	"Window frame" vertebra(e)	Nerve root compression; spinal stenosis; spondylitis
Pelvis, hip joint	Acetabular and femoral head disease with articular degeneration; protrusio acetabuli; sacroiliac joint ankylosis	Pain; end-stage arthritis; fracture
Knee	Distal femoral involvement with bone and joint deformity	Pain; arthritis; fracture
Tibia, femur, humerus	Bowing, with or without fracture; change in joint geometry	Pain; arthritis; fracture
Any site of involvement	Marked destruction of bone; extracortical extension; possible soft tissue mass	Marked increase in pain; neoplasia must be ruled out

10. Ribs, 7%.

11. Humerus, 4%.

Associated conditions are congestive heart failure (CHF) or valvular heart disease; hypercalcemia; hypercalcinuria; hyperuricemia (40%); and calcific periarthritis.

B. **Laboratory findings.** The most characteristic laboratory findings of Paget disease are **elevated serum alkaline phosphatase** and **elevated 24-hour urinary hydroxyproline (OHP)**. Alkaline phosphatase activity, as an indicator of bone formation, may be normal, mildly elevated, or markedly elevated, and tends to correlate with the extent of bony involvement. Urinary hydroxyproline, as a measure of collagen breakdown, may be a more sensitive indicator of the lytic activity of the disease. On the whole, however, alkaline phosphatase activity and urinary hydroxyproline levels correlate.

1. **Additional laboratory workup**

   a. SMA-12. Serum Ca, PO_4 usually within normal limits. Uric acid often elevated (40%).

   b. Urinalysis.

   c. 24-hour urine collection for OHP with patient on gelatin-free diet.

2. Roentgenographic workup

a. Anteroposterior and lateral x-rays of entire involved bone.

b. Bone scan. Technetium 99m–labeled diphosphonates are bone seeking and can identify multiple sites of Pagetic involvement.

c. Skeletal survey (including anteroposterior and lateral views of skull) when bone scintiscanning not available.

V. Differential diagnosis. Combined radiographic and histologic patterns are usually sufficiently characteristic to rule out other disease entities.

A. Radiographic

1. Osteoporosis circumscripta of skull.

2. "Window frame" vertebra.

3. Deformity with secondary osteoarthritis.

B. Histologic

1. Markedly increased osteoclastic resorption with secondary increase in osteoblastic activity and mosaic pattern.

2. The large number of osteoclasts in resorptive stage should not be confused with hyperparathyroidism.

VI. Therapy

A. Asymptomatic. No treatment is indicated for the patient with asymptomatic Paget disease. Documentation of the extent of skeletal involvement is prudent (e.g., bone scan). Biopsy of an involved bone is indicated only if the diagnosis is in doubt.

B. Symptomatic. Paget disease that is symptomatic is best treated at referral institutions. The two major modes of therapy are the calcitonins (porcine, salmon, or human) and the diphosphonates (primarily disodium etidronate). Mithramycin has been used experimentally in several centers. Therapy regimens seek to control the biochemical parameters (and hopefully symptoms) of the disease, although symptomatic relief has been achieved without accompanying biochemical changes. All agents now used are directed at inhibition of osteoclastic activity. Symptomatic relief often, but not always, follows the decrease in metabolic turnover and is reflected by a fall in alkaline phosphatase and urinary hydroxyproline levels. Sequential bone scanning with technetium-labeled diphosphonates has also been helpful in serial management of these patients.

1. Calcitonin

a. Rationale. Calcitonin is a polypeptide hormone found in mammals, birds, and fish. It acts to decrease bone resorption through specific osteoclastic receptors.

b. Dosage. Salmon calcitonin is the preferred agent, administered 50 to 160 units subcutaneously three times per week. Porcine calcitonin administration leads to rapid formation of neutralizing antibodies. Human calcitonin is less potent but may be used if antibodies diminish effectiveness of salmon and porcine forms.

c. Response. In almost two-thirds of patients, a fall in urinary hydroxyproline and serum alkaline phosphatase levels occurs within one month of the onset of therapy and correlates with relief of bone pain. Radiographic improvement, however, may not occur.

d. Side effects include nausea, flushing, local reaction at injection site, and urticaria. They may be treated symptomatically with antiemetics and antihistamines. If antibody formation occurs, a different form of calcitonin should be used.

2. Diphosphonates (EHDP)

a. Rationale. These pyrophosphate analogs inhibit the growth and dissolution of hydroxypatite crystals and can directly impair osteoclast function.

b. Dosage. 5 to 10 mg/kg per day orally for 6 months. No further efficacy with prolonged therapy. May be repeated in patients with more severe disease.

c. Response. Bone pain is generally relieved in most patients, although it may increase paradoxically in some as a result of osteomalacia. Significant improvement in biochemical parameters may be seen while on therapy. Improvement in bone scan may be seen.

d. Side effects include abdominal discomfort, diarrhea, increased bone pain, and increased incidence of fractures.

3. Mithramycin.

This cytotoxic agent is a DNA-inhibitor and has been used successfully to treat hypercalcemia of malignancy. Multisystem toxicity precludes its routine use in this condition.

VII. Prognosis. Sarcoma of bone has been found in association with Paget disease. The incidence of all malignant change is well below 1% of all Paget disease. Malignant tumors most commonly encountered are osteogenic sarcoma, fibrosarcoma, and chondrosarcoma. Malignant and benign giant cell tumors are also seen. The prognosis of sarcoma associated with Paget disease is poor (less than 2% five-year survival).

Bibliography

Hadjipaulou, A. G., et al.   Combination drug therapy in treatment of Paget disease of bone. *J. Bone Joint Surg.* 59-A:1045, 1977.

Jaffe, H. L.   *Metabolic Degenerative and Inflammatory Disease of Bones and Joints.* Philadelphia: Lea & Febiger, 1972. P. 240.

Krane, S. M.   Paget disease of bone. *Clin. Orthop.* 127:24, 1977.

Schmidek, H. H.   Neurologic and neurosurgical sequelae of Paget's disease of bone. *Clin. Orthop.* 127:70, 1977.

Singer, F. R., and Mills, B. G.   The etiology of Paget's disease of bone. *Clin. Orthop.* 127:37, 1977.

32. Polymyalgia Rheumatica and Temporal Arteritis

Richard Stern

Polymyalgia Rheumatica

Polymyalgia rheumatica (PMR) is a descriptive term (suggested by Barber in 1957) for an aching syndrome, usually in elderly patients with elevated erythrocyte sedimentation rates (ESRs), that cannot be attributed to more defined rheumatic, infectious, or neoplastic disorders.

PMR is estimated to affect approximately 30 per million of the U.S. population. Sixty percent of the patients are female. Most patients present after their fiftieth year and the peak incidence is between age 60 and 80. However, there are well-documented reports of PMR (usually in association with temporal arteritis) in patients in their 40s. Rarely, cases have been noted in younger patients.

I. Clinical manifestations

A. Proximal myalgias. PMR is characterized by chronic, symmetric, proximal muscle aching and stiffness. These symptoms are most prominent in the shoulder and pelvic girdles and neck, but distal muscle groups may also be involved. Aching and stiffness are worse in the morning, worse on exertion, and may be severe and incapacitating. Muscles may be tender; disuse may lead to atrophy and, occasionally, contractures may develop. Muscle strength is often difficult to evaluate because pain is present; however, it should be normal.

B. Constitutional symptoms. Patients with PMR frequently complain of malaise and fatigue. Temperature is usually low grade but may occasionally reach 102°F. Night sweats may occur. PMR may rarely present as a fever of unknown origin. Anorexia and weight loss may be prominent features and suggest malignancy; however, no direct association of PMR with neoplastic disease has been proven.

C. Neuropsychiatric manifestations such as depression, dementia, acute disorientation, and amnesia (without focal neurologic disease) may be seen and occasionally are the presenting manifestations of PMR.

D. Joints. Majority of patients have poorly localized tenderness over joints, especially prominent over shoulders and hips. The syndrome's original description excluded synovitis as a feature, but moderate effusions can be seen in the knees and, occasionally, other joints (the presence of synovitis may make differentiation from rheumatoid arthritis difficult). Interpretation of radionuclide scans has suggested the presence of synovitis in proximal joints.

E. Temporal (cranial) arteritis. A detailed discussion of this syndrome and its relationship to PMR can be found in the following section, Temporal Arteritis. The incidence of association of the two syndromes is a subject of controversy; however, in some series, 30% to 50% of patients with PMR have had temporal arteritis, and 60% to 70% of patients with temporal arteritis have had PMR.

II. Laboratory findings

A. Blood studies

1. An elevated **Westergren sedimentation rate** is the laboratory hallmark of PMR; it is usually in excess of 50 mm/hr and may exceed 100 mm/hr.

2. **Normocytic normochromic anemia** is seen in approximately 50% of patients.

3. **Immunologic studies.** Frequency of rheumatoid factors, antinuclear antibodies, and other autoreactive antibodies is not higher than that of age-matched controls.

4. **Muscle enzymes** (CPK, SGOT, LDH, aldolase) are normal.

B. **Radiographic studies** are nonspecific, although erosive lesions in the symphysis pubis, acromioclavicular, and sacroiliac joints have been observed.

C. **Electromyographic studies** are within normal limits.

D. **Muscle biopsy histology** is nondiagnostic; type II muscle fiber atrophy probably represents disuse.

E. **Synovial fluid and tissue studies**

1. **Leukocyte counts** in joint fluid range between 1,000 and 8,000 with a preponderance of lymphocytes.

2. **Synovial biopsies**, when available, reveal mild synovial proliferation with slight lymphocyte infiltration.

III. **Diagnosis.** PMR should be considered in patients over 50 who complain of proximal arthralgia and myalgia. The Westergren ESR is usually elevated above 50 mm/hr. Central to the diagnosis of PMR is a rapid and dramatic response to low-dose corticosteroid therapy (see sec. **IV.A.**).

Diagnosis requires exclusion of other syndromes associated with aching or ESR elevation, or both.

A. **Neoplasia**

B. **Infectious syndromes**

C. **Other rheumatic conditions** such as rheumatoid arthritis and systemic lupus.

D. **Muscle diseases** such as polymyositis or thyroid myopathy.

E. **Plasma cell dyscrasias**

F. **Fibromyalgia** (an ill-defined aching syndrome not associated with an elevated ESR. See Chap. 22.).

IV. **Therapy**

A. **Prednisone.** Initial therapy for PMR is usually prednisone 10 to 15 mg per day. A prompt and dramatic clinical response is considered by some to be an absolute criterion for diagnosis. Most symptoms resolve in 48 to 72 hours, and the ESR should normalize after a week to 10 days.

Following control of symptoms, the dose of corticosteroid therapy should be reduced to the lowest level required to suppress symptoms. Patients vary in how quickly the dose can be tapered (from weeks to several months) and may require a maintenance therapy (prednisone 2.5 to 7.5 mg/24 hr) for several months or more.

Because elderly patients are especially prone to corticosteroid complications (particularly osteoporosis), prednisone should not be reinstated or increased when *only* elevation of ESR values occurs, without other manifestations of active disease. It should be emphasized that PMR (without temporal arteritis) is a benign condition. For patients with chronic symptoms, the morbidity associated with therapy often exceeds that of the underlying disease.

Low-dose corticosteroid therapy used to treat PMR is not appropriate for patients with features suggestive of temporal arteritis (see Temporal Arteritis).

B. **Non-steroidal anti-inflammatory agents** may suppress rheumatic symptoms, but they do not reduce the risk of blindness if temporal arteritis is present.

Temporal Arteritis

Temporal arteritis (TA), also known as giant cell or cranial arteritis, is a vascular syndrome that affects predominantly cranial arteries. In the late nineteenth century, Jonathan Hutchinson reported the first case, a man who had difficulty wearing a hat because his temporal arteries were tender. Since that time the clinical spectrum of TA has broadened (sec **I.**). The incidence is unknown, but is probably about half that of polymyalgia rheumatica. It occurs about equally in men and women. The age distribution is similar to PMR with a peak incidence from 60 to 80 years of age, and rarely occurs in patients less than 50 years old.

I. **Clinical presentations.** TA is a strikingly heterogeneous syndrome. All of the features of PMR (myalgia, arthralgia, fatigue, malaise, fever, weight loss, and depression) are common. Whether or not PMR and TA represent different parts of a single disorder is a subject of continuing debate (see sec. **D.**).

Earlier descriptions of TA emphasized manifestations that were attributable to involvement of the ophthalmic artery and branches of the external carotid system, but it is now recognized that arterial lesions may be widespread. The varied expressions of the syndrome can be analyzed according to anatomic patterns of affected arteries.

A. **Symptoms related to involvement of external carotid artery branches**

1. **Headache** is probably the most frequent symptom of TA, occurring in 50% to 75% of patients; it is often the first manifestation of disease. It is described as extracranial, dull, boring, and burning. Classically, patients complain of temporal headaches, and the temporal arteries on physical examination may be prominent, beaded, tender, and pulseless. Patients with occipital artery involvement may have difficulty combing their hair or discomfort from pressure of a pillow on the head.

2. **Jaw claudication** occurs infrequently in TA, but its presence is highly suggestive of the syndrome. Patients with involvement of the maxillary or lingual arteries may have jaw or tongue pain on chewing or talking. There are rare case reports of tongue gangrene.

3. **Ear canal, pinna, or parotid gland pain** may occur secondary to involvement of the posterior auricular artery.

4. **Temporomandibular joint pain** may occur secondary to temporal artery involvement.

B. **Symptoms related to the internal carotid artery**

1. **Ocular damage** secondary to arteritis is the most common serious consequence of TA. While it occurs in 20% to 50% of patients and is the presenting symptom at **diagnosis** of 60% of patients with TA, ocular damage is rarely the earliest symptom. Careful history in most patients with visual loss will reveal that headache, usually specific enough to suggest the diagnosis, anteceded blindness in about 40% of patients. Symptoms characteristic of PMR are early manifestations in about 30% of patients. Since loss of vision in TA is often irreversible unless treatment is initiated within several hours following onset of ocular symptoms, special attention must be directed towards early recognition of the syndrome. Ocular manifestations vary according to the pattern of arterial branch involvement. The retina is supplied by the central retinal artery, which is the terminal branch of the ophthalmic artery. Also derived from the ophthalmic artery are the posterior ciliary arteries, which supply the optic nerve, and the muscular branches, which supply the extraocular muscles. Because the posterior ciliary arteries are the most frequently involved arteries in TA, ischemic optic neuritis is by far the most common lesion. Occlusion of the central retinal artery or its branches occurs in less than 10% of patients with eye involvement. Therefore, retinal changes such as exudates, hemorrhages, or vasculitis are infrequent. The fundoscopic evaluation will often be normal or show only mild edema of the nerve head several days after the initial symptoms. Optic atrophy is a late finding.

a. **Amaurosis fugax** occurs in about 10% of patients with TA, 80% of whom will achieve permanent visual loss if not treated.

b. **Unilateral or incomplete blindness** occurs in about 30% to 40% of patients and, if untreated, may progress to complete blindness over a period of several days.

c. **Bilateral blindness** occurs in 25% of patients with TA and, as noted in **a.** and **b.**, is often preceded by amaurosis fugax or partial blindness.

d. **Diplopia secondary to ischemic paresis** of the extraocular muscles occurs in about 5% of patients with TA.

2. **Central nervous system disease** can occur in TA secondary to involvement of any of the intracerebral arteries, producing seizures, cerebral vascular accidents, or abnormal mental status. Peripheral nerve involvement is rare. As a result of the relative inaccessibility of intracranial vessels and the high prevalence of arteriosclerotic vascular disease in older patients, the frequency with which TA leads to significant ischemic central nervous system disease is not known.

C. **Symptoms related to large artery involvement**

1. **Aortic arch and thoracic aorta.** Careful physical examination in patients with TA often reveals bruits over the carotid, axillary, or brachial arteries. Limited pathologic studies have shown giant cell arteritis in such vessels; however, since bruits secondary to arteriosclerotic vascular disease are common in elderly subjects, the frequency of aortic and aortic root involvement in TA is not known. Nevertheless, giant cell arteritis has been documented as a basis for aneurysms, dissections, and stenotic lesions of the aorta and its major branches. In isolated cases, coronary artery disease and a variety of aortic arch syndromes secondary to giant cell arteritis have been demonstrated.

2. **Abdominal aorta.** Involvement of the abdominal aorta, similar to that of the thoracic aorta, can produce symptoms secondary to aortic aneurysms and intestinal infarction. For unknown reasons renal involvement is rare. There are some clear-cut examples of leg claudication secondary to giant cell arteritis, but the relevance of this finding is not clear. There is no indication to use steroids to treat peripheral vascular disease in the usual elderly patient with leg claudication who may, for some other reason, have an elevated sedimentation rate. As will be discussed later, even in the patient with known TA, steroids should not be used to treat large vessel disease without evidence that vasculitis, rather than atheromatous disease, is responsible.

D. **Symptoms related to polymyalgia rheumatica.** The clinical picture of PMR has already been described in detail (Polymyalgia Rheumatica, sec. **I.**). Patients with TA, with or without PMR, may have similar systemic complaints such as fatigue, malaise, fever, weight loss, depression, and arthralgias or transient arthritis. Still at issue is how to predict which patient with PMR has TA. There are some physicians who advocate treating *all* patients with PMR as if they had TA. However, this approach involves unnecessary treatment of a large group of patients with high-dose steroids. Because a temporal artery biopsy is a relatively benign procedure, to biopsy *all* patients with suspected PMR, as opposed to treating them all as if they had TA, would clearly be preferable.

If a patient with polymyalgia has the classic signs or symptoms of TA, a biopsy should be done. Temporal artery biopsy can be accomplished on an ambulatory basis and, if positive, can dramatically diminish the diagnostic studies that would otherwise be needed in the evaluation of a systemically ill patient with elevated ESR. Several clinical studies have demonstrated that the chance of finding a positive temporal artery biopsy in PMR patients is greatly enhanced if temporal artery pulses are absent or diminished, even in the absence of other localizing signs. Even the presence of a nonspecific headache may increase the yield. No difference has been demonstrated in the degree of ESR elevation, the presence of minor visual symptoms, sex, age, or duration of symptoms among PMR patients with and without TA. Furthermore, about 10% of patients with PMR and localized temporal artery signs have negative biopsies (see sec. **IV.A.**). In conclusion, PMR patients without signs or symptoms of TA or histologically demonstrated arteritis should not be empirically treated with steroid regimens that are appropriate for TA.

II. Laboratory findings

A. Erythrocyte sedimentation rate. As in PMR, the laboratory hallmark of TA is the elevated ESR. The ESR (Westergren) is usually between 50 and 100 mm/hr, rarely less than 40 mm/hr, and commonly is greater than 100 mm/hr. A mild normocytic, normochromic anemia may be present. As in PMR, muscle enzymes are normal. Rheumatoid factor, ANA, and anti-DNA antibodies are negative. Complement levels are normal and cyroglobulins and monoclonal immunoglobulins are absent.

B. Radiographic procedures. Temporal artery arteriography has no value. However, arteriography of the aorta *may* be useful in differentiating giant cell arteritis from arteriosclerotic vascular disease. In the former, the vessels often show slowly tapering stenotic lesions, in contrast to the "cobblestone" pattern of arteriosclerotic disease. Unfortunately, most TA patients are in the elderly group which will have arteriosclerotic disease as well, therefore making this differentiation difficult.

III. Pathologic findings.

Always biopsy the temporal artery on the symptomatic side of the head. If a specific part of the artery is tender, beaded, or inflamed, the biopsy should include that area. There is no information as to whether the artery trunk or a distal branch specimen is best. At least 1 cm of the artery should be taken. Because the process may be segmental, multiple sections should be made. Histologically, the following are seen.

A. An inflammatory infiltrate, predominantly of mononuclear cells, usually involving the entire vessel wall. Fibrinoid necrosis is not a feature of the lesion.

B. Fragmentation of the internal elastic lamina.

C. Giant cells are almost always present and often seem to engulf parts of the internal elastic lamina. They are difficult to find in some cases, and their absence does not rule out the diagnosis.

D. Intimal proliferation is often marked, is a nonspecific feature in this age group, and cannot, if found alone, be considered evidence of past or present arteritis.

These findings are in contrast to those of the lesions in polyarteritis nodosa, which are characterized by fibrinoid necrosis of the vessel and neutrophil infiltration. When TA involves larger vessels, the lesions are indistinguishable from those seen in Takayasu arteritis (see sec. **IV.B.**).

IV. Differential diagnosis.

The diagnosis of TA is made in the patient with a compatible history and physical findings (secs. **I.–III.**). Polymyalgia need not be present, but the sedimentation rate should be greater than 50 mm/hr. (This is a highly arbitrary but clinically useful rule which should be abrogated only rarely.) A definite diagnosis requires a biopsy showing the histologic changes described in **III**. Finally, all symptoms should dramatically improve on steroids; the exception is loss of vision, which is usually irreversible.

A. Arteriosclerotic vascular disease may be responsible for some clinical signs of TA including decrease in temporal artery pulse, temporal artery thickening, and acute visual loss. Patients have been described with loss of vision, elevated sedimentation rate, and absent temporal pulses, who had only arteriosclerotic changes on temporal artery biopsy and did not respond to steroid therapy. Similarly, patients with previously documented and treated TA may develop symptoms suggesting relapse that are secondary to arteriosclerotic vascular disease (sec. **VI.E.**).

B. Takayasu arteritis is a large vessel disease and does not directly involve the temporal artery or other arteries of medium and small size. Although Takayasu is pathologically indistinguishable from TA involving large vessels, its clinical picture is different. Females predominate, and patients are usually 20 to 50 years old. While arteritic symptoms may be preceded by a "prepulseless" stage (arthralgias and fatigue), the characteristic PMR symptoms are not common. Finally, the sedimentation rate has no consistent pattern, and response to steroids is unpredictable.

C. Systemic necrotizing vasculitis. The temporal arteries may occasionally be histologically involved in patients with polyarteritis (see Chap. 42); however, these arteries are rarely abnormal on physical examination, and clinical signs of TA are rarely seen, even in patients with involvement of the temporal arteries. Finally, kidney and peripheral nervous system involvement is rare in TA, even when large vessels are involved.

V. Therapy. Management of uncomplicated temporal arteritis is prednisone 40 mg PO daily in divided doses. However, when acute visual changes thought to be secondary to temporal arteritis are present, patients should be started on methylprednisolone 80 to 100 mg IV daily and tapered to the conventional oral dose of prednisone 40 mg PO daily after 7 to 10 days. Alternate day therapy is not effective in preventing visual loss. Symptoms (e.g., PMR, headache, and lethargy) should disappear in 36 to 72 hours. Elevated ESR and ischemic manifestations such as temporal headache, jaw claudication, and localized temporal artery inflammation should diminish in several days. The temporal artery pulse may not return and visual loss may be permanent. High-dose steroids should be maintained only as long as necessary for symptoms to resolve and then should be tapered to a maintenance dose of prednisone 5 to 10 mg daily over several weeks. Both clinical signs and sedimentation rate may be used to follow the response. In patients with visual involvement, tapering should be slower. While the average patient will require continued maintenance therapy with prednisone 5 to 10 mg daily for 2 years, some patients may need treatment for as long as 5 years.

VI. Summary of diagnostic and therapeutic approach to temporal arteritis

A. Temporal arteritis suspected (no evidence of ocular involvement). Biopsy the symptomatic artery and, if positive, treat with high-dose steroids. If the biopsy is negative, do not treat with steroids unless clinical suspicion is very strong; in which case, biopsy the contralateral artery. If the biopsy is still negative, but clinical suspicion remains very strong, a short clinical trial of oral prednisone may be warranted. If clinical and laboratory parameters improve, continue therapy (sec. **V.**). If they do not improve dramatically, discontinue the therapy.

B. Temporal arteritis suspected in patient with acute visual loss. Immediately institute treatment with intravenous high-dose steroids (80 to 100 mg methylprednisolone or equivalent). If subsequent biopsy is positive, continue therapy as outlined in **V.** If biopsy is negative and picture is strongly suggestive of temporal arteritis, biopsy the ipsilateral artery and proceed as described in **VI.A.**

C. Polymyalgia rheumatica

1. TA not suspected: do not biopsy. Treat with low-dose steroids (10 to 15 mg prednisone daily).

2. TA suspected: follow procedure described in **VI.A.**; however, if biopsy is negative, low-dose steroids (10 to 15 mg prednisone daily) should be instituted.

D. Large vessel involvement suspected

1. Patient with previously proven TA

a. If involvement clinically insignificant (bruits or diminished pulses), no therapy is indicated.

b. If involvement clinically significant (claudication, coronary artery disease, or other occlusive arterial disease), and if there is other evidence of active TA, treat as described in **V.** Arteriography of the involved artery may be helpful; if it suggests that the vascular symptoms are secondary to arteritis, treat as described in **V.**

2. Patient with suspected TA. Biopsy temporal arteries as described in **VI.A.** If negative, do not institute therapy. If positive, treat as outlined in **V.**

E. Suspected relapse of temporal arteritis

1. If presentation is similar to original episode, re-treat as outlined in **V.** with 40 mg prednisone daily.

2. If presentation is not similar, rebiopsy and proceed as described in **VI.A.**

Bibliography

Fauchald, P., Rygvold, O., and Oystese, B. Temporal arteritis and polymyalgia rheumatica. Clinical and biopsy findings. *Ann. Intern. Med.* 77:845, 1977.

Hamilton, C. R., Shelley, W. M., and Tumulty, P. A. Giant cell arteritis and polymyalgia rheumatica. *Medicine* 50:1, 1971.

Healy, L. A., and Wilske, K. *The Systemic Manifestations of Temporal Arteritis.* New York: Grune & Stratton, 1979.

Hollenhorst, R. W., Brown, J. R., Wagner, H. P., and Shick, R. M. Neurological aspects of temporal arteritis. *Neurology* 10:490, 1960.

Klein, R. G., Campbell, R. J., Hunder, G. G., and Carney, J. A. Skip lesions in temporal arteritis. *Mayo Clin. Proc.* 51:504, 1976.

Klein, R. G., Hunder, G. G., Stanson, A. W., and Sheps, S. G. Large artery involvement in giant cell (temporal) arteritis. *Ann. Intern. Med.* 83:806, 1975.

Wagener, H. P., and Hollenhorst, R. W. Ocular lesions of temporal arteritis. *Am. J. Opthalmol.* 45:617, 1958.

33. Polymyositis

J. Robert Polk

Polymyositis (PM) is an inflammatory disease of striated skeletal muscle. In 40% of patients, a characteristic skin rash is present, thus the term *dermatomyositis*. Dermatomyositis (DM) was described by Unverricht in 1887. PM occurs at any age, but most cases occur between the fourth and sixth decades of life with a mild female preponderance. A childhood form of dermatomyositis has been recognized. Estimates of the *prevalence* of PM range from 0.2 to 0.6 cases per 100,000 population. Polymyositis and dermatomyositis may be associated with malignancy.

Various classification systems have been proposed. It should be remembered that patients who are weak do not all have PM. This fact has been ignored in some series, obscuring the meaning of conclusions.

The classification system of Pearson is the most widely used.

Type I. Polymyositis in adults.
Type II. Dermatomyositis in adults.
Type III. Inflammatory myositis associated with malignancy.
Type IV. Childhood myositis.
Type V. Myositis associated with other rheumatic diseases.

I. Pathogenesis

A. The etiology of PM is unknown. Evidence of infection has been sought with inconclusive results. Some PM patients give serologic evidence of recent infection with *Toxoplasma gondii*, but it is uncertain what this finding means since no other evidence for toxoplasma infection was obtained. There are also a few cases in which *T. gondii* was cultured from muscle. Tubuloreticular and crystalline structures suggestive of viral particles have been found in endothelial cells and muscle cells of some patients with DM. Vascular deposits of immunoglobulin and C3 have been found in children with DM, suggesting that altered humoral immunity may be a factor. Lymphocyte-mediated cytoxicity against muscle cells has also been demonstrated in a group of 9 patients with active PM.

B. The histologic appearance of muscle among these 5 groups is quite similar. The principal feature is an inflammatory cellular infiltrate in muscle, with an associated degeneration and necrosis of muscle fibers. Regeneration of fibers and a perivascular inflammatory infiltrate may be seen. A late finding is interstitial fibrosis. Calcinosis may be seen, especially in the childhood form. In cases that last several months, fiber size variation may occur. Not all the changes of degeneration, inflammatory infiltrate, regeneration, necrosis, and fiber size variation need be present. Ten to twelve percent of muscle biopsies will be normal.

The arteritis of childhood myositis may be seen in small arteries of muscle, skin, and gastrointestinal tract. Although this arteritis was thought not to occur in adult PM or DM, several cases are now reported. The **skin findings** in DM are quite specific clinically, but a nonspecific dermal infiltrate of inflammatory cells is seen histologically.

II. General features

A. General diagnostic considerations. Pearson has defined several criteria to classify patients with PM. PM is **definite** when four criteria are present, probable with three, and possible with two. DM must include the characteristic rash and is definite with three or four criteria present, probable with two, and possible with one. The criteria are:

1. Symmetric proximal muscle weakness with or without dysphagia or respiratory muscle involvement. (See Table 1-2 for grading of muscle weakness.)

2. **Elevation of serum enzymes:** creatinine phosphokinase (CPK), aldolase, lactic dehydrogenase (LDH), and glutamic oxaloacetic transaminase (SGOT).

3. **Typical electromyographic (EMG) triad**

    a. Small amplitude; polyphasic motor unit potentials.

    b. Pseudomyotonic high frequency pattern.

    c. Spontaneous fibrillation and positive sharp waves (sawtooth pattern) in resting muscle.

4. **Typical muscle biopsy histology** as described in sec. **I.B.**

5. **Characteristic skin rash of DM** consisting of a lilac discoloration of the upper eyelids with periorbital edema (the heliotrope rash); and an erythematous or atrophic, scaling, patchy, or linear rash involving the extensor surfaces of the joints, face, neck, back, and chest (in a V-shaped pattern). Erythematous scaling papules (Gottron papules) occur over the metacarpophalangeal and proximal interphalangeal joints.

B. **Diagnostic characteristics of PM types**

1. **Type I. PM in adults.** Proximal muscle **weakness** is the presenting feature in 90% to 95% of patients with PM. Only 25% of patients complain of muscle pain. Arthralgia, Raynaud phenomenon, and dysphagia are seen in 10% to 25%. Patients usually have an insidious onset of proximal weakness and may remain undiagnosed for several months since their complaints are vague. They may note gradually increasing difficulty in climbing steps or getting out of a chair. They may complain of not being able to comb their hair or to reach above their heads. Eventually, the patient may become bedridden and unable to raise the head from a pillow.

2. **Type II. DM in adults.** Rash is the primary presenting feature of DM, and is present initially in about 95% of patients. Only 50% to 60% of patients have proximal muscle weakness at presentation. Follow-up of patients with the rash is therefore essential since it is a rare patient who will not eventually manifest proximal weakness.

    The characteristic rash of DM has been seen in a patient with a systemic vasculitis. Arthralgia, Raynaud phenomenon, and dysphagia are seen in 10% to 25% of DM patients. As in PM, interstitial pneumonitis, cardiomyopathy, and heart block have been reported in DM, but are rare manifestations.

3. **Type III. Inflammatory myositis associated with malignancy.** Controversy exists concerning the true association of PM and DM with malignancy. Most reports indicate that DM has higher association with malignancy than does PM. Between 9% and 20% of patients with PM-DM may have an underlying malignancy. The average age of these patients is the seventh decade. An elderly patient with PM-DM is said to have a 4 times greater possibility of malignancy than his age-matched control.

    About 75% of patients with type III PM present with proximal muscle weakness. Dysphagia occurs in 15% of patients. Malignancies have not been found in childhood DM or in myositis secondary to other connective tissue diseases. In PM-DM of malignancy, the myositis precedes the malignancy in 70% of patients (by an average of 1 to 2 years) and follows it in 30%. In the 30% of patients, it may be called carcinomatous myopathy and be associated with a neuropathy.

4. **Type IV. Childhood myositis.** Childhood DM-PM presents most commonly between ages 7 and 10 years. It occurs slightly more often in females than males. Most patients have the characteristic rash of DM at presentation. About 90% present with proximal muscle weakness. Raynaud phenomenon is said to be less common in childhood DM-PM, but up to 18% of patients may have it.

Distinctive features of the myopathy are atrophy, contractures, and tissue calcifications. Calcifications usually appear after the disease has been present for a year or more.

Visceral involvement is probably more frequent in the childhood than in the adult form. Abnormal pulmonary function, esophageal motility, and gastrointestinal absorption have been reported. Some patients may present with an acute myositis with accompanying fever, malaise, and abdominal pain. Gastrointestinal ulcerations caused by a diffuse necrotizing arteritis (which may also be seen in skin and muscle) may occur.

5. **Type V. Myositis associated with other connective tissue diseases.** Overlap syndromes as defined here consist of PM or DM which fulfill the previously mentioned criteria and the presence of another connective tissue disease which fulfills diagnostic criteria of its own. Type V patients present more commonly than other PM patients with Raynaud phenomenon, sclerodactyly, arthralgia, and myalgia (in about 50% of patients). Proximal muscle weakness occurs in 40% at presentation, and the characteristic rash of DM in 20%. The presenting features reflect the underlying connective tissue disease; systemic sclerosis, systemic lupus erythematosus, and rheumatoid arthritis are the diseases most commonly associated with PM features. Sicca syndrome and necrotizing vasculitis are also associated with PM-DM.

C. **Laboratory features**

1. **White blood cell count and hematocrit** are normal.

2. **Erythrocyte sedimentation rate** (ESR) may be elevated or normal.

3. **Elevated CPK, aldolase, SGOT, and LDH**, with decreasing sensitivity as listed.

4. **Serum myoglobin** is elevated in 75% of patients.

5. **Urine** may contain myoglobin but is otherwise normal.

6. **Rheumatoid factor** is positive in 10% to 50%.

7. **Antinuclear antibodies** are positive in 5%.

8. **Total hemolytic complement** is normal except in childhood DM where it may be low.

9. **EMG triad**

   a. Short duration, small amplitude, polyphasic potentials which appear on voluntary contraction.

   b. Spontaneous high frequency potentials (called pseudomyotonic discharges), which can be triggered by movement of the electrode.

   c. Spontaneous fibrillation and positive sharp waves (sawtooth pattern) identical to the denervation pattern.

10. **Muscle biopsy** reveals inflammatory cellular infiltration of muscle with degeneration, necrosis, and regeneration of muscle fibers. Abnormalities may be focal or diffuse. In childhood DM, arteritis may also be seen.

D. **Differential diagnosis**

1. **Hypothyroid myopathy.** Features such as weight gain, constipation, hoarseness, anemia, and a slow relaxation phase of deep tendon reflexes suggest this disorder. Elevated serum CPK and cholesterol may occur.

2. **Myasthenia gravis.** Ocular symptoms and swallowing difficulties are prominent. Patients complain of increasing weakness with use of muscles and restoration of strength after rest. Muscle enzymes are normal; the edrophonium test is positive; and the EMG has a characteristic pattern (see Chap. 8).

3. **Muscular dystrophies.** A positive family history gives a clue to these disorders, and average onset age is younger than in PM. EMG, muscle biopsy, and muscle enzyme results may be similar to those of PM; however, muscle biopsy usually serves to make the distinction, especially in children (see Chap. 8).

4. **Polymyalgia rheumatica.** Serum muscle enzymes are normal, ESR is always elevated, and malaise and myalgia are prominent complaints (see Chap. 32).

5. **Fibrositis.** Pain in muscles is a prominent complaint, but weakness cannot be demonstrated clinically. Anxiety and depression are common in these patients. Muscle enzymes are normal (see Chap. 22).

6. **McArdle disease.** This disease occurs in young patients who often complain of severe cramping muscular pain after exertion. Myoglobinuria frequently occurs.

7. **Trichinosis.** The periorbital swelling and erythema may mimic those of DM. Distinguishing features include a history of ingesting undercooked pork, nausea, vomiting and abdominal pain, and eosinophilia.

III. Therapy of PM-DM

A. **Supportive therapy.** Patients are usually hospitalized in order to perform diagnostic tests and to begin rehabilitation. Range of motion and passive exercises should be done to prevent contractures, especially in childhood myositis. However, active exercises are not tolerated well early in the disease course. Resting splints are also indicated in patients with foot drop.

B. **Corticosteroids.** Once a firm diagnosis has been established, prednisone 20 mg PO QID is begun. Clinical experience indicates that alternate day steroid therapy is not effective as initial therapy but may be used as the dose is tapered. Divided doses are needed to achieve an optimal antiinflammatory effect.
Controversy exists concerning the best indicators of clinical response. Some experts believe that improvement in serum enzymes is the best indicator of response. However, it takes an average of two months to improve muscle strength by at least one numerical grade. The CPK will usually decrease to half its original value by one month but will not normalize for an average of three months. Because muscle strength often improves before CPK normalization, steroids may be tapered by 2.5-mg increments weekly, using both muscle strength and the serum enzymes as guides. If relapse occurs, then a dose of prednisone 60 to 80 mg should be resumed immediately and tapering deferred until serum enzyme values become normal. A daily dose of prednisone 5 to 15 mg is aimed for. This low dose of corticosteroid should be maintained for 6 to 12 months to allow an adequate period of observation while maintaining some antiinflammatory effect. Discontinuation of steroids should then be attempted by slowly decreasing the dose by 1-mg decrements. A few patients may never be able to discontinue steroids because disease activity remains constant. If no clinical improvement occurs after three months of daily, divided high-dose prednisone, cytotoxic drugs should be used.

C. **Cytotoxic drugs.** These are investigational drugs and should be used only by physicians familiar with their wide toxic potential. See Appendix G for detailed drug information including toxicity. Controlled comparison trials of methotrexate, azathioprine, cyclophosphamide, and plasmapheresis have not been performed.
Methotrexate is the initial drug of choice if prednisone fails to control disease. It is given intravenously at weekly intervals, beginning with a 5-mg dose. Prednisone is also continued. The methotrexate dose is increased by 5-mg increments weekly until a dose of 35 to 50 mg is reached. As improvement in strength occurs, prednisone may be slowly tapered, and methotrexate continued. A response to methotrexate should be seen in about 12 weeks. Methotrexate may be tapered when clinical and laboratory parameters have improved. Hepatic fibrosis may occur with daily methotrexate therapy but is very rare in patients receiving the

drug on a weekly schedule. If methotrexate fails, azathioprine 100 mg daily is recommended.

IV. **Prognosis.** About 75% of patients respond to steroid therapy with improved muscle strength. Long-term survival is about 90% of patients. The worst prognostic indicator is the presence of a malignancy. Patients with myositis of malignancy have about a 45% ten-year survival. These data were collected retrospectively; some neoplasms may have been missed in this series because autopsies were not performed in all deceased patients. Patients with the myositis of malignancy do not respond to steroid therapy as well as other patients with PM. The leading cause of death, excluding the malignancy group, is sepsis. Patients treated early in the course of their myositis seem to respond better than those treated late in their illness. Treatment of the underlying malignancy may occasionally improve the myositis.

Bibliography

Barnes, B. E. Dermatomyositis and malignancy. *Ann. Intern. Med.* 84:68, 1976.

Bohan, A., et al. A computer-assisted analysis of 153 patients with polymyositis and dermatomyositis. *Medicine* 56:255, 1977.

Kagen, L. J. Myoglobinemia in inflammatory myopathies. *J.A.M.A.* 237:1448, 1977.

Metzger, A. L., et al. Polymyositis and dermatomyositis: Combined methotrexate and corticosteroid therapy. *Ann. Intern. Med.* 81:182, 1974.

Packman, L. M., and Cooke, N. Juvenile dermatomyositis. A clinical immunologic study. *J. Pediatr.* 96:226, 1980.

Stevens, M. B. Polymyositis (Dermatomyositis). In A.S. Cohen (Ed.), *Rheumatology and Immunology*. New York: Grune & Stratton, 1979.

34. Pseudogout

John F. Beary III

Pseudogout is an inflammatory arthropathy caused by calcium pyrophosphate dihydrate (CPPD) crystals. Chondrocalcinosis (calcified cartilage seen on radiographs) is found in the majority of pseudogout patients. This disorder (known also as CPPD crystal deposition disease) was first recognized in 1957 by Zitnan and Sitaj who described characteristic radiographic articular calcifications. McCarty in 1962 defined the relationship of intrasynovial CPPD crystals to chondrocalcinosis.

The prevalence of pseudogout is not known, but McCarty reports that his group sees 1 case of symptomatic pseudogout for every 2 patients with symptomatic gout. Five percent of all people older than 60 years have radiographic evidence of chondrocalcinosis. The prevalence of chondrocalcinosis increases with age to involve as much as 28% of the population in the ninth decade.

The mode of inheritance of CPPD is unsettled. However, an autosomal dominant pattern has been described in some populations in which disease begins in early adulthood, progresses rapidly, and is polyarticular.

I. **Pathogenesis.** Aging, osteoarthritis, genetic defects, and certain metabolic disorders are thought to induce abnormalities in cartilage that enhance deposition of CPPD crystals. Crystals are shed into the joint and phagocytized by leukocytes which release lysosomal enzymes, resulting in an acute inflammatory response. If inflammation persists, the cellular infiltrate of the synovium changes to a mononuclear pattern with fibroblastic proliferation.

Diseases associated with CPPD include hyperparathyroidism, hemochromatosis, hypophosphatasia, hypomagnesemia, hypothyroidism, gout, neuropathic arthropathy, and osteoarthritis.

Osteoarthritis and chondrocalcinosis are both common disorders, and their exact relationship has not been established.

II. **Diagnosis**

   A. **History.** Pseudogout occurs in the following forms:

   1. **Acute pseudogout.** Acute monarthritis lasting one day to four weeks in an elderly person is the typical presentation. The knee is the most commonly involved joint. Surgical procedures, especially parathyroidectomy, and severe medical illness may precipitate acute pseudogout attacks.

   2. **Chronic pseudogout.** About 5% of pseudogout patients develop chronic polyarticular inflammation, and CPPD crystals can be demonstrated in their synovial fluids. This disease pattern may resemble either rheumatoid arthritis or osteoarthritis.

   3. **Asymptomatic pseudogout.** This term refers to the radiographic finding of chondrocalcinosis in patients without joint complaints. Knowledge of the presence of chondrocalcinosis alerts the physician to look for intrasynovial CPPD crystals in those patients who subsequently develop arthritis.

   B. **Physical examination**

   1. **Articular features.** Signs of inflammatory synovitis may be seen, particularly in the knees, hips, and wrists. Involvement of the small joints of the hands and feet is uncommon.

   2. **Extraarticular features.** Signs of diseases associated with pseudogout may be present, such as the skin pigmentation and hepatomegaly of hemochromatosis, the band keratopathy and muscle weakness of hyperparathyroidism, or the hoarseness and delayed tendon reflexes seen in hypothyroidism.

C. Laboratory features

1. **Biochemical studies.** There are no known specific biochemical abnormalities of pseudogout itself. However, associated diseases (sec. I.) may be detected by the findings of low serum levels of thyroxine, magnesium, or phosphate; and elevated levels of calcium, iron, or uric acid.

2. **Synovial fluid studies.** Study of aspirated joint fluid is required to confirm the diagnosis. The white blood cell count ranges from 3,000 to 50,000 with 70% or more neutrophils. No organisms are present on Gram-stained smear. Cultures are negative.
   CPPD crystals can be identified using a compensated polarizing microscope (see Chap. 23). CPPD crystals are rhomboid shaped and exhibit weak positive birefringence. The crystals are difficult to see; phase contrast microscopy may assist in crystal identification. The crystals are most readily identified within neutrophils but may be seen free in the synovial fluid as well.

3. **Radiographic findings.** Chondrocalcinosis may be found in about 75% of pseudogout patients when looked for carefully. Sites that are most likely to demonstrate chondrocalcinosis include knee menisci, the symphysis pubis, and the triangular cartilage of the wrist. Chondrocalcinosis is manifested as linear or punctate radiodensities within cartilage. Subchondral bone cysts may be seen.

D. Differential diagnosis

1. Disorders that resemble **acute** pseudogout follow.

   a. **Infection** may be distinguished by prominent systemic signs including fever and the identification of microorganisms by stained smear or culture.

   b. **Gout.** This diagnosis is suggested by the finding of hyperuricemia and confirmed by demonstration of urate crystals in the synovial fluid. However, gout and pseudogout may coexist.

   c. **Hydroxyapatite crystal deposition disease** may produce synovitis or tendinitis. Crystals may be seen with electron microscopy but not with routine polarizing microscopy. Therefore, the diagnosis must be made clinically. Patients with perishoulder calcifications and hemodialysis patients are prone to develop this disorder.

   d. **Other causes** of acute monarthritis are discussed in Chapter 6.

2. Disorders which may resemble **chronic** pseudogout follow.

   a. **Rheumatoid arthritis.** This disorder occurs in a younger population with a female predominance. Features that support a diagnosis of rheumatoid arthritis include subcutaneous nodules, presence of rheumatoid factor, and typical erosive changes seen in joint radiographs.

   b. **Osteoarthritis** is frequently associated with pseudogout. Distinguishing features of osteoarthritis include Heberden nodes and radiographic evidence of osteophytes and subchondral sclerosis.

   c. **Other causes** of chronic polyarthritis are discussed in Chapter 7.

III. Therapy. Any associated diseases such as hemochromatosis or hyperparathyroidism should be managed appropriately.
Chronic pseudogout may be managed with aspirin 900 mg QID. Patients who tolerate aspirin poorly may instead be given naproxen 250 mg BID.
Management of **acute** pseudogout is as follows:

A. **Joint aspiration.** This measure alone can cause an attack of pseudogout to subside. However, drug therapy is usually provided as well.

B. Nonsteroidal antiinflammatory drugs (NSAIDs)

1. **Indomethacin** 50 mg every 6 hours with tapering over 5 days is effective.

2. **Naproxen.** Patients unable to tolerate indomethacin may be treated with naproxen 500 mg initially and then 250 mg every 8 hours with gradual tapering over 5 days.

C. Intravenous colchicine. Hospitalized patients who are unable to tolerate NSAIDs as a result of peptic ulcer disease or edema can be treated with a single dose of colchicine 2 mg IV diluted in saline 15 ml.

IV. Prognosis. Pseudogout itself has no known effect on life expectancy; associated diseases carry their own prognoses.

Joint symptoms can be controlled by the therapy regimens outlined above. Patients with associated osteoarthritis may eventually require prosthetic joints if symptoms and disability become chronic and severe.

Bibliography

Ellman, M. H., Brown, N. L., and Porat, A. P.   Laboratory investigations in pseudogout patients and controls. *J. Rheumatol.* 7:77, 1980.

McCarty, D. J. (Ed.).   Conference on pseudogout and pyrophosphate metabolism. *Arthritis Rheum.* 19:275, 1976.

Tabatabai, M. R., and Cummings, M. A.   Intravenous colchicine in the treatment of acute pseudogout. *Arthritis Rheum.* 23:370, 1980.

Utsinger, P. D., Zvaifler, N. J., and Resnick, D.   Calcium pyrophosphate dihydrate deposition disease without chondrocalcinosis. *J. Rheumatol.* 2:258, 1975.

35. Psoriatic Arthritis

Joseph A. Markenson

Psoriatic arthritis (PA) is an inflammatory arthropathy occurring in 5% to 7% of patients with psoriasis (excluding subjects who are rheumatoid factor positive and presumably have coexisting psoriasis and rheumatoid arthritis). Psoriasis afflicts 1% to 2% of the general population. The pathogenesis of PA is unknown, although a genetic component is evident (see Chap. 5).

I. **Clinical presentations.** Five distinct patterns of PA are recognized.

   A. **Classic** psoriatic arthritis is an asymmetric synovitis involving any joint, most frequently the distal interphalangeal (DIP) joints of the hands and feet; digits affected often have characteristic psoriatic nail changes. This pattern occurs equally in both sexes and represents approximately 10% of all cases of psoriatic arthritis.

   B. **Arthritis multilans** is a particularly disabling form occurring in about 5% of all cases of PA. The deformity, most striking in the fingers and toes, is caused by osteolysis of the affected joints.

   C. **Symmetric polyarthritis** resembles rheumatoid arthritis, is usually rheumatoid factor negative, and comprises about 15% of all cases of PA. Constitutional symptoms such as morning stiffness and fatigue are common and tend to parallel the activity of joint disease.

   D. **Oligoarticular disease** comprises 70% of all cases of PA and is characteristically asymmetric, affecting a few scattered DIP, proximal interphalangeal (PIP), and metacarpophalangeal (MCP) joints, often in association with diffuse swelling of fingers and toes ("sausage digits").

   E. **Psoriatic spondyloarthritis** occurs in up to 5% of patients with PA and presents with clinical and radiographic features that may be indistinguishable from those of idiopathic sacroiliitis or ankylosing spondylitis. The histocompatibility antigen HLA-B27 is found in 40% of this group.

II. **Diagnosis**

   A. **Symptoms** are highly variable according to the anatomic patterns described in section I. Although interphalangeal joints of the fingers and toes are most commonly affected, larger joints such as the knee and ankles may be involved. Constitutional symptoms such as malaise, morning stiffness, and fever can occur and are more commonly seen with the symmetric polyarticular pattern. Back pain may be indicative of psoriatic spondylitis or sacroiliitis.

   B. **Physical signs** include all of the cardinal signs of inflammation in affected joints. Interphalangeal joint involvement is often associated with a sausage appearance of digits. The most common form of PA has the characteristic asymmetric "skip-hit" pattern of digit involvement. Psoriasis may be obvious or represented only as an obscure patch, dandruff, or nail pitting (onychodystrophy). PA usually follows well-established cutaneous or nail lesions, although some patients exhibit characteristic patterns of PA in the absence of such. Ocular disease such as conjunctivitis, iridocyclitis, or episcleritis is rare.

   C. **Laboratory data**

      1. **Rheumatoid factor** is seen in less than 10% of patients.

      2. **Polyclonal hypergammaglobulinemia** is occasionally present.

      3. **Serum complement** in patients with PA tends to be higher than normal;

however, this finding is of no diagnostic significance. Theoretically, elevated synovial fluid complement levels might distinguish PA from rheumatoid arthritis where such measurements are frequently subnormal.

4. **Serum uric acid.** 10% to 20% of patients with psoriasis may have elevated levels of uric acid with severe skin disease.

5. **Erythrocyte sedimentation rate** and other acute phase reactants are elevated and parallel the activity of the arthritis.

6. **Antinuclear factors (ANA)** are usually negative.

7. **Radiographic features** considered classic are the destructive lesions involving predominantly the distal interphalangeal joints of fingers and the interphalangeal joints of the toes. Bony ankylosis of the DIP joints of the hand and toes, along with bony proliferation of the base of the distal phalanx; and resorption of the tufts of the distal phalanges of hands and feet are also commonly seen. Other classic features are fluffy periostitis of large joints, "pencil-in-cup" appearance of DIP joints, absence of symmetry, and gross destruction of isolated small joints. Changes in the spine and sacroiliac (SI) joints may be similar to those seen in ankylosing spondylitis, but SI joint changes in PA are often unilateral and syndesmophytes can sometimes be distinguished from those of ankylosing spondylitis.

D. **Differential diagnosis**

1. **Reiter syndrome.** The cutaneous lesions of Reiter syndrome (RS) resemble pustular psoriasis. RS usually affects large joints in an oligoarticular fashion and rarely involves the distal interphalangeal joints or produces sausage digits. Both illnesses may be associated with spondyloarthritis. The incidence of HLA-B27 is higher in RS than in PA. Radiographically RS may demonstrate periostitis of the plantar surfaces of the calcaneus, metatarsal bones, or ankles. In PA, periostitis is limited to the long bones.

2. **Gout.** Acute psoriatic monoarthritis can resemble but should be differentiated from gout by the absence of monosodium urate crystals in the synovial fluid. Hyperuricemia may occur in up to 20% of patients with skin psoriasis but is uncommon during acute flares of PA. In contrast to monoarticular PA, acute gouty arthritis usually resolves completely in one to two weeks, even if untreated.

3. **Rheumatoid arthritis** is the most difficult entity to differentiate from PA. Distal and asymmetric interphalangeal joint involvement and the absence of rheumatoid factor supports the diagnosis of PA. The presence of skin psoriasis and onychodystrophy help distinguish PA from RA. (Patients with symmetric arthritis, positive rheumatoid factor, and psoriasis are usually considered to have coexistent rheumatoid arthritis and psoriasis.) Subcutaneous nodules are absent in PA. The radiographic features (sec **II.C.7.**) may help differentiate PA from rheumatoid arthritis.

III. **Therapy.** Management goals and therapeutic efforts applied to PA and rheumatoid arthritis are the same.

A. **Physical therapy** is used as an adjunct to drug therapy to help preserve joint range of motion and minimize muscle weakness.

B. **Drug** therapy is aimed at decreasing inflammation of synovial tissue to allow maintenance of joint function. Nonsteroidal antiinflammatory drugs (NSAIDs) are the drugs of choice. Therapeutic options follow in their order of use.

1. **NSAIDs**

a. **Aspirin.** 3.6 gm per day is the initial starting dose given in 4 divided doses with food. In patients with gastric intolerance, the addition of antacids or the substitution of other salicylate preparations may be helpful.

b. **Ibuprofen** 600 mg QID, naproxen 250 mg BID, and fenoprofen 300 mg QID are other NSAIDs which can be tried sequentially in patients who fail to respond to aspirin.

c. **Indomethacin** 75 to 200 mg per day in divided doses is usually an effective antiinflammatory agent for both spondyloarthritis and peripheral arthritis.

d. **Sulindac** 150 to 200 mg BID, a nonsteroidal antiinflammatory drug much like indomethacin, requires less frequent dosage and may be associated with less gastrointestinal intolerance.

e. **Tolmetin** 400 mg TID is chemically similar to indomethacin and sulindac, and is the only NSAID approved by the Food and Drug Administration for use in children under the age of 14.

f. **Phenylbutazone** 100 to 200 mg TID is recommended as a supplementary agent to be used for a short term (one to two weeks) in acute flares of arthritis. Concern regarding drug toxicity precludes its chronic use.

2. **Gold salts.** A course of gold aurothioglucose is indicated for the treatment of progressive severe PA, especially in those instances where the disease resembles rheumatoid arthritis. A full course usually starts with sequential weekly intramuscular injections of 10, 25, and then 50 mg until a total dose of 1,000 mg is achieved. If successful, monthly maintenance injections of 50 mg are given indefinitely.

3. **Antimalarial** therapy has been associated with exfoliative skin reaction in persons with psoriasis; however, recent studies have concluded that such drugs can be used safely and that they have the potential for inducing remission of PA. Hydroxychloroquine 400 mg per day for 1 month followed by 200 mg per day is recommended. Hydroxychloroquine therapy probably should be considered when PA fails to respond to NSAIDs or gold.

4. **Immunosuppressive drugs.** Methotrexate should be reserved for patients with the most severe form of disease who have failed all other therapy modalities. Parenteral or oral administration of methotrexate in doses of 10 to 25 mg per week (maximum dose, 50 mg per week) is usually successful in suppressing cutaneous and articular manifestations of psoriasis. A commonly employed oral regimen consists of a series of 3 doses (2.5 to 10 mg each) administered at 12-hour intervals over a 36-hour period each week. The drug is hepatotoxic; some authorities recommend a liver biopsy before starting therapy and at six-month intervals while patients receive methotrexate. Careful monitoring of liver function tests, complete blood counts to detect marrow suppression, and chest radiographs to detect methotrexate-induced infiltrates are mandatory.

5. **Reconstructive surgery** is of value in patients with end-stage joint destruction. Procedures employed and indications are similar to those for rheumatoid arthritis (see Chap. 39).

IV. **Prognosis.** The prognosis for patients with PA varies according to the anatomic patterns. The severity of arthritis tends to parallel the severity of skin disease. Most patients have mild episodic disease, affecting only a few joints. For these, the prognosis is generally favorable. Approximately 5% of patients develop severe disabling and deforming arthritis. The axial spondyloarthropathy of PA is associated with many of the same extraarticular manifestations as in idiopathic ankylosing spondylitis (uveitis, conduction defects, aortitis), and these features may significantly contribute to morbidity. Complications of therapy, especially corticosteroids, have been the largest contributing factor to mortality in several large series.

Bibliography

Katz, W. A. Psoriatic Arthritis and Reiter's Disease. In W. A. Katz (Ed.), *Rheumatic Diseases Diagnosis and Management.* Philadelphia: Lippincott, 1977, P. 540.

Kommer, G., Soter, N. A., Gibson, D. J. and Schur, P. H. Psoriatic arthritis: A clinical, immunologic and HLA study of 100 patients. *Semin. Arthritis Rheum.* 9:75, 1979.

Moll, J. M. H., and Wright, V. Psoriatic arthritis seminar. *Arthritis Rheum.* 3:55, 1978.

36. Reflex Sympathetic Dystrophy Syndrome

Stuart S. Kassan

The reflex sympathetic dystrophy syndrome (RSDS) is an excessive or abnormal response of the sympathetic nervous system in an extremity to a traumatic injury or other condition. It is first associated with swelling and pain in an affected extremity, which are often later accompanied by trophic skin changes, vasomotor disturbances, and limitation of motion in that extremity.

The entity of RSDS was first described by Mitchell in 1864. Since that time, numerous other descriptions of the syndrome have appeared (e.g., Sudek atrophy, shoulder-hand syndrome, Sudek osteodystrophy, algoneurodystrophy), which have tended to confuse the discussion of this entity.

Early reports emphasized certain isolated features of the syndrome such as its posttraumatic aspects (e.g., posttraumatic osteoporosis, traumatic vasospasm) or neurovascular aspects (e.g., peripheral acute trophoneurosis, algoneurodystrophy). More recent reports tend to support a unifying concept of the disorder which takes into account both the numerous potential causes and outward clinical presentations associated with the syndrome.

No precise **prevalence** has been given for RSDS; however, one study reports the development of the syndrome in 1 of every 2,000 accident cases. Reflex sympathetic dystrophy syndrome has been reported in 5% to 20% of coronary artery disease patients, 20% of patients with hemiplegia, and 3% of patients sustaining peripheral nerve injuries.

I. **Pathogenesis.** The exact cause for the syndrome is unclear. Numerous medical and surgical disorders (Table 36-1) have been implicated as possible etiologic factors. The ultimate development of the disorder is thought to occur by reflex neurologic mechanisms. Numerous theories have been proposed regarding the neurologic mechanisms involved, but no consensus has been reached.

II. **Diagnosis**

   A. **Clinical findings**

      1. **History** of a precipitating event is elicited in about two-thirds of patients with RSDS.

      2. **Pain** in the affected extremity.

      3. **Edema** (pitting or nonpitting).

      4. **Skin changes (trophic)**

         a. Skin atrophy.

         b. Hair loss.

         c. Desquamation.

         d. Nail changes (brittleness).

         e. Flexion contractures or thickening of the palmar fascia, or both.

      5. **Vasomotor instability** results in a warm or cool extremity, depending on whether vascular dilation or constriction predominates, and increased perspiration.

      6. **Decreased range of motion or pain,** or both, in ipsilateral shoulder (shoulder-hand syndrome).

   B. **Stages of development**

      1. **Stage I (acute stage)** is associated with edema, pain, vascular changes, and muscle wasting. It may last up to three months.

Table 36-1. Conditions Associated with the Development of RSDS

Trauma

Neurologic disease
   Central nervous system lesions with hemiplegia
   Spinal cord lesions
   Radiculopathies
   Peripheral nerve lesions
   Postherpetic neuralgia

Atherosclerotic cardiovascular disease
   Myocardial infarction
   Angina pectoris
   Postcoronary bypass surgery

Degenerative joint disease of shoulder

Pulmonary tuberculosis

Drugs
   Isonazid
   Barbiturates

    2. Stage II (dystrophic stage). Dystrophic changes with cool skin, loss of hair, loss of movement, and bone rarefaction on x-ray occur. This stage may persist up to six months.

    3. Stage III (atrophic stage). Skin and soft tissue atrophy, osteopenia, bone erosions, and proximal spread of pain are late changes with poor potential for reversibility.

  C. Radiologic changes

    1. Patchy **osteoporosis** in a diffuse or juxtaarticular distribution is usually seen alone in the extremity ipsilateral to any identifiable provocative factor.

    2. Erosions may be seen, especially in metacarpophalangeal, metatarsophalangeal, and distal interphalangeal joints. Progression of osteopenia and bone erosions usually parallels the activity of the clinical disease.

  D. Bone scan changes consist of increased uptake, often in a periarticular distribution. The bone scan is useful early in the course of RSDS when radiographs are likely to be negative.

  E. Histologic changes. Synovial histologic findings in RSDS are nonspecific and include edema, proliferation and disarray of synovial lining cells, capillary proliferation, and fibrosis of subsynovium.

  F. Laboratory data. No specific laboratory changes have been demonstrated in RSDS.

III. Differential diagnosis. Although several of the following may be inciting causes for RSDS, they may also be confused with the syndrome early in their course.

  A. Infection. Acute or chronic osteomyelitis.

  B. Inflammatory arthritis

    1. Erosive arthritis, especially rheumatoid arthritis.

    2. Nonerosive asymmetric arthritis (seronegative).

    3. Crystal-induced arthropathies such as gout or pseudogout.

  C. Central nervous system diseases

    1. Degenerative disease affecting the spinal cord, including syringomyelia, and lower motor neuron disease.

    2. Traumatic central nervous system disease.

D. Peripheral nerve diseases

    1. Systemic diseases with infiltrative metabolic or nutritional processes.

    2. Traumatic or degenerative disorders.

IV. Therapy

  A. Early mobilization of the affected extremity following a traumatic injury, herniated intervertebral disc syndrome, myocardial infarction, or surgical procedure is important.

  B. Physical therapy should include passive and active range of motion exercises. Local heat or local cooling of the involved extremity is employed depending upon whether vasospasm or vasodilation is the dominant feature.

  C. Sympathetic blockade. If physical therapy measures fail, one may try up to four nerve blocks administered on alternate days by an experienced physician. Twenty-five percent of patients will respond. Those in whom local blocks provide any relief of symptoms may then be considered candidates for surgical sympathectomy.

  D. Transcutaneous nerve stimulation is an experimental modality which has been used successfully in some patients.

  E. Systemic corticosteroids are reserved for patients who fail the measures outlined in **A.–D.** The regimen is prednisone 60 mg per day in 2 divided doses for 2 weeks followed by a rapid tapering course over the next 1 to 2 weeks to 10 mg every other day. Subsequent tapering is then guided by the clinical response. The goal is to discontinue prednisone within eight weeks.

V. Prognosis. Treatment is more successful if begun within six months of symptoms. However, 50% of patients fail to respond.

Bibliography

Kozin, F.   Painful Shoulder and the Reflex Dystrophy Syndrome. In D. J. McCarty, (Ed.), *Arthritis and Allied Conditions* (9th ed.). Philadelphia: Lea & Febiger, 1979. P. 1091.

Kozin, F., McCarty, D. J., Sims, J., and Genant, H.   The reflex sympathetic dystrophy syndrome. I. Clinical and histologic studies: Evidence for bilaterality, response to corticosteroids and articular involvement. *Am. J. Med.* 60:321, 1976.

Williams, W. R.   Reflex sympathetic dystrophy. *Rhematol. Rehabil.* 16:119, 1977.

37. Reiter Syndrome

Allan Gibofsky

The association of arthritis with urethral infection was first described by Van Forest in the sixteenth century. In 1818, 300 years later, Brodie described 5 male patients with the triad of urethritis, conjunctivitis, and polyarthritis, and in 1916, Hans Reiter, a German physician, described the triad in a cavalry officer following an episode of bloody diarrhea and ascribed the manifestations to a spirochete (which was not found in later cases). The first case in the American literature was described by Bauer and Engleman in 1942, who referred to Reiter's report and applied his name to the association of nongonococcal urethritis, arthritis, and conjunctivitis.

The exact frequency of Reiter syndrome (RS) is unknown, largely because the diversity of manifestations and their temporal dissociation often obscure or delay diagnosis. In the United States and Great Britain, most cases follow extramarital intercourse, suggesting that the disease is venereally acquired. Several large European series, however, have documented RS following epidemic dysentery. In many of these patients, no history of antecedent sexual intercourse could be obtained.

Although the disease has been reported in childhood, it is usually seen in young adults with a male-female ratio of 15 : 1. No causative organism has been conclusively identified; however, a majority of patients have the lymphocyte antigen HLA-B27 (see Chap. 5), indicating a genetic predisposition.

I. **Pathogenesis.** The disease is characterized by the clinical triad of polyarthritis, urethritis, and conjunctivitis, although incomplete forms may be seen as well. While the cause remains unknown, the appearance of symptoms following either epidemic dysentery or sexual intercourse suggests that the clinical features represent an inflammatory reaction to an infectious organism in a genetically predisposed host. Mycoplasmas, chlamydiae, and *Shigella, Salmonella,* and *Yersinia* bacteria are suspected causative organisms.

II. Diagnosis

A. Constitutional symptoms

1. **Fatigue** not prominent, but may be seen with chronic relapsing course.

2. **Weight loss** usually mild.

B. Physical findings

1. **Fever** usually low grade (less than 38°C) in most patients.

2. **Arthritis.** Large weight-bearing joints are usually involved in an asymmetric, polyarticular pattern, but finger and toe involvement may also be seen.

3. **Genitourinary**

   a. Mucopurulent or mucoid urethral discharge seen in males. Females difficult to diagnose but urethral ulcers may be present. Patients are usually asymptomatic but may complain of dysuria.

   b. Prostatitis and hemorrhagic cystitis common.

4. **Ocular**

   a. **Conjunctivitis.** Usually mild, presenting as slight burning sensation and complaints of lid adhesiveness; usually bilateral.

   b. **Iritis.** May be seen in 10% of patients initially; reported in up to 50% of chronic cases.

5. **Gastrointestinal.** Diarrhea, when it occurs, is of variable severity and is occa-

sionally bloody. In most instances, it precedes other manifestations of the syndrome by several weeks.

6. **Skin and mucous membrane** (see Chap. 10).

   a. **Balanitis circinata,** which are coalescing, shallow, superficial ulcers on the penis, are common.

   b. Similar painless ulcers may also be seen on the tongue or buccal mucosa.

   c. **Keratoderma blennorrhagica,** cornified skin lesions containing keratotic material, are common on the palms and soles, and are a self-limiting problem.

7. **Cardiologic.** Pericarditis may be seen in the active disease. Increased PR interval and nonspecific ST-T wave changes have been reported in rare cases.

C. Laboratory data

1. **Hematologic findings**

   a. **White blood cell (WBC) count** usually elevated to level of 10,000 to 18,000 cells/mm^3.

   b. **Hematocrit** usually normal acutely; normocytic or normochromic anemia may develop in patients with chronic course.

   c. **Sedimentation rate** often elevated greater than 100 mm/hr and returns to normal as patient recovers from acute attack.

2. **Urinary findings.** Pyuria and hematuria common; sterile urethral discharge contains abundant polymorphonuclear leukocytes.

3. **Joint fluid**

   a. Usually turbid to grossly purulent (2,000 to 50,000 cells/mm^3).

   b. Neutrophils are seen early, followed by predominance of lymphocytes in chronic joint effusion.

   c. Synovial fluid glucose usually normal; may be low if leukocytosis is present.

   d. Complement may be elevated but is nondiagnostic. (Serum complement is frequently increased.)

4. **Stool cultures.** Usually negative for enteric pathogens.

5. **Radiographic findings**

   a. **Painful joints** are usually normal during earlier stages; **osteoporosis** may be seen in later stages.

   b. **Periosteal proliferation** near involved joints frequent. Periostitis of the os calcis (bone spurs, "lover's heel") common but nondiagnostic.

   c. **Sacroiliitis** indistinguishable from ankylosing spondylitis is seen in up to 80% of patients with chronic disease. May be unilateral.

6. **Immunogenetics.** The lymphocyte antigen HLA-B27 has been reported in approximately 75% of patients with RS.

D. Differential diagnosis

1. When the triad of features (arthritis, conjunctivitis, urethritis) occur together in the same episode, with or without mucocutaneous manifestations, the diagnosis is established.

2. **Gonorrhea.** Acute nature of polyarthritis may suggest bacterial infection, and joint aspiration may be useful. However, it is sometimes impossible to distinguish gonococcal arthritis with a sterile joint fluid from RS. Features suggest-

ing a diagnosis of gonorrheal arthritis include tenosynovitis, pustulovesicular skin lesions, and a response to penicillin therapy.

3. Rheumatoid arthritis. While the chronic joint symptoms may suggest rheumatoid arthritis, asymmetric arthritis, sacroiliitis, and rheumatoid factor negativity support the diagnosis of RS.

4. Psoriasis. Keratoderma blenorrhagica may resemble pustular psoriasis which may also be accompanied by spondylitis. However, in contrast to those of RS, the skin lesions of psoriasis are most common on the scalp, elbows, and knees and do not resolve spontaneously.

5. Behcet syndrome. In contrast to RS, the oral and genital lesions of Behcet syndrome are painful.

III. Therapy. There is no specific treatment of RS. Antibiotics of value in RS therapy have not been documented.

A. Eye inflammation. The conjunctivitis of RS is usually mild and self-limited. However, a few patients develop chronic uveitis which should be managed by an ophthalmologist.

B. Arthritis. The disease subsides spontaneously in the majority of patients, but chronic axial or peripheral arthritis may occur.

1. Spondylitis is treated as described in Chapter 20.

2. Peripheral arthritis may be treated with one of the following nonsteroidal antiinflammatory drugs listed in their order of trial.

a. Aspirin 900 to 1,200 mg QID.

b. Indomethacin 25 to 50 mg TID.

c. Naproxen 250 mg BID.

IV. Prognosis. The majority of patients recover from the initial manifestations within several months. However, recurrences are common, with most patients having two or more episodes. The recurrent attack may present with complete triad or with a single disease feature. Chronic Reiter disease is most severe in HLA-B27 positive individuals who are often affected with spondylitis.

Bibliography

Morris, R., et al.   HLA-A W27. A clue to the diagnosis and pathogenesis of Reiter's syndrome. *N. Engl. J. Med.* 289:554, 1974.

Weinberger, H. W., et al.   Reiter's syndrome, clinical and pathologic observations: A long-term study of 16 cases. *Medicine* 41:35, 1962.

Wright, V., and Moll, J. M. H.   *Seronegative Polyarthritis.* Amsterdam: Elsevier, 1976.

38. Rheumatic Fever

Stephanie Korn

I. **Etiology and pathogenesis.** Rheumatic fever is a sequela of streptococcal pharyngitis, caused by mechanisms not well-defined despite much research. Current thinking suggests that the disease results from an unusual immunobiologic reaction of the host to streptococcal antigens.

II. **Prevalence.** Both the occurrence and severity of disease have declined dramatically over the past four decades in developing countries; this reflects a decrease primarily in recurrent rather than first attacks. In addition to antibiotics, socioeconomic factors and possibly factors of streptococcal virulence may contribute to the decline. An estimated 12,000 new cases of rheumatic fever in the age range of 5 to 14 years is expected annually in the United States. Worldwide, rheumatic fever remains a major health problem.

III. **Clinical features**

A. **Antecedent streptococcal pharyngitis** most commonly occurs two to three weeks before onset of acute rheumatic fever (ARF), although history may be negative for preceding fever and sore throat.

B. **Fever** is almost always present at onset of acute attack. It has no specific pattern. Fever may fade away in days to weeks without antiinflammatory treatment or more rapidly with treatment.

C. **Arthritis** with fever is the most common manifestation of ARF, occurring in about 75% of cases. Arthralgia without objective evidence of joint inflammation is less specific than arthritis but may be severe and, if migratory, can strongly support other evidence of ARF. Large peripheral joints are most commonly involved, but nearly any joint may be affected. Because arthritis responds dramatically to salicylates, these should be withheld during observation for joint manifestations. Without treatment, arthritis generally subsides in a few weeks and does not cause joint deformity. Arthritis usually occurs within five weeks of the streptococcal infection and this is coincident with high antistreptococcal antibody titers. Carditis occurs less frequently in cases with severe arthritis.

D. **Carditis** is the most important manifestation of ARF because it involves chronic valvular damage, although death caused by myocarditis with cardiac failure or arrythmias can occur during a severe acute episode. Carditis is said to occur in about 40% to 50% of attacks of ARF, but this incidence seems to be decreasing.

1. Symptoms of chest pain or dyspnea may occur, but complaints are often not specific to cardiac involvement.

2. **Major signs**

a. **Significant new or changing murmurs,** described below, are characteristic of acute vasculitis, often disappear with resolution of acute inflammation, and differ from the murmurs of valvular stenosis or regurgitation which may be heard later.

(1) **Mitral valvulitis murmur** is blowing, high-pitched, holosystolic, apical, and transmits to the axilla.

(2) **Carey Coombs murmur** is middiastolic, low-pitched, apical, and often associated with the mitral valvulitis murmur.

(3) **Aortic valvulitis murmur** is a soft, high-pitched, decrescendo blow, heard immediately after the second heart sound.

b. **Cardiomegaly** should be carefully monitored by serial chest x-rays.

c. **Congestive heart failure** occurs more commonly in children under six years of age and in patients without severe arthritis.

d. **Pericarditis,** when present, occurs in association with other manifestations of rheumatic carditis. Pericarditis may be expressed by chest pain, friction rub, effusions, and electrocardiogram (ECG) changes. Large effusions are rare.

e. **Other cardiac findings** may include tachycardia at rest (out of proportion to fever), and a soft, dull, first heart sound secondary to prolonged PR interval, which may be variable. The atrioventricular (AV) block is commonly seen in cases of ARF without other evidence of carditis or subsequent rheumatic heart disease; it is thought to be a toxic manifestation of ARF and not specifically indicative of carditis.

E. **Erythema marginatum** is a nonpruritic rash beginning as a pink macule that spreads outward in a sharp ring with central clearing or serpigenous coalescing lines. The rash is evanescent, rarely raised, blanches with pressure, is brought out by application of heat, and is distributed over trunk and proximal extremities, never on the face and rarely on distal extremities. The rash may appear early or late in the course of ARF or may come and go unrelated to the course of other manifestations or to treatment. Rash secondary to drug reaction or systemic juvenile rheumatoid arthritis can usually be differentiated by the characteristics just mentioned and other associated clinical manifestations.

F. **Subcutaneous nodules** are firm, nontender, nonpruritic, freely movable swellings located in crops of variable numbers over bony prominences and tendons without overlying skin discoloration. Nodules are a late and infrequent manifestation associated with severe carditis. The nodules of ARF tend to be smaller and less persistent than those of rheumatoid arthritis.

G. **Sydenham chorea** is characterized by involuntary, purposeless, abrupt, and non-repetitive movements, muscular weakness, and emotional lability. The abnormal movements subside during sleep. When subtle, chorea is demonstrated when: (1) squeezing the examiner's hand reveals an erratic "milkmaid's grip," (2) raising the arm above the head causes pronation of one or both arms, (3) extending the hands straight ahead causes spooning of the hand with wrist flexion and extension of fingers, and (4) protruding the tongue produces snakelike darting movements. A late manifestation, chorea may follow other features of ARF or may appear alone. The latent period from streptococcal infection to chorea is thought to be between one and six months; thus antistreptococcal antibodies and acute phase reactants may be normal. In Sydenham chorea patients, an antibody has been found which reacts with basal ganglia and cross-reacts with streptococcal cell membranes. Duration of chorea ranges from a week to a year with an average of three months.

IV. **Laboratory findings**

A. **Evidence of preceding streptococcal infection** may be obtained by throat culture (in about 25% of cases), by very high or rising titers of antistreptolysin O antibodies (in about 80% of cases), or by rising titers to one of the other extracellular antigens such as hyaluronidase or DNase B.

B. **Acute phase reactants.** Erythrocyte sedimentation rate (ESR) and C-reactive protein (CRP) reflect ongoing rheumatic inflammation and are useful in monitoring response to therapy.

C. **Antiheart antibodies** that cross-react with streptococcal cell membrane have been found in high titer in the serum of ARF patients but do not indicate the presence of carditis. With standardization of the technique, this test may become more readily available to clinicians.

D. **Serial chest x-rays** are important to reveal cardiomegaly as a sign of carditis.

E. Serial electrocardiograms may reveal the nonspecific AV block discussed in section **III.D.2.e.** or changes of myocarditis and pericarditis.

V. Diagnosis and differential diagnosis

A. The revised Jones criteria indicate a high probability of ARF when evidence of a preceding streptococcal infection is found with two major criteria or one major and two minor criteria.

  1. **Major manifestations** are carditis, polyarthritis, chorea, erythema marginatum, and subcutaneous nodules.

  2. **Minor manifestations** are fever, arthralgia, previous rheumatic fever or rheumatic heart disease, elevated ESR or CRP, and prolonged PR interval.

B. Differential diagnosis

  1. **Bacterial infections** including septic arthritis, osteomyelitis, and subacute bacterial endocarditis should be routinely sought by appropriate cultures.

  2. **Viral infections,** particularly rubella arthritis, arthritis associated with HB virus infection, and infectious mononucleosis, should be considered.

  3. **Collagen vascular disease,** rheumatoid arthritis, systemic lupus erythematosus (SLE), and vasculitis such as Henoch-Schönlein purpura may be differentiated on clinical and laboratory grounds.

  4. **Immune complex disease** induced by allergic reaction to drugs may be suggested by history and by clinical features such as pruritic or urticarial rash.

  5. **Sickle cell hemoglobinopathies** may superficially resemble ARF, but their differentiation is not difficult.

  6. **Malignancies,** especially leukemias and lymphomas, can present with fever and acute polyarthritis.

VI. Therapy

A. Antibiotic treatment with penicillin, or erythromycin in case of allergy, is recommended in a standard ten-day course for streptococcal pharyngitis to eradicate any residual organisms from the throat. There is, however, no evidence that such therapy significantly alters the acute or chronic phase of the disease. Daily penicillin prophylaxis (see **B.5.**) is begun after the ten-day course of treatment.

B. Antiinflammatory treatment suppresses symptoms, but evidence does not indicate that it alters the duration of the attack or the ultimate cardiac damage.

  1. **General measures** which are helpful include:

     a. Use of analgesics before initiating antiinflammatory treatment.

     b. Sodium restriction, digitalis, and diuretics for heart failure.

     c. Bed rest for three weeks if carditis is absent, and for four or more weeks if present, followed by gradual resumption of activities.

  2. **Salicylates** are highly effective in controlling fever and arthritis. If instituted before adequate observation, the expression of these symptoms may be masked, rendering the diagnosis inconclusive. A dose of about 80 mg/kg per day in divided doses with a resultant blood level of 20 to 30 mg/100 ml is usually effective in controlling the symptoms of fever, arthritis, and mild carditis when given at this dose for 2 weeks and at about 60 mg/kg per day for 6 subsequent weeks.

  3. **Corticosteroids** have not been shown to be more effective than aspirin in reducing long-term cardiac damage. Nevertheless, they are often used to treat carditis because their antiinflammatory effect is more prompt and potent. The dose of prednisone is 1 to 2 mg/kg per day in divided doses for 2 to 4 weeks with

tapering of the dose in the final week and addition of salicylates for another 4 to 8 weeks.

4. **Treatment of chorea** includes keeping the patient in a quiet protective environment and sedation with phenobarbital 3 to 5 mg/kg per day or chlorpromazine 25 to 100 mg TID as needed.

5. **Prophylaxis** with penicillin to prevent progressive cardiac damage caused by recurrent streptococcal infections and rheumatic attacks is given as penicillin G 250,000 units PO twice daily or benzathine penicillin G 1.2 million units IM every 4 weeks. For patients allergic to penicillin, either sulfadiazine 500 to 1,000 mg PO QID or erythromycin 100 to 250 mg PO BID may be given.

   Minimum recommended duration of prophylaxis is five years from the last recurrence. Recurrent attacks in adulthood are known to occur, however, and since long-term prophylaxis appears to be benign, it is probably advisable to continue prophylaxis indefinitely. All patients with evidence of chronic rheumatic heart disease, regardless of age, should be on continuous prophylaxis.

Bibliography

Markowitz, M., and Bordin, L. *Rheumatic Fever.* Major Problems in Clinical Pediatrics (second ed.), edited by A. J. Schaffer, vol. 2. Philadelphia: Saunders, 1972.

Stollerman, G. H. *Rheumatic Fever and Streptococcal Infection.* New York: Grune & Stratton, 1975.

39. Rheumatoid Arthritis

Stephen Paget and William Bryan

The term *rheumatoid arthritis* (RA), introduced by Garrod in 1859, describes a systemic disease that is characterized by a female-male predominance of 3 : 1, a symmetric inflammatory polyarthropathy with morning stiffness, and rheumatoid factor positivity in 80% of patients. Rheumatoid arthritis occurs in 1% to 2% of the U.S. population. The clinical course is highly variable: in some, manifestations are mild while in others the disease rapidly progresses to severe disability. Approximately 70% of patients manifest a chronic course, and 15% of this group develop a severe progressive crippling form of RA.

I. **Pathogenesis.** Compelling evidence implicates genetic and immunologic processes in the initiation and perpetuation of the inflammatory events characteristic of RA. Recent data indicate that susceptibility to RA is an inherited trait, determined by gene products of the major histocompatibility system. Such genes probably control the humoral and cell-mediated immune mechanisms thought to participate in the pathogenesis of RA. The source and character of the stimulus of the immunologic abnormalities are not known, but current interest is focused on atypical infectious agents. The terminal events of the pathogenesis of RA involve the generation of enzymes that cause tissue injury.

II. **Diagnosis**

   A. **Symptoms and signs.** The diagnosis of RA is based on the following criteria:

   1. **Persistent** (greater than three months), **symmetric polyarthritis** characteristically involving the small joints of the hands and feet. Quantification of joint involvement by number and severity is the primary way in which disease activity is assessed.

   2. **The presence of systemic features** such as fatigue, weight loss, and anemia.

   3. **The presence of rheumatoid nodules** (found in 20% of RA patients).

   4. **The exclusion of other systemic disorders** such as systemic lupus erythematosus, the seronegative spondyloarthropathies, and other diseases presenting as chronic polyarthritis (see Chap. 7).

   B. **Laboratory studies** that help to confirm the clinical impression of RA are:

   1. **Rheumatoid factor.** Eighty percent of RA patients have in their serum an IgM antibody (rheumatoid factor) reactive with the Fc portion of an IgG molecule. A latex fixation titer of 1 : 160 or greater is considered significant but is not specific for RA. The diagnosis of RA does not depend on the presence of serum rheumatoid factor (RF). It is not clinically useful to follow the RF once it is documented to be positive.

   2. **Elevated erythrocyte sedimentation rate (ESR).** This test is a nonspecific reflection of the amount of inflammation present. An elevated ESR and other acute phase reactants such as C-reactive protein are commonly found in active RA.

III. **Therapy.** Although no specific or curative therapy is available, most patients can benefit by a comprehensive approach using medical, rehabilitative, and surgical services. The management of RA involves the following goals: (1) education and motivation; (2) induction of a remission through the suppression of inflammation in the joints and other tissues; (3) maintenance of joint function and prevention of deformities; and (4) repair of joint damage if it will relieve pain or facilitate function.

A comprehensive therapeutic plan for the RA patient includes: (1) patient and family education, (2) systemic and articular rest, (3) physical medicine, (4) medical therapy, and (5) surgical treatment. Medical therapy, in order of usage, consists of:

Level I	Salicylates
Level IIA	Other nonsteroidal antiinflammatory drugs (NSAIDs)
Level IIB	Gold
Level IIC	Antimalarial drugs
Level III	Penicillamine
Level IV	Corticosteroids
Level V	Cytotoxic drugs

A. **Patient and family education** is important in the management of rheumatoid disease. Strong emphasis must be placed on the crucial role played by the patient in minimizing disability. Both the patient and the family must be taught what RA is and how it differs from other forms of arthritis. The patient should be told that RA can be a chronic, lifelong disease for which there are a variety of measures that can lead to disease control. Such emotional support may help the patient to maintain employment or an optimal activity schedule. In addition to familiarizing patients with the concepts of chronic disease and its management, specific points must be stressed regarding individual drug and physical medicine modalities used, nutritional information, quackery, and the social services available to the patient with arthritis. Such an educational program can take the form of frank discussions between the physician and the patient and family, supplemented by literature dispensed by the doctor. An optimum setting would be provided in an established patient education program that employed lecture and audiovisual material. Sex and vocational counseling should be part of the comprehensive approach to the RA patient.

B. **Systemic and articular rest.** It is important for the RA patient to maintain a balance between resting and exercising joints that falls short of causing significant pain or fatigue. Systemic and articular rest are both important. Although the classic recommendations for short rest periods during the day (one hour of bed rest in the midmorning and midafternoon) remain, they are incompatible with the work requirements of most individuals. At times, hospitalization may become necessary to impose a strict balance of rest and activity that cannot be followed by the patient at home. Articular inflammation may be decreased by adequate rest of the affected joints utilizing either bed rest or splints.

The purpose of **splints** is to provide rest for inflamed joints, relieve spasm, and prevent deformities or reduce deformities already present. Wrist splints are particularly useful during bouts of acute wrist synovitis and for management of carpal tunnel syndrome.

C. **Physical medicine.** Employ the following measures.

1. **Regular active exercises** with instruction by the physician or the physiotherapist. Exercise is most successful after heat application. A 15-minute early morning shower or a bath at 98°F to 100°F will help decrease morning stiffness. Unless advanced deformity, significant joint pain, or muscle wasting is present, slow and deliberate active or active-resistive exercises should be performed twice daily for approximately 15 minutes. These exercises should primarily involve the fingers, wrists, shoulders, and knees, the areas most vulnerable to deformity and functional disability (see Appendix C).

As tolerance for exercise increases and the activity of the disease decreases, progressive resistive exercises are indicated for the improvement of muscular function. Static quadriceps exercises should be performed to strengthen the muscular, ligamentous, and tendinous support of the knees. Initial therapy is 10 to 20 exercise sets in each thigh twice daily.

2. **Principles of joint protection** include maintenance of muscle strength and range of motion; avoidance of positions of deformity; the use of the strongest joints possible for a given task; the utilization of joints in the most stable anatomic planes; avoidance of continuous use of muscles and joints in a fixed position; and avoidance of activities not within the patient's muscular capacity. Active exercises in the form of activities that interest the patient should be provided (e.g., sculpting, clay modeling, weaving).

3. **Activities of daily living.** Instruction by the occupational therapist should include self-help devices, resting and functional splints, and the demonstration of alternate methods for task performance aimed at avoiding positions that cause joint deformity.

D. **Drug therapy.** Additional information on the drugs discussed below can be found in Appendix G.

1. **Salicylates** (level I) are the initial treatment of choice for RA; in some patients, no additional drug therapy is required. Aspirin (acetylsalicylic acid) is antiinflammatory in therapeutic doses of 3.6 to 7.5 gm per day (serum salicylate levels of 15 to 30 mg/100 ml) and is analgesic at lower doses. Although pain, stiffness, and swelling are diminished, salicylates and other antiinflammatory drugs are not thought to alter directly the natural course of the disease.

   a. **Indications.** Aspirin is the first-line drug for the treatment of RA as a result of its low cost and analgesic, antipyretic, and antiinflammatory effects. So effective are salicylates in the management of RA that different forms of aspirin should be tried before it is concluded that the patient is unable to take any salicylate preparation. Salicylates should remain the baseline therapy despite the addition of other forms of medical management such as nonsteroidal antiinflammatory drugs, gold, or penicillamine.

   b. **Dosage regimen.** Salicylates are administered at doses of 600 to 1,200 mg every 4 to 6 hours, usually with meals or with antacid to minimize gastric irritation. Constant serum drug levels can be achieved in most patients with this dosage interval. For an antiinflammatory effect, a blood level between 15 and 25 mg/100 ml is optimum and requires doses between 3 and 6 gm daily. The doses needed to achieve therapeutic concentrations vary widely, especially in the elderly. Salicylate levels can also be used to monitor compliance.

   Hepatic metabolic pathways may become saturated at higher dose levels. Therefore, a small dose increase can result in a very large elevation of the serum salicylate level. The maximum tolerated dose should be approached slowly because it may take as long as a week after each dose change to achieve a new, steady level. Rectal suppositories are available; however, rectal absorption is incomplete. The following oral salicylate preparations are available.

      (1) **Plain tablets.** Inexpensive; may cause gastric mucosal injury; standard tablet size 325 mg.

      (2) **Buffered tablets.** Formulated with insoluble calcium and magnesium antacids; no firm evidence of reduced gastric irritation.

      (3) **Enteric-coated tablets (Ecotrin).** Coating intact until tablet reaches small intestine, thus well-tolerated with minimal gastric bleeding; monitor serum salicylate level because absorption varies.

      (4) **Timed-release tablets.** Encapsulated aspirin particles; absorption delayed; more sustained plasma levels; some decrease in gastrointestinal (GI) bleeding but no practical advantage at high-dose levels.

      (5) **Sodium salicylate.** Enteric-coated preparations preferred; less potent analgesic than aspirin; does not inhibit platelet function; less gastric bleeding; effective antiinflammatory agent; watch total sodium intake in heart failure or hypertension.

      (6) **Choline salicylate.** Very soluble; liquid form; negligible gastric bleeding; probably somewhat less effective than aspirin; no platelet dysfunction.

   c. **Common side effects.** The most common side effects of aspirin include dyspepsia, GI bleeding, and peptic ulceration. Bleeding results from local mucosal irritation; it does not occur if the drug is given intravenously.

Taking aspirin with meals will reduce the incidence and severity of dyspepsia but does not reduce occult bleeding (2 to 10 cc/24 hr in 70% of patients taking usual aspirin doses). Guaiac-positive stools (trace to 1 plus) are common during aspirin therapy. GI evaluation is performed when clinically indicated by symptoms such as a large hemoglobin decrease, syncope, or melena.

Tinnitus or deafness are usually the earliest indications of salicylate toxicity in adults and are reversible with a small (i.e., two-tablet) decrease in daily dosage. There is an inverse relationship between plasma salicylate levels at which auditory symptoms appear and the age of the patient.

Central nervous system symptoms such as headache, vertigo, nausea, vomiting, irritability, and even psychosis can occur, especially in the elderly. At high serum levels (25 to 35 mg/100 ml), especially in juvenile patients, salicylates may cause mild, acute, reversible hepatocellular injury as demonstrated by a rise in serum enzymes. This is not an absolute indication for the discontinuation of aspirin especially if the drug is effective in disease control.

Platelet adenosine diphosphate (ADP) release, adhesiveness, and aggregation are inhibited for as long as 72 hours after a single 300 mg dose of aspirin, probably as a result of irreversible acetylation of platelet membrane proteins. This side effect should be taken into consideration before and following surgery and in the final weeks of pregnancy.

2. **Other NSAIDs (level IIA).** These agents are equipotent to aspirin and are thought to exert their antiinflammatory action by modifying prostaglandin metabolism. They cost about ten times as much as aspirin.

   a. **Indications.** Aspirin intolerance; as an adjunct to aspirin to achieve additional antiinflammatory effect.

   b. **Common adverse reactions.** Similar to aspirin including dyspepsia, GI bleeding, and platelet dysfunction. In addition, headache, dizziness, and sodium retention may occur. See formulary for detailed discussion of each drug (Appendix G). NSAIDs are not recommended in pregnant or nursing women.

   c. **Administration.** There are more than a dozen NSAIDs available. The complete list is found in Appendix G. The agents listed below have been successfully used at our institution.

      (1) **Naproxen.** Well-tolerated. BID dosage regimen encourages compliance. Tablet size 250 mg. Usual dosage is 250 mg BID.

      (2) **Fenoprofen.** Capsule sizes are 300 mg and 600 mg. Usual dosage is 600 mg QID.

      (3) **Indomethacin.** This agent is particularly effective in control of acute RA flares. Capsule sizes are 25 mg and 50 mg. Usual dosage regimen is 25 mg BID or TID. The dose may be increased by 25 mg at weekly intervals until a maximum daily dose of 150 mg is reached.

3. **Gold salts** (level IIB)

   a. **Indications.** Gold is a remittive agent which can prevent disease progression. At least two-thirds of patients with RA who receive therapeutic amounts of gold show significant improvement of synovitis. Because of toxicity, gold is not the initial therapy for RA. It is reserved for patients who continue to have active synovitis or who develop erosions on a conservative regimen of nonsteroidal antiinflammatory drugs, rest, and physiotherapy. Patients with rheumatoid nodules or strongly positive tests for rheumatoid factor (latex fixation titer greater than 1 : 320) may be candidates for earlier treatment because the prognosis implied by these findings is poor. Generally, gold is not indicated for mild disease, pauciarticular (two or three involved joints) arthritis, or end-stage noninflammatory disease.

b. **Contraindications and side effects.** Gold is contraindicated in patients with a history of previous severe skin, bone marrow, or renal reactions to gold. Significant functional impairment of the kidneys or liver is a relative contraindication to gold therapy, but toxicity to these organs is rare and, with careful clinical and laboratory monitoring, serious problems can be avoided. Leukopenia was previously considered a relative contraindication, but gold-induced improvement of leukopenia has been demonstrated in patients with Felty syndrome (RA, granulocytopenia, and splenomegaly). As a rule, phenylbutazone, oxyphenbutazone, or immunosuppressive drugs such as azathioprine or cyclophosphamide are not given concomitantly with gold because, like gold, they may suppress the bone marrow.

Toxicity usually appears after 300 to 500 mg of gold has been administered; however, undesirable reactions may occur at any time during the course of therapy. Although the incidence varies, at least 35% of patients receiving gold salts develop some toxicity:

(1) **Skin and mucous membranes.** The most common manifestation of gold toxicity is dermatitis, which may be heralded by pruritis or eosinophilia and is almost always reversible. Stomatitis is another mucocutaneous side effect and is frequently painless. The development of these side effects is an indication to withhold gold until the lesions clear. Except in the instance of exfoliative dermatitis, an uncommon but serious problem, therapy can be reinstituted at a dose lower than that used before the appearance of the skin problem. Isolated eosinophilia is also noted frequently and should merely alert the physician to watch more carefully for side effects.

(2) **Renal.** Proteinuria is detectable at some time in at least 10% of patients receiving gold therapy. Urinalyses should be performed before each gold injection. Nephritis and the nephrotic syndrome are much less common. The most common histologic lesion is a membranous glomerulonephritis with deposits of immunoglobulin and complement in the glomerulus. Renal failure is rare. If minor urinary abnormalities occur (proteinuria less than 500 mg/24 hr), therapy should be interrupted until the urine is normal, then reinstituted at small doses. If the abnormalities recur, gold must be stopped. Most reactions, particularly dermatitis and proteinuria, will clear following discontinuation of the drug. Antihistamines (hydroxyzine 25 mg TID) may be useful for pruritis. Corticosteroids (prednisone 40 to 60 mg/24 hr) are beneficial in some instances of exfoliative dermatitis and nephritis. Treatment with heavy metal chelators (dimercaprol or penicillamine) is usually unnecessary.

(3) **Hematologic.** The most serious side effects of gold therapy are hematologic disorders, which include thrombocytopenia, agranulocytosis, and aplastic anemia. These complications are rare. Granulocytopenia may be noted incidentally on routine blood tests or may present with fever and pharyngitis. Thrombocytopenia is not dose-related and may occur after very low cumulative doses of gold compounds. Aplastic anemia is a rare complication and has been reported even long after the cessation of gold therapy. For the first few months of therapy, complete blood and platelet counts should be done before each gold injection is given. If no changes have occurred after three to four months, the tests can be done at two-week intervals and, ultimately, at monthly intervals. A trend toward progressive cytopenia may be observed by making a flow sheet of the patient's laboratory data.

Management of severe hematologic gold toxicity includes the administration of prednisone 60 mg daily in 3 divided doses; anabolic steroids such as testosterone proprionate 200 mg IM, 3 times weekly; and chelating agents such as dimercaprol, penicillamine, and ethylenediaminotetraacetate (EDTA). However, it has not been proven that any of these therapies influence outcome.

252

(4) **A nitritoid reaction** consisting of flushing of the face and neck, shortness of breath, tongue swelling, nausea, and vertigo can sometimes occur after administration of gold compounds, especially gold thiomalate. Management includes switching to another gold compound or decreased dosage, and administration with the patient supine.

(5) **Miscellaneous.** A number of unusual adverse reactions have been ascribed to gold including enterocolitis, intrahepatic cholestasis, skin hyperpigmentation, peripheral neuropathy, deposits of gold in the cornea (chrysiasis), and pulmonary infiltrates.

In summary, patients with severe toxicity such as thrombocytopenia, aplastic anemia, exfoliative dermatitis, or nephropathy should not be re-treated with gold. With milder side effects, especially mucocutaneous reactions, it may be possible to reinitiate gold beginning with low doses after resolution of the skin reaction.

c. **Administration.** Gold thioglucose is given by deep IM injection. The initial dose should be small (10 mg) to test for drug idiosyncrasy (e.g., rash, thrombocytopenia). If this dose is tolerated, 25 mg should be given 1 week later, and then 50 mg weekly if tolerated. The therapeutic response begins in most patients when the cumulative dose is 300 to 700 mg. Serum gold levels do not correlate with disease activity. Improvement is gradual and continues over a period of several weeks. When improvement levels off, usually at doses ranging from 500 to 1,000 mg, the dose of gold can be decreased to 50 mg once every 2 weeks for several injections, then to 50 mg once every 3 weeks for several injections, and finally to 50 mg once a month. If gold is discontinued, the condition flares in some patients within several months. Therefore, if tolerated, it is recommended to continue gold injections indefinitely. The degree of improvement is proportional to the duration of treatment. However, if improvement does not occur after 1,000 mg, the drug should be discontinued. Future courses of gold salts in such patients are unlikely to be effective.

4. **Hydroxychloroquine** (level IIC) is an antimalarial agent with antiinflammatory effects in RA and systemic lupus patients.

a. **Indications.** Hydroxychloroquine may be used in patients with RA who fail to respond to a conservative regimen of rest, salicylates, other NSAIDs, or gold. It is especially useful in patients who have toxic reactions to gold after showing a good therapeutic response.

b. **Contraindications and side effects.** This drug is contraindicated in patients with significant visual, hepatic, or renal impairment, with porphyria, or in pregnant women and children. The most common undesirable side effects are allergic eruptions and GI disturbances, including nausea, diarrhea, and unexplained weight loss. An important toxic effect is chloroquine deposits in the cornea which may interfere with vision; this development is completely reversible if the drug is discontinued. Of even greater importance is the ability of hydroxychloroquine to damage the retina, an effect which is not reversible. Because of this potentially serious side effect, the patient must be seen by an ophthalmologist at 3-month intervals. At the first sign of any visual impairment (especially reduced sensitivity to red light), the drug should be stopped.

c. **Administration.** Tablet size is 200 mg. Six weeks to six months of therapy may be required before a therapeutic effect is evident. If objective improvement does not occur within six months, the drug should be discontinued. Initial dosage in adults is 400 mg daily taken with food to decrease gastric intolerance. When a good response is obtained (4 to 12 weeks), the dosage is decreased to a maintenance dose of 200 mg daily. Doses of 300 to 400 mg daily should not be exceeded because toxic side effects are increased at higher doses.

5. Penicillamine (level III)

 a. Indications. This drug has been shown in controlled studies to be effective in reducing inflammatory synovitis in approximately 50% of patients with RA, a response rate similar to that to gold. Some authors have suggested that penicillamine is of particular value in the therapy of extraarticular manifestations of RA such as rheumatoid vasculitis and Felty syndrome. Toxic side effects are common (60% of patients) and may be severe; therefore, penicillamine should be reserved for patients who have failed to respond to or tolerate level I or II RA therapy.

 b. Contraindications and side effects. A history of allergy to penicillin is *not* a contraindication to penicillamine, but institution of therapy in such patients should be carried out under close observation and using low dosage (125-mg tablets). Contraindications include pregnancy, renal failure, and patients who are unreliable, do not have access to a telephone, or have poor ability to communicate their symptoms.

  (1) Skin mucous membrane. Pruritis and skin rash represent the most common side effects; rashes may occur at any time during the course of therapy. These may be controlled by concomitant administration of an antihistamine (hydroxyzine 25 mg TID) or a moderate reduction in dosage. If rash persists despite these measures, the drug should be stopped for at least three months. Low-dose readministration may be possible after this period of interruption. A sudden febrile response, often associated with a generalized rash, may occur within the first three weeks of therapy; defervescence occurs when the drug is stopped, but rechallenge is not recommended. Stomatitis has been observed and often clears with decreased dosage. If oral ulcers persist, the drug should be stopped permanently. Blunting or alteration in taste perception (dysgeusia) usually occurs during the first six weeks of penicillamine therapy. It gradually disappears despite continuation of therapy.

  (2) Hematologic. Hematologic toxicity is potentially dangerous and dictates a need for close follow-up: complete blood counts, including platelet count, at two-week intervals for the first six months of therapy and at least monthly thereafter should be taken. Recording laboratory data on flow sheets will permit early detection of downward trends in white blood cell (WBC) or platelet counts. Hematologic toxicity may be sudden in onset and may occur in the interval between scheduled laboratory studies; thus patients must be alerted to report skin or mucous membrane bleeding, infection, or fever. Leukopenia of 3,000 cells/mm^3 or less or a platelet count below 100,000/mm^3 requires immediate and permanent discontinuation of penicillamine therapy. Leukopenia associated with thrombocytopenia or thrombocytopenia alone may indicate impending aplastic anemia.

  (3) Renal. Proteinuria is encountered in up to 20% of patients on long-term therapy. If proteinuria of two plus or more has persisted for 30 days and other causes of renal disease have been excluded, a 24-hour urine protein determination should be done and repeated at monthly intervals. As long as the protein excretion does not exceed 1 gm per day and creatinine clearance is stable, the drug may be continued. Proteinuria may clear completely with only a 125-mg reduction in the daily dose. Development of hypoalbuminemia, nephrotic syndrome, or hematuria requires discontinuation of the drug. Nephrosis is reversible but urinary abnormalities may persist up to one year. Rechallenge will usually lead to recurrence of proteinuria.

  (4) Miscellaneous. Uncommon side effects include autoimmune syndromes such as drug-induced lupus, Goodpasture syndrome, and polymyositis. They require discontinuance of penicillamine.

c. **Administration.** Available as 125-mg and 250-mg tablets. Up to 12 weeks may elapse between the initiation of penicillamine therapy and the observation of signs of improvement. Thus, increments in penicillamine dosage should be made at 12-week intervals. The initial regimen is a single daily dose of 250 mg which is maintained for 3 months. If no clinical or laboratory (decreased ESR) evidence of response is found, the dose is doubled to 500 mg. After the next 3 months, if there is still no evidence of response, 750 mg per day is given in 2 doses. If necessary, 500 mg twice daily for a final 3 months may be tried, but toxicity increases at high doses. Most patients demonstrate evidence of improvement at the end of the first 6 months of therapy. One should attempt to reduce the daily dose in decrements of 125 mg at 3-month intervals in order to determine the least amount of drug required to sustain a remission.

6. **Corticosteroids** (level IV). Although these drugs are the most potent of the antiinflammatory agents, they have a high incidence of toxicity and do not change the course of RA.

   a. **Indications.** Before these drugs are used, the patient and the physician must balance the desired benefits against toxic effects. A program of corticosteroid therapy is justified only after alternative treatments have been tried. The indications for **systemic** corticosteroids are:

      (1) **Active synovitis in many joints,** in spite of a good conservative regimen of antirheumatic therapy including a program of physiotherapy and levels I–III drug therapy.

      (2) **Incapacitating constitutional symptoms** such as fever, anemia, weight loss, neuropathy, or rheumatoid vasculitis. Intraarticular corticosteroids are useful when only a few joints are affected and are the source of significant disability. This form of steroid administration may be used to supplement levels I–III therapy since systemic side effects do not occur when used properly.

   b. **Contraindications and side effects.** As a result of disease chronicity in a majority of RA patients, a large number of rheumatoid patients develop chronic steroid dependency. Such patients, especially when treated with prednisone doses of more than 7.5 mg daily for long periods, are likely to develop the serious and multiple side effects outlined in Appendix G.

   c. **Administration**

      (1) **Intraarticular corticosteroid.** The risk of introducing infection, although slight, is always present; careful aseptic technique is required. (For dosage and preparations, see Chap. 3.) An evanescent postinjection flare may occur from inflammation induced by leukocyte ingestion of corticosteroid microcrystals. This possibility should be brought to the patient's attention. Within 24 to 48 hours, joint pain should improve, and relief may persist anywhere from a few days to a few months. Frequent intraarticular corticosteroid injections (more than once in a two- to three-month period or more than three times per year) are not advised because there is evidence that accelerated cartilage destruction may occur.
      Remember: One should suspect sepsis in RA patients who have an isolated joint inflamed out of proportion to other joints. This possibility especially holds for joints that have received previous injections.

      (2) **Systemic corticosteroid.** Prednisone is the preferred agent because its cost and mineralocorticoid activity are low. Tablets are available in 1-mg and 5-mg sizes. When used to suppress synovitis, the regimen is 5.0 to 7.5 mg of prednisone, preferably in a single morning dose although divided dose schedules may be required. The total dose should be the smallest possible needed to ameliorate symptoms. The physician

should attempt to decrease steroid requirement by using NSAIDs. RA patients tolerate alternate day corticosteroid therapy poorly because synovitis tends to flare on the "off" day. At times, an acute flare of RA may require in-hospital management with the institution of prednisone 20 to 30 mg daily for 3 to 5 days with tapering, but only if more conservative therapy has failed.

Rheumatoid vasculitis, if manifested by mesenteric and other internal organ ischemia, is an indication for prednisone 40 to 60 mg per day because of its malignant, life-threatening nature.

7. **Cytotoxic drugs.** Two types of cytotoxic drugs, the purine analog azathioprine and the alkylating agent cyclophosphamide, have been studied in patients with RA. There is accumulating evidence that these experimental drugs are effective in controlling rheumatoid disease. Cyclophosphamide has been shown to minimize the development of joint erosions.

   a. **Indications.** Azathioprine or cyclophosphamide may be used in patients with severe RA who continue to have active, incapacitating inflammatory synovitis in spite of therapy with NSAIDs, gold, penicillamine, and corticosteroids. Because of their toxicity, they should be used as a last resort in patients who are significantly disabled by active synovitis or by systemic manifestations of rheumatoid disease. Patients must be informed, cooperative, and willing to permit meticulous follow-up by the physician. The responsible clinician must be familiar with all of the toxic effects of each drug and be prepared to monitor both short- and long-term toxicity.

   In general, we favor the initial use of azathioprine to cyclophosphamide because incidence of severe side effects is lower and patient's tolerance is better. In severe life- or organ-threatening vasculitis, cyclophosphamide is the preferred drug.

   b. **Contraindications and side effects.** These drugs are contraindicated in pregnant women. They should be used with great caution and at reduced doses in patients with hepatic or renal impairment and should not be administered to patients with a history of malignant tumors. Undesirable side effects of both agents include bone marrow suppression (more common with cyclophosphamide) and hepatotoxicity (more common with azathioprine). The incidence of malignant tumors, especially involving the hematopoietic system, is increased in patients receiving immunosuppressive drugs. Additional undesirable side effects of cyclophosphamide are alopecia, amenorrhea, irreversible sterility in both men and women, hemorrhagic cystitis, and carcinoma of the bladder.

   If these agents are used, it is imperative that complete blood counts (CBCs) and urinalyses (with cyclophosphamide therapy) be done at frequent intervals. The intervals should be weekly at first; then, after the first two months, CBC, differential, platelet counts, and urinalyses should be done once every two to four weeks. A persistent decrease or rapid fall in leukocyte count dictates a decrease in dosage or temporary discontinuance of the drug.

   c. **Administration.** Because these drugs are experimental and have potentially severe toxicity, informed consent should be obtained from the patient.

   With both azathioprine and cyclophosphamide, it is desirable to begin therapy with relatively small doses to minimize the chances of bone marrow suppression. This side effect is more common with cyclophosphamide than with azathioprine. With either azathioprine or cyclophosphamide, objective improvement, if it occurs, does not appear until several weeks of therapy have elapsed. If there is no response after 16 weeks, the drugs should be discontinued. If synovitis has been controlled for several months, it is desirable to taper these agents slowly and attempt to discontinue use. Tapering may result in a disease flare, but this risk must be compared to the increased risk of malignancy with long-term therapy.

(1) Azathioprine is available in 50-mg tablets. Therapy is begun with 50 mg daily and the dose is increased by weekly 50-mg increments until a 2 to 3 mg/kg maintenance dose is reached (if weekly CBC, differential, and platelet counts remain stable). If GI symptoms occur following administration of the drug, it may be given in a single dose at bedtime to minimize this effect.

Caution: In patients receiving allopurinol, azathioprine should be employed with great caution and only at reduced doses.

(2) Cyclophosphamide is supplied as 25- and 50-mg tablets. It should be started in relatively small oral doses of 1.5 to 2.0 mg/kg. This dose can be raised to 2.5 to 3.0 mg/kg over a few weeks if complete blood counts and platelet counts remain normal and no other toxicity appears. For patients with RA, the maximal dose is 3 mg/kg. Cyclophosphamide must be given in the morning and a large urine volume should be maintained. Patients should be encouraged to void frequently and to urinate in the middle of the night to prevent prolonged bladder contact with drug metabolites.

IV. Surgical treatment. Orthopedic surgeons have a major role in the management of RA. Traditional techniques of joint fusion and synovectomy remain in the orthopedist's armamentarium while total joint arthroplasty is achieving an even higher level of acceptance.

Surgical reconstruction in RA patients must be regarded as part of a comprehensive care plan and judiciously balanced with medical management. The pattern of joint involvement and eventual functional goals of the patient must be considered.

A. Criteria for surgery. Many factors enter into the choice and timing of an operation. More than 40 years ago, Dr. Philip Wilson, Sr. of the Hospital for Special Surgery listed these questions to assist in forming a surgical plan.

1. Is the arthritis still active?

2. Is the patient in adequate physical condition to permit extensive surgical procedures?

3. Considering the age and physical state of the patient, and the number of operations required, is the expected gain in function from the operation worth the effort?

4. Should the operation be delayed in order that other therapy may be instituted?

5. Will the patient cooperate in postoperative care with the proper morale and willingness to endure some pain?

6. Are the comprehensive facilities necessary for successful treatment present in the hospital?

7. Will the patient be able to receive proper postoperative care on leaving the hospital?

8. Will the patient's financial status permit independent undertaking of the entire treatment, or have community resources been mobilized to care for such treatment?

In the final analysis, either intractible pain or disability requires the patient to request the operation.

B. Surgical procedures

1. **Cervical spine.** Cervical spine instability should be considered in all patients with cervical neck pain, occipital or lower cervical radiculopathy, patient-reported neck crepitance, instability on active motion, or signs of cervical myelopathy. Radiographic signs of cervical spine instability may be seen in 40% of RA patients, but only 10% of these will develop neurologic symptoms.

Important lesions include atlantoaxial subluxation, superior migration of dens, and subaxial subluxation. Subluxation of lower cervical vertebrae is most common at the C3-C4 level. These lesions can be expected to progress in 30% of patients. Lateral cervical spine films in extension and flexion are mandatory for evaluation of instability.

Cervical orthotics can serve as temporary stabilizing devices but little evidence exists to suggest that they enhance autofusion. Surgical intervention is reserved for those with incapacitating pain related to spine instability or neurologic signs of cord or root entrapment. All levels of instability should be included in a posterior cervical fusion procedure. Along with traditional wiring and autogenous bone grafting techniques, methylmethacrylate cement has proved of great value in achieving stabilization of osteoporotic bone, especially where long fusions are needed for multiple levels of instability. Postoperative care should include a rigid orthotic device until bony consolidation appears on x-ray.

2. **Shoulder.** Evaluation of shoulder pain in RA requires differentiating soft tissue pain from that of articular origin. Bursitis, bicipital tendinitis, and rotator cuff tears can be discerned with a careful history, examination, diagnostic xylocaine injections, and arthrograms when indicated (see Chap. 13). Rotator cuff tears are difficult to repair in this group as a result of degenerated tissue. The presence of severe articular destruction and refractory pain and disability is an indication for total joint replacement. Shoulder prostheses are in a state of evolution as problems of restoring rotator cuff power in the face of degenerated tissue and loosening of the glenoid component have required design adjustment.

3. **Elbow.** Elbow synovectomy and radial head excision can be expected to provide good pain relief in those with persistent elbow synovitis and minimal bone loss. Total elbow replacement is reserved for patients with severe articular destruction and moderate activity expectations because lifting heavy objects on a repetitive basis will cause prosthesis loosening.

4. **Wrist and hand.** Severe wrist synovitis and bony destruction are amenable to surgical therapy; the degree of involvement dictates the choice of a synovectomy and ulnar head resection (dorsal stabilization procedure), a total wrist arthroplasty, or wrist fusion. Total wrist arthroplasty retains wrist motion while providing pain relief. While ten-year follow-up data are not available, early results are encouraging.

Wrist synovitis can attenuate and rupture extensor tendons. Wrist synovectomy is indicated in the presence of persistent boggy dorsal swelling to prevent rupture of extensor tendons.

Silastic implants (Swanson prostheses) continue to play an important role in the management of thumb and metacarpophalangeal (MCP) joint disease. Critical to success are soft tissue balancing and prolonged dynamic postoperative splinting to prevent recurrence of ulnar drift. This procedure results in pain relief with only slight decrease in grip strength. While fusions are not indicated for finger MCP joints, they are often useful in advanced proximal interphalangeal joint disease to reestablish a functional hand. Thumb reconstruction requires careful consideration of tendon imbalance and articular destruction. A combination of tendon repositioning and joint fusion is often needed.

5. **Hip.** Total hip replacement has provided consistent success in treating end-stage RA hip disease. Early problems with materials and designs, infections, and pulmonary emboli have diminished, and clinical results are steadily improving. Present areas of clinical research include techniques of managing deficient acetabuli and the improvement of acrylic-cementing technique. Presently under investigation are porous metals and plastics which may be superior to acrylic cement in the prevention of latent stem loosening. Concern for femoral stem loosening has led to enthusiasm for surface replacement pro-

cedures in which the femoral neck is capped with a hollow metal hemisphere. Results are too preliminary to endorse this procedure as an alternative to total hip replacement.

6. **Knee.** Knee synovectomy can be expected to provide pain relief in those with persistent boggy synovitis, recurrent large painful effusions unresponsive to medical therapy, and minimal articular destruction. Long-term studies have shown that while pain relief is good, synovectomy does not prevent progression of cartilage loss. Regrowth of the synovial membrane often occurs within three to five years.

   Total knee replacement can give results as good as those in total hip replacement if patients are properly selected. A variety of nonarticulated condylar prostheses are available and allow for the resurfacing of the femoral, tibial, and patellar surfaces. Preexisting alignment deformities (varus-valgus) or flexion contractures require experienced surgical attention for soft tissue balancing, proper bony cuts, and component choice.

7. **Ankle and foot.** Ankle pain may be due to talotibial or subtalar disease. This differentiation is important in selecting the proper surgical procedure.

   a. **Talotibial pain** that is intractible is treated by ankle fusion. Rates of latent loosening in total ankle replacements have been too high to gain general acceptance.

   b. **Subtalar pain,** elicited by hindfoot inversion or eversion, is a result of destructive changes in the talocalcaneal, talonavicular, and calcaneocuboid joints. Triple arthrodesis which fuses three joints is a highly successful procedure.

   c. **Forefoot pain** in RA is the result of synovitis, capsular destruction, and joint subluxation giving rise to hallux valgus (bunion) or metatarsalgia. Carefully placed shoe inserts can redistribute weight and provide pain relief (see Chap. 18). Surgery is reserved for those who fail conservative treatment. Excision of the first metatarsal exostosis and the proximal one-half of the proximal great toe phalanx (Keller procedure) is a time-honored procedure for correction of hallux valgus in RA. Excision of the metatarsal heads (Hoffman procedure) is successful in relieving plantar metatarsal pain.

V. Prognosis. In general, 70% of patients with RA experience chronic disability with alternating incomplete remission and exacerbation. While 10% to 20% have sustained remissions, a similar number will develop a severe, crippling disorder. The potential for disease remission is greatest within the first year. The following, in a statistical sense, are unfavorable prognostic features: (1) female sex, (2) insidious onset, (3) *early* detection of rheumatoid factor positivity, erosions, subcutaneous nodules, multiple joint effusions, and constitutional symptoms, (4) initial severe disease activity, and (5) extraarticular features such as neuropathy, pericarditis, scleritis, and vasculitis.

Diseases Associated with Rheumatoid Arthritis

I. **Sicca syndrome.** See Chapter 41.

II. **Felty syndrome** consists of RA, splenomegaly, and granulocytopenia; hematologic abnormalities may also include anemia and thrombocytopenia. Recurrent infections and chronic leg ulcers are common complications. The response of granulocytopenia to high-dose corticosteroids is usually disappointing. Recurrent systemic infections or pancytopenia are indications for splenectomy, although the results of this procedure are variable. Gold (see preceding sec. **III.D.** for dose regimen) and lithium carbonate (300 mg BID) are experimental therapies.

III. **Rheumatoid vasculitis** occurs in approximately 5% to 10% of patients with RA and can be life-threatening. In its mildest form, it is manifested as systemic fatigue, weight loss, fever, peripheral neuropathy, and necrotic skin lesions. Mortality is high in patients with digital gangrene and peripheral neuropathy as a result of frequent involvement of the mesenteric and coronary arteries and the central nervous system. There are no certain successes in the management of RA vasculitis. Therapy employed includes prednisone (40 to 60 mg/24 hr), penicillamine (up to 1,000 to 1,500 mg/24 hr), and cytotoxic drugs (azathioprine or cyclophosphamide, each 2 to 3 mg/kg/24 hr). Of these, only prednisone can be expected to have an immediate suppressive effect; hence it is the recommended treatment for patients with life-threatening visceral vasculitis. In very high risk situations, prednisone may be combined with a slower acting agent (penicillamine or a cytotoxic drug) in the hope that the latter will permit earlier reduction of steroid treatment. Reports regarding the efficacy of plasmapheresis, leukopheresis, and thoracic duct drainage are too preliminary to judge these measures' roles in the treatment of RA vasculitis.

IV. **Pulmonary and other systemic manifestations of RA.** Several patterns of pulmonary disease are infrequent but significant manifestations of RA: solitary or multiple nodules, pleuritis or pleural effusions, interstitial pneumonitis, and diffuse granulomatous pneumonitis. Granulomatous pneumonitis is sometimes associated with similar lesions affecting the eye (scleromalacia), heart, and other organ systems. The frequency of these problems is higher in patients with Felty syndrome and vasculitis than with RA; no generalizations can be made regarding management, but the same principles associated with RA vasculitis (sec. **III.**) apply to patients with life-threatening patterns of illness.

Bibliography

Bunch, T. W., and O'Duffy, J. D.   Disease-modifying drugs for progressive rheumatoid arthritis. *Mayo Clin. Proc.* 55:161, 1980.

Christian, C. L., and Paget, S. A.   Rheumatoid Arthritis. In M. Samter (Ed.), *Immunological Diseases* (3rd ed.). Boston: Little, Brown, 1978.

Ferguson, R. H., and Polley, H. F.   Treatment of the complications of rheumatoid arthritis. *Clin. Rheum. Dis.* 1:429, 1975.

Paget, S. A., and Gibofsky, A.   Immunopathogenesis of rheumatoid arthritis. *Am. J. Med.* 67:961, 1979.

Pearson, C. M., et al.   Diagnosis and treatment of erosive rheumatoid arthritis and other forms of joint destruction. *Ann. Intern. Med.* 82:241, 1975.

40. Scleroderma and Undifferentiated Connective Tissue Syndromes

H. Hallett Whitman III

Scleroderma (systemic sclerosis) is a syndrome characterized by excessive fibrosis and vascular changes in multiple organ systems. The incidence ranges between 4 to 12 cases per 1 million population, and is higher if overlap syndromes with other rheumatic diseases are included. There is a 4 : 1 female-male predominance.

I. **Pathogenesis.** Vascular damage occurs in most involved organ systems and is the hypothetical unifying pathologic feature of scleroderma. The recognized small arterial pathology is intimal proliferation, medial thinning, adventitial collagen cuffing, and chronic inflammation. This lesion is classically seen in the kidney and peripheral vasculature. Other organ systems show varying degrees of arterial damage. It is unclear whether vascular pathology leads to abnormal collagen metabolism or vice versa. In a recent study, sera of scleroderma patients was specifically cytotoxic for human endothelial cells, and the partially purified cytotoxic factor was free of immunoglobulin. Despite the known association of scleroderma with other autoimmune diseases, and the recent demonstration of antinuclear antibodies in a high percentage of scleroderma patients, the exact role of the humoral or cellular immune system in the pathogenesis of the disease has not been elucidated.

II. **Diagnosis.** The hallmark of systemic sclerosis is taut, hidebound skin (scleroderma) with thinning of the overlying epidermis. Scleroderma usually occurs first on the extensor surface of the fingers and hands, with swelling and puffiness, followed later by a more indurative or atrophic appearance (sclerodactyly). The syndrome, with characteristic visceral patterns, may occur in the absence of scleroderma.

   A. **Vascular** involvement, which occurs in 95% of patients at some time in their course, usually presents as Raynaud phenomenon. (See Chap. 11 for the description and differential diagnosis of Raynaud phenomenon.) Physical examination may also show periungual telangiectasia, decreased pulses, and digital ulceration or infarction. Fingernail fold capillary microscopy reveals capillary dilation and decreased flow. Doppler examinations are usually normal, unless there is an existent large vessel atherosclerotic disease, but extremity pulse wave tracings may show decreased pulse amplitude and intermittent spasm.

   B. **Skin** involvement is present in 95% of patients. Physical examination may reveal only edematous hands in the early stage. Later, hidebound skin commonly affects the hand, face, trunk, and extremities, occasionally with either increased pigmentation or vitiligo. Telangiectasias are commonly found on the nail fold, extensor surfaces of the forearms, and the face. Increased weight of a 4- or 7-mm punch biopsy plug when trimmed of subcutaneous tissue as compared to normal controls may be helpful in documenting thickened skin and following disease progression (normal weights: 4-mm punch = 20 mg ± 4 mg; 7-mm punch = 35 mg ± 7 mg). Skin biopsy histology may appear normal, even with increased weight, but it usually shows evidence of increased dermal collagen, fibrosis, and loss of skin appendages.

   C. **Gastrointestinal** (GI) symptoms are present in 50% of patients. Complaints include dysphagia, reflux, vomiting, abdominal pain, constipation or diarrhea, and weight loss. The esophagus may be dilated with or without gastroesophageal stricture, and there may be hypomotility of the lower two-thirds of the esophagus. Cricopharyngeal muscle weakness or spasm caused by myositis may be a separate cause of dysphagia. A combination of manometric and cineradiographic evaluation of the upper gastrointestinal tract is the most sensitive and reliable method for diagnosis of GI involvement. Mobility disorders and abnormal thickened mucosa are also found in the stomach, small bowel, and colon. Colonic sacculations are relatively characteristic of the disorder. Malabsorption of fat, fat-soluble vitamins (A, D, E, K), vitamin B12, folic acid, and iron may complicate bowel involvement with scleroderma. Acquired lactose intolerance and bacterial overgrowth are also relatively common. Serious rare gastrointestinal complications include hemorrhage from septic esophagitis and perforation.

D. Renal involvement is present in approximately 50% of patients. Hypertension is the most serious complication of scleroderma. Headaches, diplopia, retinopathy, and nausea may signal the onset of malignant or accelerated hypertension and renal insufficiency. Renal involvement is usually abrupt in onset and is accompanied by encephalopathy, multiple organ system involvement, and a microangiopathic peripheral blood smear. In most cases, plasma renin activity is increased. Angiographic studies reveal decreased cortical perfusion. Histologic changes include intimal hyperplasia of the interlobular and intralobular arteries, with fibrinoid necrosis, medial thinning, and adventitial fibrosis. These abnormalities may antedate the onset of hypertension, suggesting that arterial damage in some cases leads to hyperreninemia, angiotensin II–mediated vasoconstriction, and hypertension. Patients with occult renal disease can sometimes be identified by close examination of renal markers (proteinuria, urine sediment, and clearance measurements), changes in plasma renin levels, and examination of the peripheral blood smear.

E. Cardiopulmonary symptoms of dyspnea, chest pain, palpitation, and cough are present in at least 25% of patients. Signs of heart failure, pericardial friction rubs, irregular rhythms, rales, cyanosis, and clubbing can be varying manifestations of myocarditis, pericarditis, interstitial lung disease, and pulmonary hypertension. All are significant complications of the syndrome. Electrocardiogram, chest radiographs, Holter monitoring, echocardiography, radionucleotide cineangiography, and pulmonary function tests are all useful techniques to document the extent of cardiopulmonary involvement. Recent reports suggest that creatine phosphokinase (CPK) isoenzyme MB fraction of greater than 5% may indicate the presence of myocarditis.

F. Musculoskeletal symptoms, which are present in 25% of patients, include morning stiffness and muscle weakness. Physical examination may reveal soft tissue swelling, joint effusions, tendon crepitation or rubs, and soft tissue calcinosis which may be confirmed by radiographs. Muscle enzymes are elevated in some patients. Severe myopathic weakness is an infrequent but significant feature of systemic sclerosis.

III. Differential diagnosis. Entities to consider in the differential diagnosis of scleroderma include Raynaud disease (Chap. 11), other connective tissue diseases, overlap syndromes, localized scleroderma (morphia or linear scleroderma), and eosinophilic fasciitis.

A. Undifferentiated connective tissue syndromes. Patients with varied clinical features of several rheumatic diseases are said to have overlap syndromes. Clinical and serologic features of systemic lupus erythematosus, systemic sclerosis, polymyositis, rheumatoid arthritis, and sicca syndrome may occur in several combinations. One such syndrome complex has been termed *mixed connective tissue disease* (MCTD). The common clinical and laboratory findings in MCTD include:

1. Positive ANA (speckled) and high titer antibodies to nuclear ribonucleoprotein (nRNP).
2. Polyarthralgia.
3. Raynaud phenomenon.
4. Hyperglobulinemia.
5. Polyarthritis.
6. Puffy hands (sclerodactyly).
7. Esophageal disease.

8. Myositis.
9. Renal disease (previously thought to be mild but now recognized as serious in some patients).

MCTD is more common in women than in men; the male-female ratio is similar to that in SLE, while the prevalence is estimated to be slightly less. The long-term natural history of MCTD has not yet been determined. Some observations suggest that it is a phase of scleroderma or other "better defined" rheumatic syndrome.

B. Localized scleroderma (see also Chap. 10). There are two forms of localized scleroderma, morphea and linear scleroderma. Morphea refers to localized areas of skin thickening of the trunk, extremities, or face, which appear waxy and may be as large as several centimeters. There is an associated inflammatory reaction. Histologic differentiation from systemic sclerosis may be impossible. The lesions may be multiple, but usually heal rather than progress, and there are no systemic signs or symptoms.

Linear scleroderma usually occurs in children as a linear patch of sclerosis on an extremity. Occasionally it may produce hemiatrophy and deformity of the face and one extremity, giving the impression of coup de sabre, a traumatic injury.

C. Eosinophilic fasciitis, an illness recently described by Shulman, is characterized by marked inflammation and thickening of fascia. Eosinophilic, plasmocytic, and lymphocytic exudation are common. Puckering of the skin secondary to fascial involvement may superficially resemble scleroderma. The illness often presents insidiously after strenuous physical exercise and is associated with musculo-skeletal pain, swelling, tenderness, flexion contractures, and nerve entrapment syndromes. Raynaud phenomenon and sclerodactyly are always **absent**. Elevated erythrocyte sedimentation rate, hypergammaglobulinemia, and eosinophilia (up to 30% of the total leukocyte count) are common features. Deep wedge biopsy that includes skin fascia and muscle reveals the characteristic inflamed and thickened fascia. Prednisone 5 to 20 mg daily usually causes dramatic improvement, and the disease is usually self-limited with remission occurring after almost 2 years. Several patients with the syndrome have developed aplastic anemia, but the overall frequency of the association is not known.

IV. Therapy. There is no specific therapy for systemic sclerosis. Current treatment is largely aimed at recognizing and treating complications of organ system dysfunction.

A. Peripheral vasculature involvement with Raynaud phenomenon and cutaneous ulcerations is usually refractory to vasodilator therapy; however, the major classes of vasodilators and the dosages commonly used for the treatment of Raynaud phenomenon follow.

1. Presynaptic sympathetic blockers

a. Guanethidine, up to 35 mg PO daily.

b. Alphamethyldopa, up to 500 mg PO TID.

c. Reserpine, up to 0.50 mg PO daily.

2. Postsynaptic alpha blockers and vascular smooth muscle vasodilators

a. Phentolamine, up to 50 mg PO every 4 hours.

b. Phenoxybenzamine, up to 15 mg PO every 6 hours.

c. Hydralazine, up to 100 mg PO QID.

d. Prazosin, up to 2 mg PO QID.

e. Tolazoline, up to 25 mg PO QID.

f. Nitrates, isosorbide dinitrate, and nitropaste. Increase dose until therapeutic effect occurs or headache prevents increased dosage.

3. Experimental drugs

a. Captopril (angiotensin-converting enzyme inhibitor), up to 50 mg PO QID.

b. Verapamil (calcium antagonist), up to 40 mg PO TID.

Our approach to therapy is to try one or more agents from each group for one month to see if a response without unacceptable side effects can be obtained. All vasodilators are potentially dangerous drugs in that they may produce hypotension, syncope, severe flushing, or aggravation of digital ischemia by a steal phenomenon. Guanethidine, prazosin, and captopril have been the most effective vasodilators in our experience.

B. Skin. Treatment of skin involvement has been disappointing. It falls into three general categories.

1. Antifibrotic therapy. Potassium *p*-aminobenzoate 2 gm PO QID. Some patients claim benefit.

2. Antiinflammatory or anticollagen linking. Penicillamine 250 mg PO daily or BID. May be useful in early cases. Prednisone 5 to 15 mg PO daily. Useful largely if myositis coexists. Colchicine 0.6 mg PO daily.

3. Experimental therapy. Dimethyl sulfoxide (DMSO), topical or IV (we have not used this).

C. Gastrointestinal system. Treatment of gastrointestinal complaints is shown in Table 40-1.

D. Renal system. Renal complications of hypertension and kidney failure are often sudden in onset (scleroderma renal crisis) and particularly refractory to therapy. Careful monitoring of plasma renin activity and blood pressure for sudden rises, peripheral smear for the appearance of microangiopathy, and urinalysis for the appearance of renal markers are essential.

Therapy of hypertension without evidence of microangiopathy or renal markers

Table 40-1. Therapy for Gastrointestinal Complaints

Complications	Therapy
Reflux esophagitis	Antacids, especially Gaviscon (combination of aluminum hydroxide and magnesium trisilicate), while awake
Dysphagia	
Stricture	Dilation
Cricopharyngeal weakness	Trial of prednisone 40 mg daily if symptoms are severe
Cricopharyngeal spasm	Surgical myotomy
Intestinal hypomotility	Cholinergic stimulants
Malabsorption	
Vitamins, minerals	Multivitamins, vitamin B12, folate, iron
Calories	Elemental diet
	Nutritionally complete dietary preparation with medium chain triglycerides and lactose free.
	Intravenous hyperalimentation
Diarrhea	
Lactose intolerance	Remove lactose
Bacterial overgrowth	Tetracycline
Hemorrhage	Lavage, vasoconstrictors, surgery

should be guided by plasma renin activity and the presence or absence of Raynaud phenomenon and heart failure.

Since excessive stimulation of the renin angiotensin system may be involved in triggering scleroderma renal crisis, treatment with drugs that suppress or do not stimulate the renin system is probably desirable. Beta blockade with metoprolol up to 100 mg PO BID, except when contraindicated by heart failure or asthma, is the drug measure of first choice. If an additional agent is needed or if Raynaud phenomenon is significantly worsened by metoprolol, prazosin up to 3 mg PO TID should be utilized. The combination of metoprolol and prazosin is particularly effective but may cause salt retention. Diuretics are used only when there is heart failure, fluid retention, or failure to control blood pressure.

Once markers of scleroderma renal crisis appear, maximum doses if necessary of metoprolol, prazosin, and diuretics should be employed to control blood pressure swiftly. Patients should be monitored carefully in intensive care settings where nitroprusside can be administered when conventional agents fail to lower blood pressure. Captopril (in doses up to 100 mg PO QID) has aborted scleroderma renal crisis and averted renal failure in 50% of patients and may replace other forms of antihypertensive therapy in scleroderma.

Some patients may progress to renal failure despite all therapies and have persistent unmanageable hypertension. In these patients, nephrectomy and subsequent support by hemodialysis or renal transplantation may be the only recourses.

E. Cardiopulmonary system. Cardiopulmonary complications such as heart failure, dysrhythmias, and pericarditis are treated by standard measures. There is no established treatment for pulmonary fibrosis or pulmonary hypertension. Vasodilator therapies described in section **IV.A.** have all been tried for pulmonary hypertension. None is predictably effective, but phentolamine, hydralazine, prazosin, nitrates, and captopril may improve exercise tolerance in a few cases. Right heart catheterization during sequential vasodilator administration, searching for a significant fall in pulmonary artery pressure or a rise in cardiac output (signifying falling pulmonary vascular resistance), may be helpful in picking an effective agent.

F. Musculoskeletal system. Musculoskeletal aching or synovitis is best treated with aspirin 600 mg PO QID or nonsteroidal medications in doses customarily used for osteoarthritis (see Chap. 27). If there are significant muscle weakness and elevated muscle enzymes, prednisone 15 to 20 mg daily in tapering dosage may result in improvement. Physical therapy, pool therapy, bed rest, and heat can be effective in improving joint function and relieving symptoms (see Appendixes A–C).

V. Prognosis is extremely difficult to estimate in systemic sclerosis. Some studies quote a 45% survival at 7 years, but some patients have rapidly progressive disease and die within 2 to 3 years after onset. The clinical course is extremely variable but cases usually divide into two groups: slow progression over more than 15 years, or a rapid downhill course over 1 to 2 years with death occurring from renal failure, malignant hypertension, or cardiac arrhythmias. Patients with the CREST syndrome (calcinosis, Raynaud phenomenon, esophageal disease, sclerodactyly, and telangiectasia) seem to comprise the majority of patients with a slowly progressive course. Spontaneous remissions are extremely rare but do occur. Hypertension, the presence of renal disease, or cardiopulmonary involvement are poor prognostic features. Patients with CREST syndrome have increased survival but may die from complications related to pulmonary hypertension or gastrointestinal disease.

Bibliography

Cannon, P. J., et al. The relationship of hypertension and renal failure in scleroderma (progressive systemic sclerosis) to structural and functional abnormalities of the renal cortical circulation. *Medicine* 53:1–46, 1974.

Gavras, H., et al. Is elevated plasma renin activity of prognostic importance in progressive systemic sclerosis? *Arch. Intern. Med.* 137:1554–1558, 1977.

Kahaleh, M. B., Sherer, G. K., and LeRoy, E. C. Endothelial injury in scleroderma. *J. Exp. Med.* 149:1326–1335, 1979.

Kovalchik, M. T., et al. The kidney in progressive systemic sclerosis: A prospective study. *Ann. Intern. Med.* 89:881–887, 1978.

Maricq, H. R., Green, G., and Leroy, E. C. Skin capillary abnormalities as moderators of organ involvement in scleroderma (systemic sclerosis), Raynaud's syndrome, and jermatomyositis. *Am. J. Med.* 61:862–870, 1976.

Meddsger, T. A., et al. Survival with systemic sclerosis (scleroderma). A life-table analysis of clinical and demographic factors in 358 male U.S. veteran patients. *J. Chronic Dis.* 26:647–660, 1973.

Mitnick, P. D. and Feig, P. U. Control of hypertension and reversal of renal failure in scleroderma. *N. Engl. J. Med.* 299:871–872, 1978.

Oliver, J. A. and Cannon, P. J. The kidney in scleroderma. *Nephron* 18:141–150, 1977.

Wasner, C., Cooke, C. R., and Fries, J. F. Successful medical treatment of scleroderma renal crisis. *N. Engl. J. Med.* 229:873–875, 1978.

Whitman, H. H., et al. Variable response to oral converting enzyme blockade in hypertensive scleroderma patients (Abstract). *Arthritis Rheum.* 23:762–763, 1980.

41. Sicca Syndrome

Stuart S. Kassan

The sicca syndrome (SS) is a chronic inflammatory disease associated with lymphocytic infiltration of exocrine glands. Certain clinical, serologic, and genetic differences are found between patients with SS alone (or primary [first-degree] sicca syndrome) and those with SS and other connective tissue diseases (or secondary [second-degree] sicca syndrome). These differences suggest varying etiologies for similar clinical manifestations of disease. The most commonly accepted definition of the sicca syndrome has been the presence of two of the following findings: (1) keratoconjunctivitis sicca, (2) xerostomia, and (3) one of the connective tissue disease syndromes. This definition takes into account the existence of patients with keratoconjunctivitis and xerostomia in the absence of any other definable connective tissue disease (first-degree SS). Of the connective tissue diseases associated with secondary SS (SS with another connective tissue disease), rheumatoid arthritis is the most common, but others have been well-documented and include lupus erythematosus, scleroderma, polymyositis, mixed connective tissue disease, and juvenile rheumatoid arthritis. As a result of the obvious shortcomings of the above purely clinical definition, most recent investigators have included pathologic criteria (see sec. III.) as supporting evidence for the presence of primary or secondary SS.

The clinical manifestations of the disease were first described in 1888. In 1933, Henrik Sjögren published a monograph describing in great detail the histologic and clinical components of this syndrome, which has often been referred to as Sjögren syndrome. Confusion later arose between Sjögren syndrome and a disease previously reported by Mikulicz in the late 1800s. In 1927, Schaffer and Jacobsen defined two main categories: (1) *Mikulicz disease* proper, of unknown etiology and following a benign course, and (2) *Mikulicz syndrome,* caused by a variety of disorders such as leukemia, lymphosarcoma, tuberculosis, sarcoidosis, and iodide poisoning. Later, Morgan and Castleman concluded, on the basis of pathologic descriptions, that Mikulicz disease and Sjögren syndrome were identical.

Much of the interest in SS over the past decade has focused on the opportunity to study the interrelationships among the autoimmune disorders, lymphoproliferative malignancies, and dysproteinemias, all of which may be features of the syndrome.

I. Prevalence

- **A. Sex.** Women comprise at least 90% of the patients with sicca syndrome (first- or second-degree) in most studies.

- **B. Age.** Most with the disease are over 40 years of age, but the disease may be encountered in the second and third decades of life.

- **C. Other connective tissue diseases in patients with SS**

   1. When various populations of patients with SS are evaluated for the presence of other connective tissue diseases, the results have been as follows:

      a. Rheumatoid arthritis: 30% to 55%.

      b. Scleroderma: 5% to 8%.

      c. Systemic lupus erythematosus: 5% to 10%.

      d. Polymyositis: 2% to 4%.

   2. Alternatively, when evidence of SS is specifically sought in patients with other connective tissue diseases, the results are quite different. Evidence for SS in patients with:

      a. Systemic lupus erythematosus: greater than 50%.

      b. Rheumatoid arthritis: 20% to greater than 50%.

      c. Scleroderma: 40% to 50%.

D. Glandular involvement in SS. Eighty percent of SS patients have major salivary gland enlargement. Focal lymphocytic infiltration with linear destruction may be seen in minor salivary glands in labial, nasal, and hard palate mucosa. Involvement of the exocrine glands of the upper and lower respiratory tracts, gastrointestinal tract, vagina, pancreas, and skin have all been found in SS.

E. Extraglandular involvement

1. **Hepatic** disorders in patients with SS have included:

   a. Primary biliary cirrhosis.

   b. Chronic active hepatitis.

   c. Cryptogenic cirrhosis (15% of SS patients in one study).

2. **Renal** disorders have been found in as many as one-third of SS patients and include:

   a. Renal tubular acidosis type I.

   b. Nephrogenic diabetes insipidus.

   c. Chronic interstitial nephritis.

   d. Immune complex glomerulonephritis.

3. **Pulmonary** disorders may be found in 4% to 15% of SS patients and may range from pulmonary infiltrates (pseudolymphoma) to mild fibrosing alveolitis.

4. **Myositis,** often of an indolent nature, may be encountered in SS. Up to 50% of patients have been found to exhibit on random muscle biopsies abnormalities consisting of interstitial and perivascular fibrosis, or inflammatory infiltrates, or both.

5. **Vasculitis** is present in less than 10% of SS patients. It is often seen in association with myositis, mononeuritis multiplex, immune complex glomerulonephritis, and purpura.

F. Malignancy in SS

1. **Non-Hodgkin lymphoma** has been found to occur more often in patients with SS (first- or second-degree); the relative risk is 44 times the expected incidence. Patients with a history of parotid enlargement, splenomegaly, and lymphadenopathy are those at greatest risk of developing lymphoma.

2. **Waldenström macroglobulinemia** appears to be more frequent in SS but the risk is unknown.

3. **Pseudolymphoma** is a condition in SS associated with extraglandular extension of lymphoproliferation which is clinically and histologically benign. The incidence is not known.

II. Genetics
Histocompatibility testing of patients with SS has demonstrated a genetic dichotomy between patients with primary SS (sicca syndrome alone) and those with secondary SS (sicca syndrome with another connective tissue disease, generally rheumatoid arthritis).

A. Primary sicca syndrome has a significantly increased association with HLA-B8, HLA-DW3, and certain B-lymphocyte alloantigens.

B. Secondary sicca syndrome patients usually do not show the above HLA associations. In the case of patients with sicca syndrome and rheumatoid arthritis, there is an increased incidence of the HLA-DR4 antigen (that antigen found most often in seropositive rheumatoid arthritis alone).

III. Pathogenesis
Studies in SS pertaining to pathogenesis may be classified into:

A. Abnormalities of humoral immunity

1. **Antisalivary duct antibody** is present more frequently in secondary SS (70% positive) than in primary SS (10% positive).

2. **Antibodies to soluble acidic nuclear antigens** extracted from lymphoid cell lines.

   a. SS-B (or Ha,La) antibodies are present in (1) primary SS, 50% to 70%, (2) SS with RA, 3% to 5%, and (3) SS with SLE, 73%.

   b. SS-A (or Ro) antibodies are present in (1) primary SS, 70%, (2) SS with RA, 1%, and (3) SS with SLE, 33%.

B. Abnormalities of cellular immunity and immunoregulation in primary SS

1. There are normal absolute numbers and proportions of peripheral B- and T-cells. No increase of circulating B-cells has been found despite high incidence of autoantibodies, hypergammaglobulinemia, and circulating immune complexes. Evidence suggests the presence of a serum-blocking factor that may decrease the percentage of T_γ-cells.

C. Viral studies.
Tubuloreticular structures have been identified in labial salivary gland tissue and renal endothelium from SS patients. No successful viral isolation from salivary gland tissues has been accomplished.

D. Immune complexes.
Elevated levels of immune complexes and abnormal clearance of these complexes by the reticuloendothelial system have been demonstrated in active SS. Their role in the pathogenesis of disease is unclear but may be important in vasculitic states and glomerulonephritis.

E. Graft-versus-host disease.
Initiated SS resembling spontaneous SS suggests a possible pathophysiologic mechanism for the development of SS and other connective tissue diseases in man, and extends previous observations limited to animal models.

IV. Clinical features

A. Ocular symptoms
may not be present in one-third to one-half of patients at any one time in their course of disease despite definite pathologic changes. However, approximately 95% of SS patients will have ocular symptoms at some time in their course.

B. Xerostomia
is an infrequent presenting sign of SS but about 90% of patients will have sialographic abnormalities of the parotids. Salivary gland enlargement, primarily parotid gland, is present in one-third of SS patients and is usually bilateral. Lacrimal gland enlargement is unusual (4%).

V. Laboratory abnormalities

A. Specific tests

1. **Tests of functional abnormalities**

   a. **Schirmer test.** 5 mm of unstimulated wetting of filter paper in 5 minutes (17% false positive and 15% false negative results).

   b. **Parotid salivary flow rate**

   c. **Radionuclide scan** of parotid glands (^{99m}Tc pertechnetate). The scan may be falsely abnormal as a result of other abnormalities of the parotid gland (see sec. **VI.**).

   d. **Parotid gland sialography** is performed by introducing radioopaque dye into the parotid duct system. The abnormalities seen in SS include acinar and duct atrophy with puddling of dye, main duct enlargement, and retention of contrast material. All of above may be seen in chronic parotitis from causes other than SS.

2. Tests of anatomic abnormalities

a. **Rose Bengal staining** of the cornea may be helpful in confirming the diagnosis but is not specific (4% false positive and 5% false negative results).

b. **Parotid gland sialography** (see sec. **V.1.d.**).

3. Biopsy

a. **Minor salivary glands** of lip and palate. A correlation may be made with severity of disease and degree of focal lymphocytic infiltration in the minor salivary glands.

b. **Lacrimal glands and parotid glands.** Abnormalities are similar to those found in the minor salivary glands of the lip. Because of the relative lack of morbidity associated with lip biopsies, this procedure is preferred over lacrimal or parotid gland biopsies as a diagnostic tool.

B. Nonspecific laboratory abnormalities. These changes are often seen in other states of inflammation and in many autoimmune diseases.

1. **Elevated erythrocyte sedimentation rate:** 60% to 80%.

2. **Anemia:** 30% to 40%.

3. **Leukopenia:** less than 30%.

4. **Hypergammaglobulinemia:** 50%.

5. **Positive rheumatoid factor:** 70%.

6. **Positive antinuclear antibodies:** 50% to 70%.

VI. Differential diagnosis
The salivary gland involvement in SS may be confused with numerous other conditions. These may include:

A. Infection of salivary glands.

1. **Viral.** Coxsackie, mumps, cytomegalic inclusion disease.

2. **Bacterial.** Acute sialadenitis is often seen in dehydrated, debilitated patients. Chronic bacterial sialadenitis is often associated with obstruction of the salivary ducts by inspissated saliva.

3. **Fungal.** Actinomycosis or histoplasmosis.

4. **Tuberculosis.** Rare.

B. Granulomatous disease. Sarcoidosis.

C. Other infiltrative disorders.

1. Primary neoplasms of the parotid gland.

2. Leukemia.

3. Lymphoma of the intraparotid lymph node.

4. Burkitt lymphoma.

5. Pseudolymphoma.

D. Systemic diseases

1. Cirrhosis.

2. Diabetes mellitus.

3. Hyperlipoproteinemias (types III, IV, V).

4. Obesity.

5. Pregnancy and lactation.

6. Gouty parotitis (rare).

7. Cushing disease.

8. Cystic fibrosis.

E. Nutritional deficiency

1. Starvation.

2. Vitamin B6 deficiency.

3. Vitamin C deficiency.

4. Vitamin A deficiency.

F. Drugs associated with the development of dry mouth

1. Sedatives.

2. Hypnotics.

3. Narcotics.

4. Phenothiazines.

5. Atropine.

6. Propantheline.

7. Antiparkinsonian drugs.

8. Antihistamines.

9. Ephedrine.

10. Epinephrine.

11. Amphetamines.

VII. Therapy
No controlled trials have been undertaken in the therapy of the systemic manifestations of SS. In general, the approach to treatment has been empiric. Vasculitis, renal disease (immune complex–mediated or otherwise), myositis, alveolitis, cryoglobulinemia, and other manifestations have mostly been treated in the past with corticosteroids or immunosuppressive agents, or both, depending on the severity of disease. Because the cytotoxic drugs are immunosuppressive and renal transplant patients and others treated with these agents have an increased incidence of lymphoma (as do untreated SS patients), it is advisable to avoid their use in SS.

A. Ocular abnormalities. Artificial tears are the mainstay of treatment. Solutions consisting of methylcellulose and polyvinyl alcohol are useful. The dose varies from 2 drops QID to every 15 minutes depending on the clinical state. Inserts placed into the conjunctival sac that release small amounts of methylcellulose over many hours are presently in the experimental stage.

B. Xerostomia. Unfortunately, very little in the way of therapy for xerostomia is available. Lubrication of the mouth with mild secretagogues, such as lemon flavored juice or lubricating agents proper (water, methylcellulose), is useful. More potent secretagogues (e.g., supersaturated potassium iodide [SSKI]) are of no benefit and may exacerbate the signs and symptoms of parotitis. Prevention of states of dehydration in SS is very important since dehydration may enhance parotid ductal calculus formation. Avoidance of drugs that may aggravate oral dryness (e.g., narcotics, antihistamines, anticholinergics) is also important.

C. Parotid enlargement. In the past, numerous modes of therapy have been employed to treat parotid enlargement.

1. Parotid irradiation has been associated with an increased incidence of lymphoma in SS patients. Because of its oncogenic potential, this form of therapy should not be used in SS.

2. **Surgical removal** is often technically difficult, and resultant nonhealing fistulas and facial nerve damage preclude this mode of therapy.

3. **Drug therapy** for symptomatic inflammatory parotid enlargement.

   a. **Nonsteroidal antiinflammatory drugs.** Aspirin 600 to 900 mg QID. Alternative regimens for those with aspirin intolerance are indomethacin 25 to 50 mg QID or ibuprofen 400 mg QID.

   b. **Corticosteroid therapy** should be limited to those with severe, recalcitrant disease because of the risk of corticosteroid toxicity. The regimen is 20 to 40 mg per day with dose tapering as soon as a clinical response is obtained.

4. **Cytotoxic therapy** (specifically azathioprine, cyclophosphamide, chlorambucil, methotrexate) does not seem to offer any significant benefit unless one is treating a true malignancy (lymphoma) or an invasive form of pseudolymphoma in SS.

Bibliography

Kassan, S. S., and Gardy, M.   Sjögren's syndrome: An update and overview. *Am. J. Med.* 64:1037–1046, 1978.

Moutsopoulos, H. M. (Moderator).   Sjögren's syndrome (sicca syndrome): Part 1. Current issues. *Ann. Intern. Med.* 92:212–226, 1980.

42. Vasculitis

Ted Parris

The term *necrotizing vasculitis* refers to a heterogeneous group of clinicopathologic conditions having in common inflammation and necrosis of blood vessel walls. Differing clinical manifestations of the various vasculitis syndromes depend on the nature and magnitude of the underlying (often immunologic) insult and the size and distribution of affected blood vessels. Necrotizing vasculitis may be the most significant lesion in several clinical disorders, such as classic polyarteritis nodosa or temporal arteritis, or it may be a minor or unusual complication of a number of other diseases, such as bacterial endocarditis or lymphoreticular malignancies.

For nearly a century after the original pathologic description of polyarteritis nodosa in 1866 by Kussmaul and Maier, all disorders manifesting necrotizing vasculitis were designated *polyarteritis (periarteritis) nodosa*. Subsequently it became clear that the spectrum of vasculitis syndromes was diffuse and heterogeneous, and that specific entities carried different prognoses and required different therapy. Many previous classification systems were based entirely on pathologic material and were quite rigid, not allowing for the significant clinical overlap present in these disorders. Certain syndromes, such as Wegener granulomatosis or temporal arteritis, have emerged as well-defined entities because they present distinctive clinicopathologic features (see Group III, Group IV, and Chap. 32). Other disorders, especially some of those designated in groups I and II, may not have such distinctive features but may manifest necrotizing vasculitis involving vessels of different sizes and different locations. For example, necrotizing vasculitis accompanying systemic lupus, rheumatoid arthritis, and hepatitis B antigenemia may vary from a purely cutaneous (leukocytoclastic) vasculitis to a fulminant systemic vasculitis indistinguishable from classic polyarteritis nodosa. To call all these various syndromes *polyarteritis nodosa* would be a gross oversimplification and would fail to yield useful clinical or prognostic implications.

At present, no standard classification of the various vasculitis syndromes exists. The ideal classification would be based on immunoetiology with definable antigen(s) leading to well-characterized vasculitis syndromes. Unfortunately, the etiology of the majority of vasculitis syndromes in humans remains unknown. Given this fact, the goals of an adequate classification system at present should include a synthesis of both clinical and pathologic information that has clinical utility, prognostic value, and allows rational therapeutic intervention. Such a classification system is presented in Table 42-1, while Figure 42-1 schematically represents the vessel sizes affected in the various vasculitis syndromes.

I. **Pathogenesis.** The theory that immune mechanisms are involved in the pathogenesis of vasculitis syndromes is supported by studies in animals as well as by clinical observations in humans. Central to this theory is the deposition of soluble immune complexes (ICs) in vessel walls, with subsequent activation of complement leading to inflammation and vessel necrosis. Alternatively, circulating antigen may be deposited in vessel walls with in situ formation of antigen-antibody complexes, complement activation, and further developments. Figure 42-2 schematically depicts events felt to be involved in the pathogenesis of IC-mediated vasculitis caused by circulating, soluble ICs.

Animal data derive largely from the study of acute serum sickness in rabbits, the prototype experimental IC disease (Fig. 42-3). Seven to ten days after injection of heterologous protein, immune elimination of antigen occurs and the lesions of acute serum sickness are observed in the arteries, joints, and kidneys. These findings coincide with serum hypocomplementemia and the presence of circulating ICs. The arterial lesion is a necrotizing vasculitis with an intense polymorphonuclear leukocyte infiltrate identical to that seen in human syndromes. Immune reactants (antigen, antibody, complement) are detectable in the vessel wall during the first one to two days but are rapidly removed by phagocytosis (which may in part account for

Table 42-1. Classification of the Necrotizing Vasculitides

Group I. Systemic Necrotizing Vasculitis Affecting Medium and Small Arteries (Polyarteritis Nodosa Group)
  Classic polyarteritis nodosa (PAN)
    Hepatitis B surface antigen–related
    Following serous otitis media
    Infantile polyarteritis (Kawasaki disease)
    Associated with drug (methamphetamine) abuse
  Allergic angiitis and granulomatosis (Churg-Strauss syndrome)
  Vasculitis complicating rheumatic disease
    Systemic lupus erythematosus
    Rheumatoid arthritis
    Childhood dermatomyositis
Group II. Necrotizing Vasculitis Affecting Small Vessels (Leukocytoclastic Vasculitis)
  Primary cutaneous vasculitis
  Distinct clinical subgroups
    Henoch-Schönlein purpura
    Essential mixed cryoglobulinemia
    Vasculitis associated with rheumatic diseases, e.g., systemic lupus erythematosus, rheumatoid arthritis, sicca syndrome
    Vasculitis associated with hematologic malignancies, e.g., Hodgkin disease, non-Hodgkin lymphoma
    Vasculitis associated with infectious endocarditis
    Drug-induced vasculitis
    Hypocomplementemia, urticaria, vasculitis syndrome
Group III. Giant Cell Arteritides
  Temporal arteritis
  Takayasu arteritis
Group IV. Wegener Granulomatosis
  Limited
  Generalized
Group V. Lymphomatoid Granulomatosis

---

some of the negative immunofluorescent data in humans). While classic serum sickness rarely occurs presently in humans, it has nevertheless served as a valuable experimental model to study the events involved in IC-mediated disease.

The evidence that ICs are responsible for vasculitis syndromes in humans is less direct, with the possible exception of the hepatitis B virus syndromes discussed subsequently. However, the occurrence of vasculitis in diseases such as systemic lupus erythematosus, rheumatoid arthritis, and infectious endocarditis, in which ICs are known to cause other manifestations, makes it quite likely that ICs are also connected with the vascular inflammation seen in these illnesses. The reasons why some patients manifest vasculitis and others do not are probably multifactoral, depending on physicochemical properties of the complexes themselves, functional status of the reticuloendothelial system (responsible for removing ICs from the circulation), and, ultimately, the specific host's immune response to the offending antigen(s).

Group I. Systemic Necrotizing Vasculitis Affecting Medium and Small Muscular Arteries (Polyarteritis Nodosa Group)

Pathologically these disorders are characterized by necrotizing vasculitis of medium and small muscular arteries. The lesions tend to be segmental with a predilection for bifurcations, and lesions of all stages (acute, subacute, chronic) are seen in pathologic specimens. The finding of multiple, small aneurysms on abdominal angiography is quite specific for this group of disorders (see sec. **II.B.**).

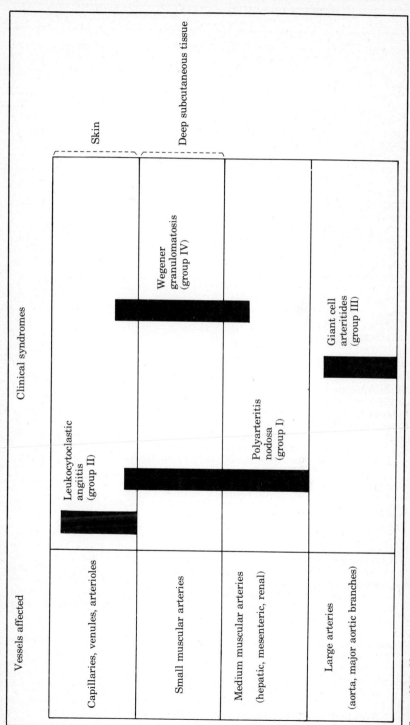

Figure 42-1. Classification of the necrotizing vasculitis syndromes by vessel size.

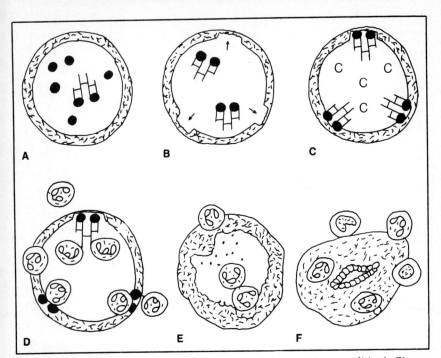

Figure 42-2. Pathogenesis of immune complex-mediated necrotizing vasculitis. A. Circulating soluble immune complexes in antigen excess. B. Increased vascular permeability through platelet-derived vasoactive amines and IgE-mediated reactions. C. Trapping of immune complexes along basement membrane of vessel wall and activation of complement components (C). D. Complement-derived chemotactic factors (C3a, C5a, and C567) cause accumulation of PMNs. E. PMNs release lysosomal enzymes (collagenase and elastase). F. Damage and necrosis of vessel wall, thrombosis occlusion, and hemorrhage. (From A. S. Fauci, et al., The spectrum of vasculitis. *Ann. Intern. Med.* 89:660, 1978.)

I. **Clinical features.** The clinical hallmark for these disorders is their propensity for major organ involvement, with frequent marked morbidity and mortality. Associated features such as hepatitis B antigenemia, previous serous otitis media, or coexistent rheumatic disease may be present or absent. A previous history of asthma is always obtainable in patients with Churg-Strauss syndrome.

A. **Classic polyarteritis nodosa (PAN)** presents as an acute to subacute febrile (75%) illness of a nonspecific nature or, more commonly, a febrile illness with clinical involvement of one or more organ systems. The organs most commonly involved are the kidneys, heart, gastrointestinal tract, nervous system, and musculoskeletal system. Skin involvement occurs in only 5% to 20% of patients; when present, it consists of painful nodular lesions as opposed to the "palpable purpura" which characterizes leukocytoclastic vasculitis (see Group II).

In recent series of patients with PAN-like illnesses, 20% to 30% are carriers of the hepatitis B surface antigen (Hb$_s$Ag). Much evidence that ICs containing Hb$_s$Ag and antibody participate in the pathogenesis of these vasculitis syndromes exists, including (1) demonstration of Hb$_s$Ag in arterial walls by immunofluorescence, (2) demonstration of Hb$_s$Ag in the circulating ICs, and (3) known participation of hepatitis B antigen-antibody complexes in other extrahepatic manifestations of hepatitis B virus infection (e.g., arthritis-urticaria syndrome, glomerulonephritis).

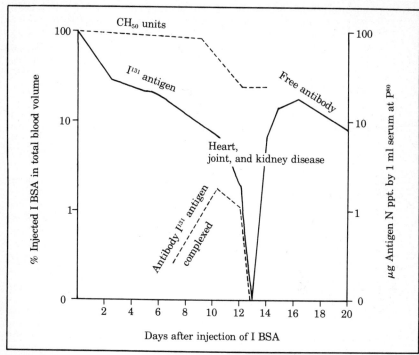

Figure 42-3. Elimination of I^{131} BSA from circulation of a rabbit. The relationship of detection of immune complexes to appearance of lesions is shown. (From C. Cochrane and D. Koffler, Immune complex disease in experimental animals and man. *Adv. Immunol.* 16:187, 1973.)

Clinical syndromes indistinguishable from classic PAN have also been reported following a bout of serous otitis media in adults; complicating rheumatic diseases such as systemic lupus erythematosus, rheumatoid arthritis, and childhood dermatomyositis; and occurring in intravenous methamphetamine abusers. However, the role of the Hb_sAg in the latter group was not determined.

The mucocutaneous lymph node syndrome (Kawasaki disease) is a recently described disease of infants and young children characterized by prolonged fever, with temperature greater than 39°C for more than seven days; conjunctivitis; pharyngitis, dry fissured lips, and strawberry tongue; truncal rash, with polymorphous exanthem; nonpurulent cervical lymphadenopathy; and erythema of palms and soles, with indurative edema and subsequent desquamation over the fingertips and toes. Sudden cardiac death is reported to occur in 1% to 2% of patients, usually during the convalescent phase of the illness. Pathologic study of the hearts of these infants reveals coronary arteritis, histologically identical to that seen in infantile PAN (which is characterized by coronary arteritis and aneurysms). The histologic similarities between the two diseases have led to speculation that Kawasaki disease and infantile PAN may be slightly different clinical expressions of the same disorder.

B. Major organ system involvement

1. **Renal** involvement occurs in approximately 70% to 75% of patients and can result from either a necrotizing glomerulitis (30%) or necrotizing vasculitis of the medium-sized renal vessels (70%). Clinical manifestations vary from mi-

crohematuria and proteinuria to fulminant acute renal failure. Renal papillary necrosis, perirenal hemorrhage, and renal infarction have also been reported. Hypertension is present in approximately 60% of patients.

2. **Cardiac** involvement is demonstrable in approximately 50% to 70% of patients at autopsy, but clinical cardiac disease is less frequent. Manifestations include congestive heart failure, angina pectoris, arrhythmias, and myocardial infarction. Cardiac involvement consisting of diffuse coronary arteritis is a characteristic feature of infantile PAN.

3. **Gastrointestinal tract** involvement occurs in approximately 60% to 70% of patients. Most commonly it presents as diffuse abdominal pain which may progress to intestinal infarction. Upper or lower gastrointestinal bleeding, pancreatitis, cholecystitis, and hepatic and gallbladder rupture have also been reported.

4. **Neurologic** involvement occurs in 50% to 80% of patients. The most characteristic manifestation is mononeuritis multiplex, which can be quite disabling. Less common manifestations include hemiplegia, seizures, myelopathy, and brainstem or cerebellar signs. Peripheral nervous system involvement occurs much more frequently than central nervous system involvement.

5. **Musculoskeletal** signs and symptoms are one of the most frequent nonspecific complaints in these patients, occurring in 50% to 75%. Diffuse arthralgias and myalgias are common; frank arthritis is not.

C. **Churg-Strauss syndrome (allergic granulomatosis and angiitis)** is a systemic necrotizing vasculitis of unknown etiology occurring against a background of chronic asthma of variable duration and severity. The typical patient with Churg-Strauss syndrome has chronic asthma and then presents with a systemic illness with multisystem involvement, accompanied by blood eosinophilia and pulmonary involvement.

1. **Comparisons and contrasts between PAN and Churg-Strauss syndrome**

a. Gastrointestinal tract, renal, neurologic, and musculoskeletal **system involvement** is identical clinically (although some groups report less frequent renal disease in Churg-Strauss syndrome).

b. **Clinical pulmonary disease** *sine qua non* of Churg-Strauss syndrome and is rare in classic PAN.

c. **Pathology** of Churg-Strauss syndrome reveals necrotizing vasculitis with a predominantly eosinophilic infiltrate and extravascular granulomas (the latter two findings do not occur in classic PAN).

d. **Natural history and reponse to therapy** are similar in the two disorders. Many cases previously designated polyarteritis with lung involvement may well fall into the category of Churg-Strauss syndrome.

II. **Diagnostic investigations.** Occasionally, Group I necrotizing vasculitis is discovered serendipitously in pathologic material removed at surgery (e.g., gallbladder, appendix, infarcted bowel) for acute abdominal emergencies. More commonly, one is faced with a severely ill patient with a multisystem illness in whom rapid and appropriate diagnosis and institution of therapy may be life saving. The following diagnostic measures should be undertaken.

A. **Tissue biopsy.** Adequate histologic documentation (if possible) is crucial in these disorders before institution of potentially life-threatening therapy. Initially, deep biopsy of any involved skin or muscle biopsy is the procedure of choice. Muscle biopsy will be positive in 40% to 50% of patients, and biopsy of involved skin should always be positive (although skin involvement is not common). Sural nerve biopsy should be performed if neuropathic signs or symptoms occur.

B. **Abdominal angiography.** In the absence of a positive tissue biopsy, if the diagnosis is still being strongly considered, abdominal angiography should be undertaken. This procedure should include the celiac axis, mesenteric, renal, and hepatic circulations. The presence of multiple, small aneurysms is highly specific for group I disorders. The sensitivity of this procedure is unknown, although one group reported a 60% incidence of angiographically documented aneurysms in their PAN patients (10 of 17 patients).

C. **Nerve conduction studies and electromyography** are helpful in diagnosing mononeuritis multiplex. The presence of mononeuritis multiplex serves as corroboration of the presence of vasculitis, especially if other disorders producing this lesion (e.g., diabetes, uremia, sarcoidosis) are absent.

D. **Screening for the presence of HB$_s$Ag** and evaluation for evidence of **underlying rheumatic disease** such as systemic lupus erythematosus, rheumatoid arthritis, or childhood dermatomyositis should be undertaken.

E. Determination of the **pattern of organ involvement** in a given individual is necessary, as this feature will have a major impact on the magnitude and aggressiveness of therapy.

F. Occasionally, the diagnosis of systemic necrotizing vasculitis is still considered when all diagnostic procedures are negative. Severe visceral vasculitis may exist even when skin and muscle biopsy, angiography, and other measures are negative. In this situation, consultation with a physician experienced in the diagnosis and management of these disorders is strongly advised before instituting therapy.

III. Therapy

A. **Corticosteroids** are the mainstay of therapy in patients with Group I disorders and major organ involvement. High-dose parenteral corticosteroids (prednisone 60 to 80 mg per day in four divided doses) are the initial treatment of choice in patients with active vasculitis and major organ involvement (i.e., renal, cardiac, gastrointestinal, neurologic). Although no prospective study has been done, a good deal of retrospective evidence combined with favorable clinical experience suggest that steroid therapy improves outcome. One retrospective study from the Mayo Clinic reported a five-year survival of 48% in steroid-treated patients versus a 13% five-year survival in untreated patients.

B. **Cytotoxic drugs** have also been used recently, in addition to corticosteroids, to treat patients with Group I disorders. Cyclophosphamide (1 to 2 mg/kg/24 hr PO or IV) and azathioprine (2 to 3 mg/kg/24 hr PO) are the drugs most commonly used. Recent literature suggests that cyclophosphamide is more efficacious than azathioprine. The onset of action for these drugs is delayed for 10 to 14 days, and thus they cannot serve as substitutes for systemic corticosteroids in acutely ill patients. In patients severely ill with major gastrointestinal disease, cardiac disease, or progressive renal or neurologic deterioration, the addition of cytotoxic drugs to corticosteroids is indicated. They may also be useful in patients with chronically active vasculitis requiring continued high-dose corticosteroids for control in an attempt to reduce the steroid dose and thus minimize the complications associated with long-term, high-dose corticosteroid therapy. It is imperative to monitor hematologic indices carefully in patients on these drugs, with the aim of keeping the total white blood cell count greater than 3,000 cells/mm^3 and the absolute neutrophil count greater than 1,500/mm^3.

Group II. Necrotizing Vasculitis Affecting Small Vessels (Leukocytoclastic Vasculitis)

This group of disorders is characterized pathologically by necrotizing vasculitis of small vessels, especially the postcapillary venule. The characteristic lesion consists of infiltration of a necrotic vessel wall with polymorphonuclear leukocytes and scattered nuclear debris (hence the term *leukocytoclasis*). Leukocytoclastic vasculitis (venulitis) may be a primary disorder (primary cutaneous vasculitis) or be associated with a number of other disease processes, including Henoch-Schönlein purpura, essential mixed cryoglobulinemia, rheumatic diseases (systemic lupus erythematosus, rheumatoid arthritis, sicca syndrome), hematologic malignancies, drug reactions, infectious endocarditis, and the syndrome of hypocomplementemia, urticaria, and vasculitis (see Chap. 10).

I. **Clinical features.** The clinical hallmark of all these disorders is cutaneous vasculitis, with variable amounts of systemic disease. Skin lesions accompanying these illnesses are pleomorphic. However, the classic lesion is so-called **palpable purpura,** often occurring on the lower extremities and other dependent areas. Papular, vesicular, ulcerative, urticarial, or infarctive lesions may also be manifestations of leukocytoclastic vasculitis.

A. **Henoch-Schönlein purpura (HSP)** refers to a syndrome occurring predominantly in children and young adults that is characterized by nonthrombocytopenic purpura, arthralgias or mild arthritis (especially ankles and knees), abdominal pain, gastrointestinal hemorrhage, and nephritis. Leukocytoclastic vasculitis is found in all affected organs. The renal lesion may vary from a mild glomerulitis to severe crescentic glomerulonephritis with a rapidly progressive course. Intussusception from active gastrointestinal tract vasculitis is a problem in young children.

HSP occurs most commonly in spring and frequently follows an upper respiratory tract infection. Although most patients recover, there is a strong tendency for several relapses to occur before complete resolution. A small percentage of patients develop severe, progressive renal disease.

IgA is the predominant immunoglobulin found in skin and renal tissue in patients with HSP. Since IgA can activate complement only through the alternative pathway, HSP may represent an immune complex–mediated vasculitis operating through this mechanism. In support of this theory is the known occurrence of HSP in several C2-deficient patients, as well as recent preliminary data documenting circulating IgA-containing immune complexes.

B. **Essential mixed cryoglobulinemia** is a clinical syndrome characterized by arthralgias, weakness, purpura (leukocytoclastic vasculitis) and varying degrees of glomerulonephritis. Prognosis depends to a large degree on the severity of the renal lesion. Mixed cryoglobulins (often containing IgM rheumatoid factor and its antigen, IgG) are seen in a variety of infectious and rheumatic diseases. However, in patients with essential mixed cryoglobulinemia, no primary disease can be found. It was recently shown that a large proportion of patients with this syndrome had either Hb_sAg or hepatitis B surface antibody in their serum or cryoprecipitates. This finding may be yet another manifestation of hepatitis B virus infection in humans.

C. **Systemic lupus erythematosus, rheumatoid arthritis, and sicca syndrome** may have necrotizing vasculitis as an associated feature. Rarely, this is a severe visceral vasculitis of the Group I type. Usually, however, it is a dermal vasculitis that is histologically identical to other leukocytoclastic vasculitides. Common manifestations include purpura, cutaneous infarcts, ulcers (often nonhealing), cold sensitivity, and occasional digital gangrene. Rheumatoid arthritis patients with vasculitis generally have strongly seropositive, erosive disease with rheumatoid nodules.

D. **Other disorders** frequently complicated by cutaneous vasculitis include hematologic malignancies (especially Hodgkin disease and non-Hodgkin lymphoma), infectious endocarditis, and drug hypersensitivity reactions.

II. **Diagnostic investigations.** The key to diagnosis in these disorders is biopsy of the skin lesions, which will show leukocytoclastic vasculitis. Histologically, one cannot differentiate the various disorders by means of biopsy. Next, an attempt should be made to identify one of the aforementioned syndromes (sec. I.) with which leukocytoclastic vasculitis is associated. Additional investigations should include the following.

A. Attempt to identify an exogenous antigen such as a **drug** or **infectious agent.**

B. Search for an associated **rheumatic disease** or, if clinically indicated, an associated **hematologic malignancy.**

C. Attempt to identify **cryoglobulins** in serum if clinical illness is compatible with essential mixed cryoglobulinemia.

D. Determination of presence and extent of **systemic disease,** especially in patients with essential mixed cryoglobulinemia, rheumatoid arthritis, systemic lupus erythematosus, or Henoch-Schönlein purpura.

III. Therapy. Therapy for Group II disorders should be individualized depending upon the primary disorder responsible for the vasculitis.

A. Occasionally, **no therapy** of the vasculitis per se is indicated. Such a situation occurs in vasculitis complicating infectious endocarditis or hematologic malignancies where treatment of the underlying disease will result in resolution of the vasculitis. Specific therapy may not be necessary in drug-related vasculitis, once the offending agent is withdrawn; however, a short course of moderate-dose corticosteroid therapy (20 to 40 mg/24 hr PO) may be needed if the vasculitis is severe.

B. Efficacy of **corticosteroid therapy** has not been definitively proven in HSP. However, most clinicians will employ moderate- to high-dose steroid therapy (prednisone 40 to 60 mg/24 hr) in patients with very active disease, especially if significant gastrointestinal tract or renal involvement is present. Musculoskeletal symptoms may respond to nonsteroidal antiinflammatory agents.

C. No controlled study of treatment in **essential mixed cryoglobulinemia** has been reported. Therapeutic modalities employed have included corticosteroids, cytotoxic drugs, and plasmaphoresis. Results have been variable.

D. **Vasculitis complicating rheumatoid arthritis** should be managed with both moderate-dose oral prednisone (20 to 40 mg/24 hr) and a remittive agent. Indications for treatment include severe, active vasculitis as manifested by ulcers of the extremities, distal extremity cyanosis or gangrene, infarctive lesions of the fingers or nail pulp, or evidence of visceral vasculitis. Penicillamine or cytotoxic drugs (azathioprine or cyclophosphamide) are the rheumatoid arthritis remittive agents of choice here, as opposed to chrysotherapy. The dosage regimens for these drugs are discussed in Chapter 39. Uncontrolled studies have reported improvement of rheumatoid vasculitis with plasmapheresis.

E. **Cutaneous vasculitis accompanying systemic lupus erythematosus,** if mild, can be managed with low to moderate doses of corticosteroids (prednisone 10 to 30 mg/24 hr). For very mild lesions, no therapy is needed. More severe forms of dermal vasculitis or visceral vasculitis, or both, require high-dose corticosteroids occasionally combined with cytotoxic drugs.

Group III. Giant Cell Arteritides

The two disorders included in this category are temporal arteritis and Takayasu arteritis. Although quite similar histologically, they are markedly different clinically. Pathologically, both are panarteritides involving large vessels, characterized by disruption of the internal elastic lamina, intimal proliferation, and infiltration with mononuclear cells. Giant cells are seen more commonly in temporal arteritis.

I. Clinical features

A. Temporal arteritis is discussed in Chapter 32.

B. **Takayasu arteritis** is a disease of unknown etiology manifesting inflammation of the aorta and its major branches, with varying degrees of secondary stenosis or occlusion. It is most common in young females (80% of patients under 30 years of age), especially of Oriental background. Presenting symptoms and signs are either **systemic,** such as fever, arthralgias, weakness, and weight loss, or **ischemic,** relating to occlusion of major vessels. The latter group may include absence of peripheral pulses (hence the name *pulseless disease*), claudication, renovascular hypertension, and pulmonary hypertension secondary to involvement of the major pulmonary arteries. The clinical course is quite variable: the patient usually deteriorates gradually but may achieve remission, temporarily stabilize, or abruptly deteriorate.

II. Diagnostic investigations

A. Temporal artery biopsy is discussed in Chapter 32.

B. Diagnosis of **Takayasu arteritis** depends on a compatible clinical picture (see sec. **I.B.**) corroborated by the angiographic demonstration of multiple stenoses or occlusions of the aorta and its major branches. Because of the location of the lesions, biopsy is rarely feasible.

III. Therapy

A. Therapy of temporal arteritis is discussed in Chapter 32.

B. **Corticosteroid therapy** has been used in Takayasu arteritis with variable results. No controlled studies have been done. Some authors feel that steroids are beneficial early, when evidence of marked inflammation exists as manifested by an elevated sedimentation rate and constitutional symptoms. Late in the disease, when vessel occlusion is significant and no indication of active inflammation exists, corticosteroid therapy does not seem beneficial.

Group IV. Wegener Granulomatosis

I. Clinical features

A. **Wegener granulomatosis (WG)** is characterized by necrotizing granulomatous vasculitis of the upper and lower respiratory tract, glomerulonephritis, and various degrees of vasculitis of other organs. Limited forms of the illness involving only the upper and lower respiratory tract have also been described.

Typically, patients present with symptoms or signs referable to the sinuses, nasopharynx, ears, or lungs. Less commonly, constitutional symptoms, musculoskeletal complaints, or signs referable to vasculitis of other organs (e.g., skin, heart, central nervous system) predominate. When renal disease becomes clinically apparent, it is rapidly progressive if untreated. Table 42-2 lists the salient features in a group of patients followed at the National Institute of Health.

The radiographic manifestations of the pulmonary disease in WG are diverse. Most commonly seen are solitary or multiple nodular densities or infiltrates, varying in size from less than 1 cm to more than 9 cm. Cavitation of the nodular lesions is common. Pulmonary involvement is usually bilateral. Rarely, focal atelectasis and small pleural effusions are seen.

II. Diagnostic investigations. Definitive diagnosis rests upon demonstrating the typical granulomatous necrotizing vasculitis on pathologic material.

A. Tissue biopsy

1. Lung biopsy (generally through thoracotomy) is the diagnostic modality of choice in the majority of cases.

2. Occasionally, biopsy of a necrotic, ulcerative nasal or skin lesion will be adequate in a patient with a classic clinical presentation (i.e., upper and lower respiratory tract and renal disease).

3. Renal biopsy

a. To distinguish WG, which presents as a focal, necrotizing glomerulitis, from **Goodpasture syndrome,** which presents as a diffuse, crescentic glomerulonephritis. Clinically, it is sometimes difficult to differentiate these two diseases.

b. To assess the **severity** of the renal lesion.

c. Occasionally, **occult renal involvement** will be found on biopsy in a patient with a normal urine sediment and normal renal function. The finding of occult glomerulitis will influence therapy (see sec. **III.**).

Table 42-2. Organ System Involvement in Wegener Granulomatosis

Organ System	Typical Features	Approximate Frequency (%)
Nasopharynx	Necrotizing granuloma with mucosal ulceration; saddle nose deformity	75
Paranasal sinuses	Pansinusitis; necrotizing granuloma; secondary bacterial infection	90
Eyes	Keratoconjunctivitis; granulomatous sclerouveitis	60
Ears	Serous otitis media; secondary bacterial infection	35
Lungs	Multiple nodular cavitary infiltrates; necrotizing granulomatous vasculitis	95
Kidneys	Focal and segmental glomerulitis; necrotizing glomerulonephritis later in course	85
Heart	Coronary vasculitis; pericarditis	15
Nervous system	Mononeuritis multiplex; cranial neuritis	20
Skin	Dermal vasculitis with secondary ulcerations	40
Joints	Polyarthralgias	50

III. Therapy

A. Limited forms of WG (i.e., upper and lower respiratory tract; no clinical or histologic renal involvement) may be treated with **corticosteroids** alone, the dose depending on the severity of the symptoms and signs.

B. Cyclophosphamide is clearly the drug of choice for generalized WG. Before the use of cytotoxic drugs, generalized WG was a highly aggressive and almost uniformly fatal disease. Untreated, WG pursued a rapidly fatal course with mean survival of five and one-half months. Ninety percent of patients died within two years. Corticosteroid therapy alone did not appreciably alter the course of generalized WG. The dose of cyclophosphamide is 1 to 2 mg/kg daily for 2 weeks. If a clinical response occurs, the dose is kept at this level with readjustments to keep the total leukocyte count above 3,000 cells/mm³. If no clinical response is obtained within 2 weeks, the dose is increased by 25 mg and kept at this level for an additional 2 weeks. This rate of increase in therapy is continued until a clinical response occurs or drug toxicity is manifest.

Patients with fulminant vasculitis or rapidly progressing renal insufficiency, or both, are initially treated with cyclophosphamide at 4 mg/kg daily for 3 days and then rapidly tapered to 1 to 2 mg/kg daily. Concomitant corticosteroid therapy is used in patients with fulminant renal or pulmonary disease, severe skin involvement, eye involvement, or pericarditis.

With the above regimen, a remission rate of over 90% is reported, with many patients showing improvement in renal function. A small proportion of patients have been able to discontinue therapy and have been free of disease for up to seven years. Therapy is continued until the patient has shown no traces of disease for one year.

Group V. Lymphomatoid Granulomatosis

Lymphomatoid granulomatosis (LG) is a necrotizing, granulomatous pulmonary vasculitis with features similar to Wegener granulomatosis but sufficiently distinct to be designated a separate clinicopathologic entity. Pathologically it is an angiocentric and angiodestructive granulomatous disorder, characterized by an infiltrate of normal lymphocytes, plasma cells, and atypical plasmacytoid cells. Whether or not this infiltrate constitutes pulmonary lymphoma is unsettled, but a significant proportion (10% to 15%) of patients develop clearcut nodal lymphoma during the course of their disease.

I. **Clinical features.** Lung involvement is present in all patients. Multiple, bilateral, nodular pulmonary infiltrates are the usual x-ray finding. Skin (40%), kidney (45%), and nervous system (30%) are also frequently involved.

A. **Comparisons and contrasts between lymphomatoid granulomatosis and Wegener granulomatosis**

1. **Atypical plasmacytoid cell infiltrate** is seen only in lymphomatoid granulomatosis.

2. **Renal involvement** in lymphomatoid granulomatosis is characterized by nodular infiltration of the **kidney** parenchyma by the plasmacytoid cell infiltrate. Necrotizing glomerulitis or arteritis are the renal lesions of Wegener granulomatosis.

3. **Sinus and upper airway disease** is absent in lymphomatoid granulomatosis but is characteristic of Wegener granulomatosis.

4. **Response to therapy** is markedly different in the two diseases.

II. **Therapy.** Lymphomatoid granulomatosis is a highly aggressive, often fatal disease, for the most part refractory to therapy. Median survival in the largest group of patients reported was only 14 months. Response to various therapeutic modalities, including corticosteroids, cytotoxic drugs, and radiotherapy, has been uniformly poor.

Bibliography

General Reviews
Christian, C. L., and Sergent, J. S.   Vasculitis syndromes. Clinical and experimental models. *Am. J. Med.* 61:385, 1976.

Fauci, A. S. (Moderator).   The spectrum of vasculitis. Clinical, pathologic, immunologic and therapeutic considerations. *Ann. Intern. Med.* 89:660, 1978.

Group I Disorders
Churg, J., and Strauss, L.   Allergic granulomatosis, angiitis, and periarteritis nodosa. *Am. J. Pathol.* 27:277, 1951.

Melish, M. E., Hicks, R. M., and Larson, E. J.   Mucocutaneous lymph node syndrome in the United States. *Am. J. Dis. Child.* 1308:599, 1976.

Sergent, J. S., Lockshin, M. D., Christian, C. L., and Gocke, D. J.   Vasculitis with hepatitis B antigenemia. *Medicine* 55:1, 1976.

Group II Disorders
Meltzer, M., et al.   Cryoglobulinemia. A clinical and laboratory study. II. Cryoglobulins with rheumatoid factor activity. *Am. J. Med.* 40:837, 1966.

Sams, W. M., et al.   Leucocytoclastic vasculitis. *Arch. Dermatol.* 112:219, 1976.

Soter, N. A.   Clinical presentations and mechanisms of necrotizing angiitis of the skin. *J. Invest. Dermatol.* 67:354, 1976.

Group III Disorders
Nakao, K., et al.   Takayasu's arteritis. Clinical report of eighty-four cases and immunologic studies of seven cases. *Circulation* 35:1141, 1967.

Group IV Disorders
Wolff, S. M. (Moderator).   Wegener's granulomatosis. *Ann. Intern. Med.* 81:513, 1974.

Group V Disorders
Katzenstein, A. A., Carrington, C. C., and Liebow, A. A.   Lymphomatoid granulomatosis. A clinicopathologic study of 152 cases. *Cancer* 43:360, 1979.

IV. Appendixes

Appendix A
Physical Therapy

Judith M. Kurtz, R.P.T.

The **goals** of physical therapy include the restoration of function and the prevention of injury or disability.

The **methods** by which goals are achieved include evaluation; therapeutic exercises; ambulation training; modalities of heat, cold, electrical stimulation, mechanical traction, and transcutaneous nerve stimulation; activities of daily living; and patient education.

I. Evaluation

Baseline evaluation should be made for all patients either preoperatively or prior to initiating therapy. The evaluation profiles the functional level at which the patient is first seen. Periodic reevaluations give valuable information regarding the patient's progress. Relevant information should include:

A. **Range of motion (ROM)**

B. **Manual muscle grade**

C. Description of any **gait deviation**

II. Therapeutic exercises

A. **Active** exercises are performed by the patient without assistance from any source. The patient is instructed carefully in specific exercises performed to the limit of pain.

B. **Active-assisted** exercises are performed by the patient with the assistance of another person. Available ROM and limit of pain should be used as therapeutic guidelines.

C. **Passive** exercises are performed entirely by another person. The guidelines of available ROM and limit of pain are most important in this type of exercise. Conditions such as osteoporosis and recent surgery require caution.

D. **Resisted** exercises are performed by the patient for the purposes of increasing strength and endurance. These exercises should be carefully graded by pounds of weight and number of repetitions. It is important not to fatigue the muscle too quickly.

E. **Isometric** exercises may also be used to increase strength without producing motion at the joint. The number of repetitions of muscle contraction should be carefully graded.

III. Ambulation training

A. **Non–weight–bearing** ambulation is performed with axillary crutches. Weight bearing is shared between the upper extremities and the unaffected lower extremity. The patient should be instructed to push with the upper extremities in order to establish a smooth gait pattern.

B. **Partial weight-bearing** (three-point gait) ambulation may be performed with either axillary or Lofstrand crutches. The **gait pattern** is such that both crutches and the affected lower extremity come forward at the same time. The amount of weight placed on the affected lower extremity is controlled by the upper extremities pushing on the crutches.

C. **A four-point gait** is extremely slow and used with a patient who requires crutches for balance and some decrease in weight bearing of the lower extremity joints. The **gait pattern** begins with one crutch forward and then the opposite foot; second crutch forward, other foot.

D. **A two-point gait** most closely approximates a normal gait pattern. The **gait pattern** is crutch and opposite foot forward at the same time. The patient may use crutches or two canes with this gait.

IV. **Ambulation devices.** Careful selection is important in order to give the patient the opportunity to relearn as normal a gait as possible.

A. **Axillary crutches** are measured with the patient in the standing position. The crutches are placed under the patient's arms with the tips 6 to 8 in. from the anterolateral borders of the feet. The hand pieces are adjusted so that the elbows are at 15 to 20 degrees of flexion. The axillary pads should reach no closer than the width of two fingers from the patient's axillae. Axillary crutches may be used for all gaits.

B. **Lofstrand crutches (Canadian canes)** are aluminum and adjustable. The height is adjusted so that the patient's elbow is in 15 to 20 degrees of flexion. The cuff is open and should encircle the middle of the forearm. These crutches can be used for all gaits except non–weight bearing.

C. **A cane** may or may not be adjustable. The height should be such that the patient's hand is at the level of the greater trochanter of the hip joint. The patient is instructed to use the cane in the hand opposite to the affected lower extremity. Many canes are made with flat handles that are easier for patients with decreased hand function to use. Two canes may be used to teach a partial weight-bearing gait, if the patient cannot manage crutches.

D. **Standard walkers** vary in size according to the patient's height. The **height** should be adjusted so that the patient's elbows are in 15 to 20 degrees of flexion. There are modifications and attachments that may be added to the walker. For example, some walkers may be opened more to accommodate the abducted gait of the patient with total hip replacement. Wheels and platform attachments can also be added for a patient with severe rheumatoid arthritis. The walker can be used for all gaits.

E. **A platform walker** is basically a standard walker with attachments for weight bearing on the forearms. It is used when the patient cannot bear weight directly on the hands. This walker may or may not have wheels attached to it. It may be used for all gaits.

V. **Modalities**

A. **Moist heat** modalities include **hot packs, whirlpool,** and **pool.**

1. **Hot packs** may be applied before each session of therapeutic exercise to provide increased circulation and muscle relaxation. Individual patients may not respond well to moist heat, in which case application of ice packs may be more beneficial.

   a. **Indications.** Muscle spasm, joint contracture.

   b. **Contraindications.** Sensory loss, malignant tumors, open lesions.

2. **Whirlpool** is beneficial for cleaning open wounds and in conjunction with mild exercises of the foot and hand. Care must be taken not to put the limb in a dependent position, thus increasing the potential for edema. If a patient sits in a whirlpool, there is little room for exercising a joint such as the hip or knee.

   a. **Indications.** Open lesions, muscle spasm.

   b. **Contraindications.** Patients with poor heat tolerance, debilitated patients, cortisone withdrawal.

3. The **therapeutic pool** is an excellent modality for therapeutic exercises and ambulation because the forces of gravity are eliminated in deep water. The temperature should be maintained between 94°F and 96°F. Patients should progress from deep to shallow water, as tolerated. Exercises and ambulation

should then be continued out of the water, again with progression to the patient's tolerance.

   a. Indications. Muscle spasm; muscle weakness; postoperative pain; pain and deformity resulting from a disease process such as generalized rheumatoid arthritis; difficulty with initial ambulation.

   b. Contraindications. Open lesions, debilitated patients, patients with poor heat tolerance, urinary tract infection, tracheostomy, and diarrhea.

B. Dry heat modalities include **diathermy** and **infrared.** They may be used before an exercise program to obtain increased circulation and muscle relaxation. However, most patients with rheumatoid arthritis find a modality such as diathermy to be extremely uncomfortable.

   1. Diathermy may be either short-wave or microwave. Microwave is usually preferred because the equipment does not come in direct contact with the patient.

   a. Indications. Muscle spasm, joint contractures, chronic pain as in low back pain, adhesive capsulitis.

   b. Contraindications. Metallic implants, coagulation defects, sensory loss, open lesions, bone deformities, malignant tumors.

   2. Infrared should be applied approximately 20 in. from the area to be treated and perpendicular to that area.

   a. Indications. Relief of muscle spasm, relief of pain, and promotion of healing of open lesions.

   b. Contraindications. Sensory loss, excessive scar tissue, and circulatory disease are relative contraindications.

C. Other modalities that can be used effectively are paraffin baths, ultrasound, intermittent traction, cold packs, electrical stimulation, and transcutaneous nerve stimulation.

   1. Paraffin baths are beneficial for the patient with disability of the hands or feet. The mold conforms closely to the joints and produces some increased circulation and muscle relaxation. It may be used before exercise of the hands and feet. The home units that are available are usually too difficult and dangerous for the patient with severe hand involvement to manage.

   a. Indications. Joint pain, contractures.

   b. Contraindications. Open lesions, skin rash, loss of sensation.

   2. Ultrasound is a form of deep heat that may be used before exercise. It is very effective in treatment of joints covered by thick layers of tissue, such as the hip. In contrast to diathermy, metal reflects rather than absorbs ultrasound and can therefore be used in patients with prosthetic joints. When prescribed, a specific dose and duration of application should be indicated. Dosage is expressed in watts per square centimeter; time is expressed in minutes. The size and cost of equipment limit its use to the office or rehabilitation department.

   a. Indications. Joint contractures, scarring of periarticular and capsular tissues, relief of muscle spasm.

   b. Contraindications. Direct application to the eyes, abdominal application during pregnancy, malignant tumors. **Special precautions** should be taken in the area of the spinal cord following laminectomy.

   3. Intermittent traction is used for disorders of the spine. Its application should be preceded by some form of heat. The amount of traction prescribed ranges from 5 to 60 pounds, depending on the area treated and the patient's tolerance. This form of traction is usually tolerated better than static traction as a result of the periods of relaxation.

    a. Indications. Vertebral osteoarthritis, correction of mild contractures, relief of muscle spasm.

    b. Contraindications. Damaged ligaments, unstable vertebrae, local malignancy, osteoporosis, spinal cord disease, osteomyelitis, pregnancy, debilitation.

4. Cold packs are very effective in the treatment of conditions such as low back pain, postoperative pain after joint replacement, and soft tissue injury associated with swelling. Application of ice can also take the form of water frozen in a small, round plastic cup which is rubbed over the painful area. Packs may be purchased for home use.

    a. Indications. Prevention of posttraumatic hemorrhage, reduction of edema and inflammatory reaction, sprains, bruises, contusions, acute bursitis, post-manipulation, traumatic arthritis.

    b. Contraindications. Raynaud phenomenon, sensitivity to cold.

5. Electrical stimulation is used most often as an adjunct to muscle reeducation in peripheral nerve injuries. It should never be used as a substitute for active exercises.

6. Transcutaneous nerve stimulation is used to promote pain inhibition in postoperative and chronic pain states. The patient is instructed to use the unit and may wear it for long periods throughout the day. The unit may be rented or purchased for use at home.

VI. Activities of daily living (see also Appendix B)

A. Transfer activities are important for patients to learn during the course of their rehabilitation program. Assistive devices such as walkers, crutches, canes, sliding (transfer) board, raised toilet seat, grab bars, and bathtub seat should be utilized when needed. Ability to perform the following transfers should be emphasized.

    1. Bed to chair (wheelchair); chair to bed.

    2. Bed to standing; standing to bed.

    3. Wheelchair to toilet; toilet to wheelchair.

    4. Chair to bathtub (stall shower); bathtub to chair.

    5. Chair to car; car to chair.

B. Positioning of the patient is important, particularly when the patient is in bed for prolonged periods. For example, the patient with rheumatoid arthritis should *not* be allowed to place pillows under the knees. The cervical spine should always be maintained in a neutral position with a small flat pillow under the head for comfort. If the fingers are in flexion, a **small, rolled towel** should be placed in the palm of the hand. When **lying on the side,** a pillow should be placed between the legs to maintain a neutral position of the hips and provide comfort. When **prone,** a small, flat pillow may be placed under the lower abdomen for comfort, without allowing the hips to flex. A **footboard** or firm padding should be used to maintain the ankles in a neutral position.

C. Posture. All patients should be given instruction in correct posture when sitting, standing, and ambulating. Many patients with postoperative or chronic pain acquire the habit of functioning in a flexed position or position of most comfort. In the long run, poor posture may produce back pain and tightness or contractures of major muscle groups.

D. Body mechanics. The key point in proper body mechanics is to keep the knees and hips slightly flexed and the trunk straight when moving or lifting objects.

VII. Patient education. Such programs should be multidisciplinary, involving all members of the health team. They should strongly emphasize the role that patients must play in the execution of a successful program.

Bibliography

Krusen, F. (Ed.). *Handbook of Physical Medicine and Rehabilitation.* Philadelphia: Saunders, 1971.

Licht, S. (Ed.). *Therapeutic Exercise.* Baltimore: Elizabeth Licht, 1958.

Licht, S. (Ed.). *Therapeutic Heat and Cold.* Baltimore: Elizabeth Licht, 1965.

Licht, S. (Ed.). *Arthritis and Physical Medicine.* Baltimore: Elizabeth Licht, 1969.

McCarty, D.J. (Ed.). *Arthritis and Allied Conditions.* Philadelphia: Lea & Febiger, 1979.

Appendix B
Occupational Therapy

Ellen Rader, O.T.R.

Occupational therapy (OT) provides assistance to persons whose functional level of performance has been affected by physical, psychologic, or developmental disabilities. Carefully selected modalities and activities are used to promote an optimal level of independence in activities of daily living.

I. Indications and modalities in orthopedics and rheumatology

A. Indications

1. Maintain or increase upper extremity (UE) range of motion (ROM), strength, and endurance.
2. Improve functional abilities in activities of daily living (ADL).
3. Provide patient education.
4. Explore adaptations or alternatives in vocational and avocational interests.
5. Facilitate psychosocial adjustment to the impact of disability.

B. Modalities

1. Instruction in adaptive ADL methods, including the use of assistive devices.
2. Functional hand and UE training.
3. Instruction in joint protection, energy conservation, and work simplification techniques.
4. Fabrication of splints.
5. Therapeutic exercise.
6. Psychosocial support through verbalization and problem solving.

II. Activities of daily living (ADL)

A. ADL includes the tasks of feeding, dressing, personal hygiene, bathing, transfers, and homemaking (cooking, laundering, shopping, housecleaning, and child care), which are all basic to **self-care**.

B. **Evaluation** is necessary to determine a patient's past and present ADL skills. The potential for maximum independent performance is considered, along with other evaluative findings including ROM, strength, endurance, fatigue, pain, stiffness, deformity, motivation, and overall medical status. Changes in disease status may cause fluctuations in functional abilities, indicating the necessity for periodic ADL reevaluation.

C. **The American Rheumatism Association (ARA) functional classification** is a general classification system for rheumatic disease patients.

Class I	Complete functional capacity with ability to carry on all usual duties without handicaps.
Class II	Functional capacity adequate to conduct normal activities despite handicap of discomfort or limited mobility of one or more joints.
Class III	Functional capacity adequate to perform only few or none of the duties of usual occupation or of self-care.
Class IV	Largely or wholly incapacitated with patient bedridden or confined to wheelchair, capable of little or no self-care.

D. **ADL treatment** includes instruction in **alternative methods** of performance, that is, substitution or compensation skills. **Adaptive equipment** and **assistive devices** which may be provided follow.

1. **Feeding.** Long, built-up or angled utensil handles; universal cuff; and lightweight utensils.

2. **Dressing.** Long-handled shoe horn, reacher, dressing stick, or sock aid; button hook; zipper pull; Velcro closures; and loose-fitting or front-fastening clothing.

3. **Hygiene and bathing.** Long-handled comb, brush, or sponge; shower hose; bathroom grab bars; bathtub transfer bench; and raised toilet seat.

4. **Miscellaneous hand devices.** Zim jar opener, Dycem matting, book holder, doorknob extension, key holder, and felt-tip pens.

III. Patient education. Patient education includes instruction in joint protection and energy conservation.

A. **Joint protection** concepts help preserve joint integrity and reduce stress to involved joint structures, especially those stresses that can further contribute to deformity.

Patients are encouraged to use pain as a signal to moderate activity. They are advised to avoid positions of deformity, tight grasp, and pinch, and static or holding positions. Patients should change positions frequently, utilize larger and stronger joint structures when possible, and use assistive devices and splints as applicable.

B. **Energy conservation** techniques encourage task accomplishment with a minimum amount of energy expenditure. A balance of rest and work is essential and requires careful daily scheduling. Proper body mechanics, posture, and positioning are important. Environmental adaptations at home and work, along with the use of modern, lightweight electrical appliances, should be employed. These principles can be applied as follows.

1. **Rheumatoid arthritis** patients need to avoid stress to all joints, especially the hand and inflamed joints.

2. **Osteoarthritis** patients need to avoid stress to weight-bearing joints.

3. **Back** patients must avoid stress due to improper positioning, bending, and carrying.

IV. Splinting

A. **A splint** is a temporary orthosis used to support, immobilize, position, or mobilize a specific joint.

1. **Static splints** contain no movable parts and maintain the affected part in the desired position.

2. **Dynamic splints** allow movement in specific directions by the application of a nearly constant force. They may utilize hinges, springs, or outriggers with elastic tension.

Splints must be chosen with a specific intent in mind. They should be **custom-made** for each patient to assure proper fit and maximum therapeutic benefit (commercial splints are not recommended). Splinting in rheumatoid arthritis is a **controversial** issue since adverse effects from immobilization can occur. It does play an important role in helping to reduce inflammation, pain, and muscle spasm by providing support to inflamed joints. Splints cannot prevent deformity, but they can help to position the hand, provide counteractive forces, and eliminate stresses to which the hand is subject during normal daily usage.

B. **Careful evaluation** of the hand or affected part is required before splint fabrication. Considerations include anatomic and skeletal structures, skin, wound, and sensory status. The patient's willingness to wear the splint and understanding of its purpose are also important.

Table B-1. Commonly Prescribed Splints

Problem	Splint	Rationale
Rheumatoid hand inflammation	Volar wrist cock-up	Provides wrist support; extends to distal palmar crease and thenar eminence
	Full resting hand	Provides support to wrist, MCP and IP joints, and thumb by resting hand in functional position; for night use or acute flare
Carpal tunnel syndrome	Volar or dorsal wrist	Relieves pressure on median nerve; generally for night wear
DeQuervain tenosynovitis	Volar wrist with thumb support	Immobilizes wrist and thumb CMC and MCP joints; maintains thumb in palmar abduction for pinch
Lateral epicondylitis	Dorsal or volar wrist	Prevents sudden and forceful wrist movements during work or sport activities

C. Splint indications and types

1. Immobilization or rest of a joint (for inflammation, wound or fracture healing, or pain).

2. Positioning and maintenance of optimum joint alignment.

3. Prevention or correction of deformity or contracture.

4. Positioning of joints for optimum function.

5. Assistance in weak movement; substitution for absent movement; and assistance in muscle reeducation and exercise.

6. Maintainence of surgical correction.
Table B-1 lists common problems that may require splinting and the types of splints used. Specific splints can be constructed and designed for numerous other orthopedic and rheumatologic problems including stiffness, contracture, edema, peripheral nerve injuries, fracture healing, myopathies, and postsurgical care.

V. Exercise treatment. Therapeutic exercise and functional activities are utilized to maintain or increase hand, elbow, and shoulder ROM, strength, coordination, dexterity, and endurance.

A. Evaluation is the first step in treatment. Evaluation includes goniometry, individual and functional muscle testing, objective strength measurements (dynamometer, sphygmomanometer, or pinch gauge), sensory testing, edema assessment, and specific hand function tests.

B. Therapeutic exercise includes the use of active, assisted, and passive ROM exercises as well as isometric and resistive exercises. In conjunction with occupational therapy, physical therapy modalities of heat, ultrasound, and paraffin are often used to augment treatment.
Hand exercises should strive to maintain ROM. When exercising specific hand joints, adjacent joint structures should be protected. Resistive hand exercises in rheumatoid arthritis are *contraindicated* since they provide additional stress to already weakened joint and tendon structures (e.g., squeezing a rubber ball only contributes to ulnar and volar forces). See Appendix C for specific exercise prescriptions.

C. Functional activities include the active involvement of the patient in graded and goal-directed activities. Specific crafts such as weaving, macrame, leather working, and copper tooling are carefully structured to supplement a formal exercise program.

   1. Shoulder problems. Pulleys, skateboards, rolling pins, wall climbing, and dowel stick exercises are useful.

   2. Hand therapy. Prehension activities employ a variety of large and small objects to develop grasp and pinch. Pegboards, cones, Velcro checkers, rubber bands, and theraplast are utilized to enhance fine motor coordination and dexterity skills.

Bibliography

Hopkins, H., and Smith, H. *Willard and Spackman's Occupational Therapy* (5th ed.). Philadelphia: Lippincott, 1978.

Melvin, J. *Rheumatic Disease: Occupational Therapy and Rehabilitation.* Philadelphia: Davis, 1977.

Sweezy, R. *Arthritis: Rational Therapy and Rehabilitation.* Philadelphia: Saunders, 1978.

Appendix C
Therapeutic Exercises

Judith M. Kurtz, R.P.T.
and Ellen Rader, O.T.R.

Table C-I lists therapeutic exercise prescriptions for some of the rheumatic disorders. Additional exercise regimens are noted in chapters dealing with individual anatomic areas.

General Instructions to Patients

1. **Use pain as your guide.** Pain or discomfort should not last longer than one hour after exercise.

2. Make the exercises part of your **daily routine.**

3. Try to do a complete set of exercises at least twice a day at a time convenient to you.

4. Prescribed medication and heat or cold applications may precede exercises to enhance relaxation.

5. Perform only those exercises given to you by your physician or therapist. Do only the **prescribed number** of repetitions. The average initial regimen is 5 repetitions. The average maximum exercise regimen is 25 repetitions. If pain occurs, exercise is stopped temporarily and increased gradually, as tolerated.

6. Perform exercises on a **firm surface.**

7. **Exercise slowly** with a smooth motion. Do not rush.

8. Avoid holding your breath.

9. **Moderate the exercise** regimen during an acute attack.

10. Contact your physician or therapist if you have any problems with the exercises.

Exercises

1. **Pendulum exercise for shoulder** (Fig. C-1)

   Position. Standing, lean forward, bending from the waist, with knees slightly flexed. Allow arm to hang loosely with shoulder relaxed. (One arm may hold on to a chair or table for additional support if necessary.)

   a. Swing arm forward and backward. Repeat ____ times.*

   b. Swing arm from side to side. Repeat ____ times.

   c. Swing arm in gradually widening circles, in both clockwise and counterclockwise directions. Repeat ____ times.

2. **Assisted shoulder forward flexion exercise** (Fig. C-2)

   Position. Supine, sitting, or standing. Arms at side.

   a. Grasp arm at wrist, with palm facing you.

   b. Use "grasping" arm to raise affected arm (overhead if possible). Holding a broomstick or a cane in both hands may help assist in performance of this exercise.

*____ represents the number of repetitions prescribed by physician or therapist.

Table C-1. Exercise Prescriptions

Problem	Exercises (see text)	Goals	Precautions
Rheumatoid arthritis and other inflammatory arthritides	1–28; for scleroderma, include gentle stretch at end of range	Maintain joint mobility, range of motion, and strength	Generalized fatigue, increased pain, acute flare
Osteoarthritis			
Cervical spine	1, 2, 26, 27	Maintain optimal head alignment and posture	Muscle spasm, increased pain, edema
Knee	14, 16, 19, 20	Maintain or increase range of motion and strength	Increased pain, edema
Ankylosing spondylitis	1–6, 14–18, 23–27	Maintain or increase range of motion; maintain posture; avoid hip immobility	Increased pain or muscle spasm
Polymyositis	3–7, 9, 10, 14–19, 21, 22, 24, 25; add graded resistance to tolerance	Maintain or increase range of motion and muscle strength, particularly of proximal muscle groups; prevent contractures	Muscle fatigue
Shoulder periarticular disorders	1–6; include gentle stretch at end of range	Maintain or increase shoulder range of motion	Increased muscle spasm, pain, or inflammation
Chronic low back pain	14, 19, 23–25	Maintain or increase strength of trunk musculature; decrease pain; maintain posture	Increased pain, radiation to lower extremities

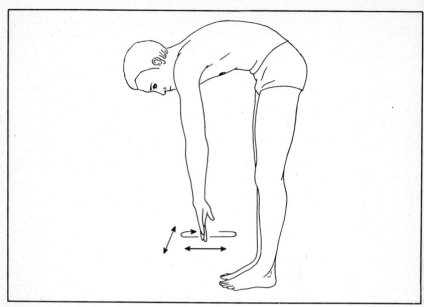

Figure C-1. Pendulum exercise for shoulder.

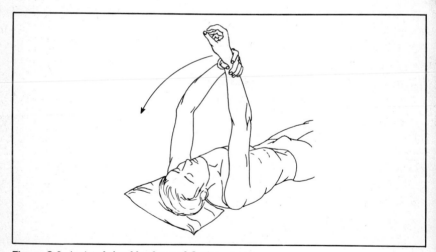

Figure C-2. Assisted shoulder forward flexion exercise.

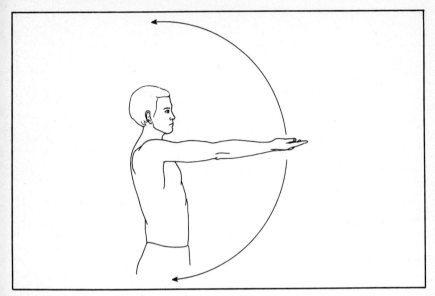

Figure C-3. Active shoulder forward flexion exercise.

  c. Hold to count of 5.

  d. Return to starting position.

  e. Relax.

  f. Repeat _____ times.

3. Active shoulder forward flexion exercise (Fig. C-3)

 Position. Supine, sitting, or standing. Arms straight at sides.

  a. Raise arm(s) over head, as high as possible, with palms up. Avoid shrugging your shoulders.

  b. Hold to count of 5.

  c. Return to starting position.

  d. Relax.

  e. Repeat _____ times.

4. Shoulder abduction exercise (Fig. C-4)

 Position. Supine, sitting, or standing. Arms straight at sides.

  a. Bring arm(s) away from you and out to side, with palms up. Avoid shrugging your shoulders. (Moving a broomstick from side to side can be used as well.)

  b. Hold to count of 5.

  c. Return to starting position.

  d. Relax.

  e. Repeat _____ times.

5. Shoulder external rotation exercise (Fig. C-5)

 Position. Supine, sitting, or standing. Arms at sides. Keep head straight.

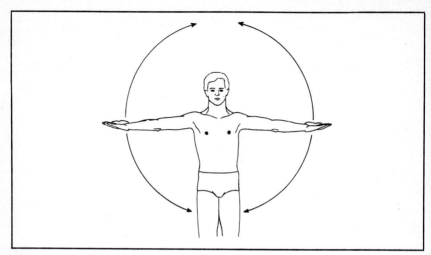

Figure C-4. Shoulder abduction exercise.

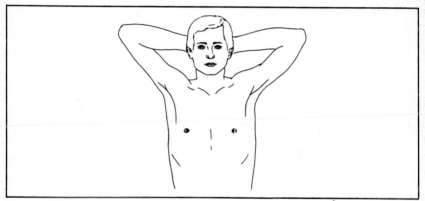

Figure C-5. Shoulder external rotation exercise.

a. Raise arm(s) to touch hands behind head. Avoid tucking your chin or leaning to one side. Try to keep elbows as wide apart as possible.

b. Hold to count of 5.

c. Return to starting position.

d. Relax.

e. Repeat ____ times.

6. Shoulder internal rotation exercise (Fig. C-6)

Position. Prone (on stomach) or standing. Arms at sides.

a. Raise arm(s) to touch hands behind back, reaching for waist and up to shoulder blades if possible. (One hand may assist the other, or a broomstick can be used to assist both arms.)

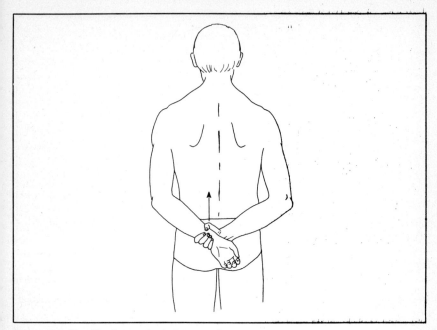

Figure C-6. Shoulder internal rotation exercise.

    b. Hold to count of 5.

    c. Return to starting position.

    d. Relax.

    e. Repeat ____ times.

7. Elbow flexion and extension exercise

    Position. Supine, sitting, or standing. Arms straight at sides with palms up.

    a. Bend elbow(s), trying to touch finger tips to shoulder.

    b. Hold to count of 5.

    c. Return to starting position.

    d. Relax.

    e. Repeat ____ times.

8. Forearm pronation and supination exercise (Fig. C-7)

    Position. Sitting, elbow tucked at side and flexed to 90 degrees (at right angle). Thumbs up. Forearm may be supported by table top.

    a. Turn forearm palm up.

    b. Hold to count of 5.

    c. Turn forearm palm down.

    d. Hold to count of 5.

    e. Return to starting position.

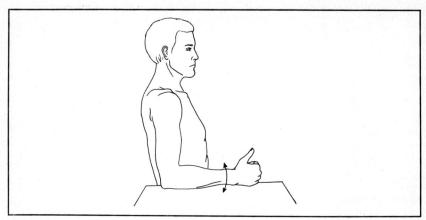

Figure C-7. Forearm pronation and supination exercise.

    f. Relax.

    g. Repeat ____ times.

9. Wrist extension exercise

Position. Sitting, hand resting flat on table or over table edge.

    a. Raise hand off table, keeping forearm flat on table. Fingers should be loosely flexed and in a relaxed position.

    b. Hold to count of 5.

    c. Return to starting position.

    d. Relax.

    e. Repeat ____ times.

10. Finger flexion and extension exercise

Position. Sitting.

    a. Make a fist, trying to bring all finger tips into palm.

    b. Open hand to spread and extend fingers fully. (This can also be done with hands squeezing a soft small sponge in a basin of warm water.)

    c. Relax.

    d. Repeat ____ times.

11. Intrinsic muscle stretching exercise (Fig. C-8)

Position. Sitting, palm up. Place a Bunnell block (a smooth rectangular piece of plywood which is ¼ in. thick, 2 in. wide, and 4 in. long) in palm of hand over knuckles, to keep knuckles straight and prevent them from moving.

    a. Curl finger tips into palm of hand to touch block. Only the two end finger joints should bend. (This exercise can be done without a block; be sure to support knuckles with opposite hand to prevent any motion at this level.)

    b. Hold to count of 5.

    c. Straighten fingers fully.

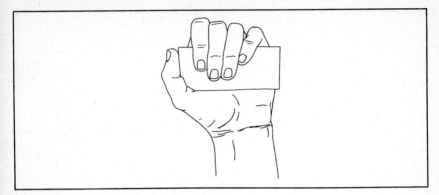

Figure C-8. Intrinsic muscle stretching exercise.

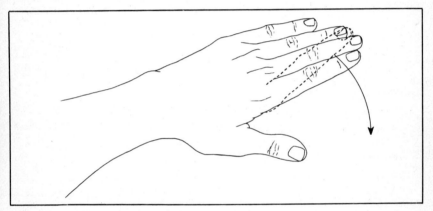

Figure C-9. Radial correction exercise.

    d. Relax.

    e. Repeat _____ times.

12. Radial correction exercise (Fig. C-9)

    Position. Sitting. Hands palm down on table.

    a. Lift each finger up and over in direction of thumb.

    b. Lift entire hand to return to starting position.

    c. Relax.

    d. Repeat _____ times.

13. Thumb exercises

    Position. Sitting. Palm up. Thumb resting against index finger.

    a. Touch thumb tip to each finger tip, making circles with each finger.

    b. Touch thumb tip to base of little finger.

    c. Move thumb sideways and away from palm and index finger.

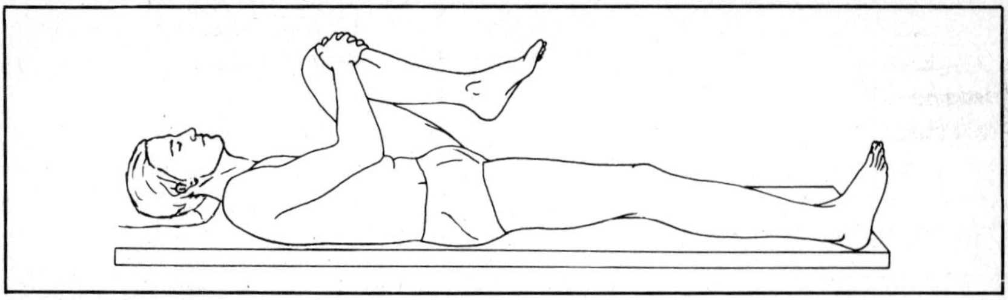

Figure C-10. Hip flexion and extension exercise.

    d. Lift thumb straight up (perpendicular to) the palm and index finger.

    e. Hold to count of 5 at the end of each motion.

    f. Relax.

    g. Repeat ____ times.

14. Hip flexion and extension exercise (Fig. C-10)

    Position. Supine.

    a. Bring one knee to chest.

    b. Straighten opposite leg until back of knee is flat.

    c. Hold to count of 5.

    d. Return to starting position.

    e. Relax.

    f. Repeat ____ times.

15. Hip abduction-adduction exercise (Fig. C-11)

    Position. Supine.

    a. Bring entire leg, from hip, out to side.

    b. Do not bend at waist.

    c. Keep hip and knee straight.

    d. Hold to count of 5.

    e. Return to starting position.

    f. Relax.

    g. Repeat ____ times.

16. Hip abduction-adduction exercise (Fig. C-12)

    Position. Side-lying (on uninvolved side, knee straight).

    a. Bring entire leg, from hip, back and up toward ceiling.

    b. Do not bend at waist.

    c. Keep knee straight.

    d. Hold to count of 5.

    e. Lower leg slowly.

    f. Relax.

    g. Repeat ____ times.

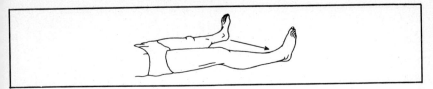

Figure C-11. Hip abduction-adduction exercise (supine).

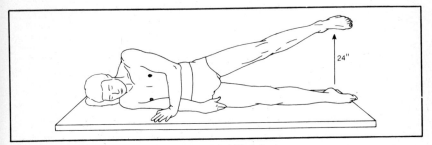

Figure C-12. Hip abduction-adduction exercise (side-lying).

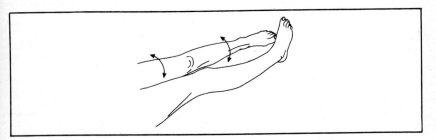

Figure C-13. Hip internal rotation exercise.

17. Hip internal rotation exercise (Fig. C-13)

   Position. Supine, with legs slightly apart, knees straight.

   a. Roll entire leg, from hip, inward.

   b. Do not bend knee.

   c. Do not move upper part of body.

   d. Hold to count of 5.

   e. Return to starting position.

   f. Relax.

   g. Repeat ___ times.

18. Hip external rotation exercise (Fig. C-14)

   Position. Supine, with legs slightly apart, knees straight.

   a. Roll entire leg, from hip, outward.

   b. Do not bend knee.

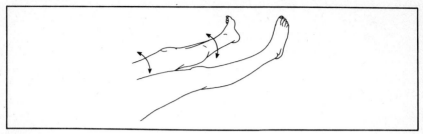

Figure C-14. Hip external rotation exercise.

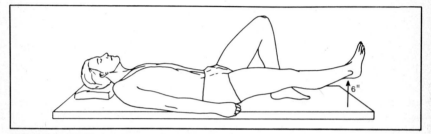

Figure C-15. Knee-straight leg raising exercise.

    c. Do not move upper part of body.

    d. Hold to count of 5.

    e. Return to starting position.

    f. Relax.

    g. Repeat ____ times.

19. Knee-straight leg raising exercise (Fig. C-15)

    Position. Supine with one knee bent, foot on surface.

    a. Raise opposite leg 6 to 8 inches off surface.

    b. Keep knee straight.

    c. Hold to count of 5.

    d. Lower slowly.

    e. Relax.

    f. Repeat ____ times.

20. Knee-quadriceps strengthening exercise (Fig. C-16)

    Position. Sitting with legs hanging freely.

    a. Lean back slightly, using arms to stabilize.

    b. Lift thigh toward chest.

    c. Keep knee bent.

    d. Hold to count of 5.

    e. Lower thigh slowly.

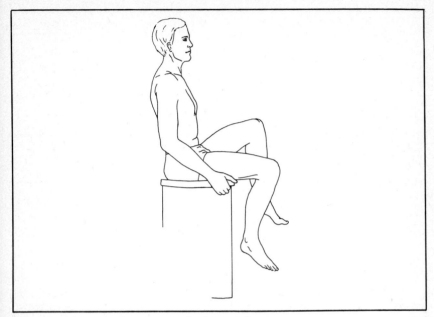

Figure C-16. Knee-quadriceps strengthening exercise.

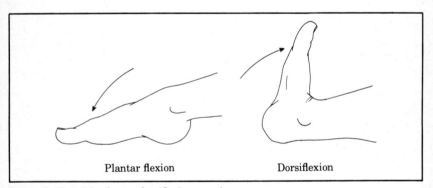

Plantar flexion   Dorsiflexion

Figure C-17. Ankle plantar-dorsiflexion exercise.

 f. Relax.

 g. Repeat ____ times.

 h. Progress to weight, as tolerated.

21. Ankle plantar-dorsiflexion exercise (Fig. C-17)

 Position. Supine, with knees straight.

 a. Point foot downward (motion at ankle).

 b. Hold to count of 5.

 c. Bring foot slowly back to neutral position.

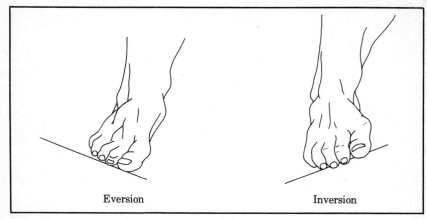

Figure C-18. Ankle eversion-inversion exercise.

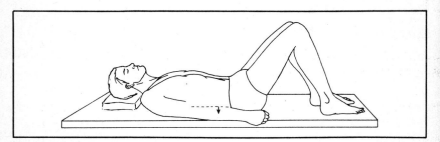

Figure C-19. Pelvic tilt exercise.

    d. Pull foot toward body.

    e. Hold to count of 5.

    f. Bring foot slowly back to neutral.

    g. Relax.

    h. Repeat ____ times.

22. Ankle eversion-inversion exercise (Fig. C-18)

    Position. Supine, with knees straight. Motion is at ankle.

    a. Turn foot out.

    b. Return to starting position.

    c. Relax.

    d. Turn foot in.

    e. Return to starting position.

    f. Relax.

    g. Repeat ____ times.

23. Pelvic tilt exercise (Fig. C-19)

    Position. Supine with hips and knees bent, feet flat on surface, arms at sides.

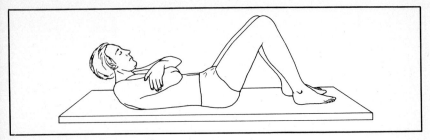

Figure C-20. Abdominal strengthening exercise.

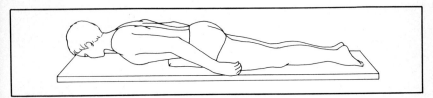

Figure C-21. Gluteal setting exercise.

    a. Flatten small of back against surface.

    b. Tighten stomach and buttocks at the same time.

    c. Hold to count of 5.

    d. Relax.

    e. Repeat ____ times.

24. **Abdominal strengthening exercise** (Fig. C-20)

    Position. Supine, with knees and hips bent, feet flat on surface, arms across chest.

    a. Tighten abdominal muscles.

    b. Raise head and shoulders up from surface, toward knees.

    c. Hold to count of 5.

    d. Lower head and shoulders slowly.

    e. Relax.

    f. Repeat ____ times.

25. **Gluteal setting exercise** (Fig. C-21)

    Position. Prone (on stomach), with hips and knees straight, arms at sides, pillow under stomach.

    a. Squeeze buttocks together tightly.

    b. Hold to count of 5.

    c. Relax.

    d. Repeat ____ times.

26. **Neck range of motion exercise**

    Position. Seated in a firm-back chair, hands resting at sides. Head erect and facing forward. Perform exercise in a smooth circular motion, including each position listed below.

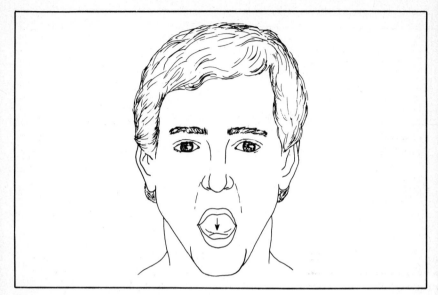

Figure C-22. Temporomandibular joint exercise.

    a. Tuck chin to chest.

    b. Turn (rotate) chin to right shoulder.

    c. Turn chin towards ceiling.

    d. Turn (rotate) chin to left shoulder.

    e. Return to starting position.

    f. Relax.

    g. Repeat in opposite direction.

27. Neck isometric exercises

Position. Seated in a firm-back chair, hands resting at sides. Head erect and facing forward. Use your hand(s) to provide resistance. There is *no* motion involved in these exercises.

    a. Place hand(s) under chin. Push chin down. Hold for count of 5. Relax. Repeat ____ times.

    b. Place right hand over right cheek. Push head against chin. Hold for count of 5. Relax. Repeat ____ times.

    c. Place left hand over left cheek. Push head against hand. Hold to count of 5. Relax. Repeat ____ times.

28. Temporomandibular joint exercise (Fig. C-22)

Position. Supine or sitting.

    a. Open mouth as widely as possible.

    b. Hold to count of 5.

    c. Close mouth slowly.

    d. Relax.

    e. Repeat ____ times.

Appendix D
Desirable Weights of Adults[a]

Table D-1. Desirable Weights of Men, Ages 25 and Over (in Indoor Clothing)

Height in Shoes[b]			Small Frame[c]		Medium Frame[d]		Large Frame[e]	
Ft	In.	Cm	Lb	Kg	Lb	Kg	Lb	Kg
5	2	157.5	112–120	50.8–54.4	118–129	53.5–58.5	126–141	57.2–64.0
5	3	160.0	113–123	52.2–55.8	121–133	54.9–60.3	129–144	58.5–65.3
5	4	162.6	118–126	53.5–57.2	124–136	56.2–61.7	132–148	59.9–67.1
5	5	165.1	121–129	54.9–58.5	127–139	57.6–63.0	133–152	61.2–68.9
5	6	167.6	124–133	56.2–60.3	130–143	59.0–64.9	138–156	62.8–70.3
5	7	170.2	128–137	58.1–62.1	134–147	60.3–66.7	142–161	64.4–73.0
5	8	172.7	132–141	59.9–64.0	138–152	62.5–68.9	147–166	66.7–75.3
5	9	175.3	136–145	61.7–65.8	142–156	64.4–70.3	151–170	68.5–77.1
5	10	177.8	140–150	63.5–68.0	146–160	66.2–72.6	155–174	70.3–78.9
5	11	180.3	144–154	65.3–69.9	150–165	68.0–74.8	159–179	72.1–81.2
6	0	182.9	148–158	67.1–71.7	154–170	69.9–77.1	164–184	74.4–83.3
6	1	185.4	152–162	68.9–73.5	158–175	71.7–79.4	168–189	76.2–85.7
6	2	188.0	156–167	70.3–75.7	162–180	73.5–81.6	173–194	78.5–88.0
6	3	190.5	160–171	72.6–77.6	167–185	75.7–83.5	178–199	80.7–90.3
6	4	193.0	164–175	74.4–79.4	172–190	78.1–86.2	182–204	82.7–92.5

[a]Weights of insured persons in the United States associated with lowest mortality.
[b]1 in. heels for men.
[c]10.7 in. or less chest width at nipple line; 10.8 in. or less hip width.
[d]10.8–11.8 in. chest width at nipple line; 10.9–12.9 in. hip width.
[e]Chest and hip widths are wider than the criteria for a medium frame.
Source: From New weight standards for men and women. *Statist. Bull. Metrop. Life Insur. Co.* 40:3, 1959.

Table D-2. Desirable Weights of Women, Ages 25 and Over (in Indoor Clothing)[a]

Height in Shoes[b]			Small Frame		Medium Frame		Large Frame	
Ft	In.	Cm	Lb	Kg	Lb	Kg	Lb	Kg
4	10	147.3	92–98	41.7–44.5	96–107	43.5–48.5	104–119	47.2–54.0
4	11	149.9	94–101	42.6–45.8	98–110	44.5–49.9	106–122	48.1–55.3
5	0	152.4	96–104	43.5–47.2	101–113	45.8–51.3	109–125	49.4–56.7
5	1	154.9	99–107	44.9–48.5	104–116	47.2–52.6	112–128	50.3–58.1
5	2	157.3	102–110	46.3–49.9	107–119	48.5–54.0	115–131	52.2–59.4
5	3	160.0	105–113	47.6–51.3	110–122	49.9–55.3	118–134	53.5–60.3
5	4	162.6	108–116	49.0–52.6	113–126	51.3–57.2	121–138	54.9–62.6
5	5	165.1	111–119	50.3–54.0	116–130	49.0–59.0	125–142	59.4–64.4
5	6	167.6	114–123	51.7–55.8	120–135	54.4–61.2	129–146	58.5–66.2
5	7	170.2	118–127	53.5–57.7	124–139	56.2–63.0	133–150	60.3–68.0
5	8	172.7	122–131	55.3–59.4	128–143	58.1–64.9	137–154	62.1–69.9
5	9	175.3	126–135	57.2–61.2	132–147	59.9–66.7	141–158	64.0–71.7
5	10	177.8	130–140	59.0–63.5	136–151	61.7–68.5	145–163	65.8–73.9
5	11	180.3	134–144	60.3–65.3	140–155	63.5–70.3	149–168	67.6–76.2
6	0	182.9	138–148	62.6–67.1	144–159	65.3–72.1	153–173	69.4–78.5

[a]Frame sizes correspond to those for men after a 20% reduction in chest width and 5% increase in hip width.
[b]2 in. heels for women.
Source: From New weight standards for men and women. *Statist. Bull. Metrop. Life Insur. Co.* 40:3, 1959.

Appendix E
Neurologic Dermatomes

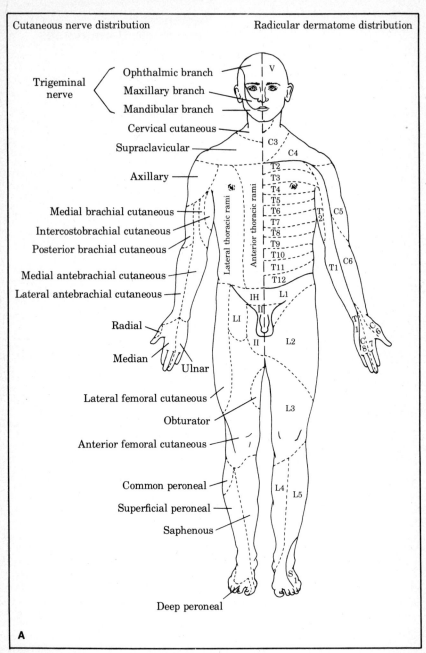

Figure E-1. A. Radicular dermatomes and cutaneous nerve distribution, anterior view. B. Radicular dermatomes and cutaneous nerve distribution, posterior view. IH = iliohypogastric; II = ilioinguinal; LI = lumboinguinal.

Radicular dermatome distribution   Cutaneous nerve distribution

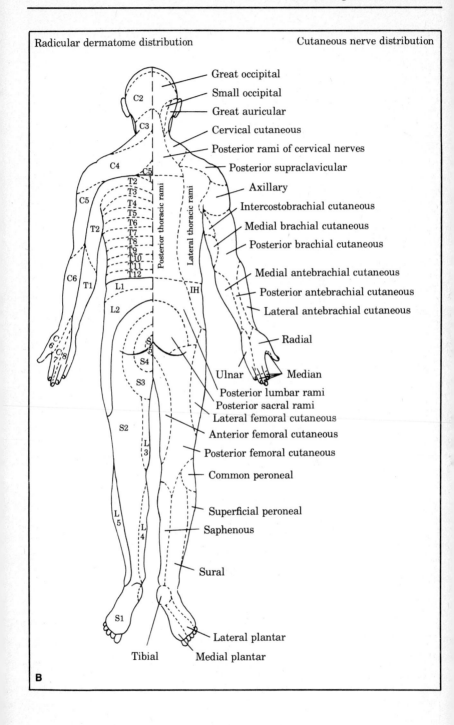

B

Appendix F
Basic Rheumatology Library

Textbooks

Aegerter, E., and Kirkpatrick, J. A. *Orthopedic Diseases.* Philadelphia: Saunders, 1975.

Cohen, A. S. *Rheumatology and Immunology.* New York: Grune & Stratton, 1979.

Dubois, E. L. *Lupus Erythematosus* (2nd ed.). Los Angeles: University of Southern California, 1974.

Katz, W. A. *Rheumatic Diseases: Diagnosis and Management.* Philadelphia: Lippincott, 1977.

Kelley, W. N., Harris, E. D. Jr., Ruddy, S., and Sledge, C. B. *Textbook of Rheumatology.* Philadelphia: Saunders, 1981.

McCarty, D. J. *Arthritis* (9th ed.). Philadelphia: Lea & Febiger, 1979.

Samter, M. *Immunological Diseases.* Boston: Little, Brown, 1971.

Wyngaarden, J. B., and Kelly, W. M. *Gout and Hyperuricemia.* New York: Grune & Stratton, 1976.

Journals

Arthritis and Rheumatism. Atlanta, Ga: Arthritis Foundation.

Bulletin of Rheumatic Diseases. Atlanta, Ga: Arthritis Foundation.

Clinics in Rheumatic Diseases. London: Saunders.

Journal of Rheumatology. Toronto: J. Rheum. Publishing Co.

Seminars in Arthritis and Rheumatism. New York: Grune & Stratton.

Appendix G
Formulary

Jane E. Salmon and Robert P. Kimberly

Medications used in management of the rheumatic diseases may be grouped into several broad categories: nonsteroidal antiinflammatory drugs (NSAIDs), slow-acting remittive agents for rheumatoid arthritis (gold compounds and penicillamine), antimalarial agents, corticosteroids, cytotoxic agents and hypouricemics. While the clinical situation may define the need for a given therapeutic category, the use of a specific agent is often determined by an empiric trial of patient response, tolerance, and compliance, as well as by drug expense.

General Considerations

NONSTEROIDAL ANTIINFLAMMATORY DRUGS (NSAIDS)

NSAIDs (aspirin, fenoprofen, ibuprofen, indomethacin, naproxen, phenylbutazone, salicylates, sulindac, tolmetin) exhibit antipyretic, antiinflammatory, and analgesic activity. All act by interrupting the arachidonic acid metabolic cascade, but therapeutic effects may involve actions other than, or in addition to, the inhibition of prostaglandin synthesis. With the exception of phenylbutazone, NSAIDs are essentially equipotent, although individual responses may vary among patients. All have similar side effects. Individual patient tolerance may vary between preparations. If an inadequate therapeutic response or intolerance occurs with aspirin or another agent, a trial of an additional agent is often worthwhile. Although aspirin is occasionally used in conjunction with other NSAIDs, two or more nonaspirin NSAIDs are not used concurrently. Side effects common to most NSAIDs include gastrointestinal intolerance, tinnitus, fluid retention, platelet abnormalities, and hepatic and renal dysfunction. Asthmatic attacks, urticaria, and angioedema may be related to enzymatic inhibition of prostaglandin synthesis in susceptible individuals or to IgE-mediated reactions, which usually occur with pyrazolone-type drugs.

SLOW-ACTING REMITTIVE AGENTS

Slow-acting remittive agents (gold salts, penicillamine) are used primarily in rheumatoid and rheumatoidlike arthritis. Their mode of action is unknown. Their clinical effect becomes apparent only after several weeks to months. Although their potential for renal and hematologic side effects necessitates careful monitoring, they appear capable of ameliorating the course of disease in a significant percentage of patients.

ANTIMALARIALS

Antimalarials (hydroxychloroquine) are used primarily for management of rheumatoid arthritis and the skin disease associated with systemic lupus erythematosus. Their mode of action is unclear. The toxicity of greatest concern involves the rare deposition of pigment in the macula of the retina. This side effect is more likely to occur after prolonged continuous usage.

CORTICOSTEROIDS

Corticosteroids (prednisone and others) are potent antiinflammatory agents capable of suppressing many disease manifestations, both articular and systemic. They have been used in all inflammatory arthritides and systemic inflammatory diseases. However, their ability to modify the ultimate course of the disease is controversial, and their side effects with prolonged use are incontrovertible. Corticosteroids should play a minor role in the management of inflammatory arthritis.

CYTOTOXIC AGENTS

The cytotoxic agents (azathioprine, chlorambucil, cyclophosphamide, methotrexate) are reserved for severe destructive inflammatory arthritis and severe systemic inflammatory disease unresponsive to more conventional forms of therapy. Evidence for efficacy is often lacking, partly because of the difficult clinical situations in which these agents are employed. In addition to specific short-term toxicities, the possibility of late malignancies favors the use of these agents only in serious clinical situations and preferably in older age groups.

HYPOURICEMIC AGENTS

Hypouricemic agents lower serum uric acid, either by decreasing production (allopurinol) or by increasing renal excretion (probenecid, sulfinpyrazone). Neither type of agent is indicated for management of an acute attack of gout. Hypouricemic agents are used primarily in patients with chronic, recurrent gouty arthritis, tophaceous gout, nephrolithiasis, gouty nephropathy, or significant hyperuricemia.

Specific Therapeutic Agents

ALLOPURINOL

Action. Allopurinol, an analog of the purine hypoxanthine, inhibits the enzyme xanthine oxidase, which converts hypoxanthine to xanthine and xanthine to uric acid. Plasma and urine concentrations of uric acid are lowered. Hypoxanthine, a more soluble product, and other purine metabolites are excreted in the urine rather than uric acid. Allopurinol also acts by a feedback mechanism to inhibit de novo purine synthesis. Allopurinol is effective in patients with renal failure. However, efficacy decreases when the creatinine clearance falls below 20 ml/min.

Metabolism. 20% excreted in urine unchanged with the remainder excreted in urine as alloxanthine. Half-life of major metabolite oxipurinol, which also inhibits xanthine oxidase, is 30 hours.

Adverse reactions. Maculopapular rash is the most common side effect and occurs in 3% of patients. Immune complex dermatitis and hepatitis, occasionally with vasculitis and nephritis, can occur; pruritis is an important warning symptom. Side effects from allopurinol are increased in the presence of marked renal failure (creatinine clearance less than 20 ml/min).

Caution. Allopurinol inhibits the oxidation of 6-mercaptopurine. Since 6-mercaptopurine is the active metabolite of azathioprine, either concomitant azathioprine or 6-mercaptopurine should be avoided with allopurinol or appropriate dosage reductions should be made. Allopurinol inhibits hepatic microsomal enzymes for drug metabolism; coumadin derivatives and other drugs metabolized by these enzymes should be given in lower doses. Concurrent administration of ampicillin and allopurinol leads to a three-fold higher incidence of drug rash. The toxicity of cytotoxic agents, such as cyclophosphamide, appears to be enhanced by concomitant administration of allopurinol. Dose of allopurinol should be reduced in renal failure.

Supply. Tablets, 100 and 300 mg.

Dose. For mild disease, 200 to 300 mg daily is usually adequate, but dosage should be individualized to achieve the desired serum urate level. It is advisable to start with 100 mg per day and gradually build toward full dosage in order to lessen the probability of acute gout attacks that may be precipitated by sudden lowering of the serum uric acid. *Allopurinol is counterproductive in acute attacks of gout.* For severe tophaceous gout, 400 to 600 mg can be used. The maximum single dose should be 300 mg. Total daily doses in excess of 600 mg are associated with increased toxicity. It is advisable to prescribe colchicine (0.6 mg PO daily or BID) during the first three months of therapy as prophylaxis for acute gout.

To prevent uric acid nephropathy when treating neoplastic disease, a daily dose of 600 to 800 mg may be required, with the maintenance of large volumes of an alkaline urine.

ASPIRIN

Action. Inhibits prostaglandin synthesis.

Metabolism. It is metabolized in the liver and excreted by the kidney. Half-life increases with increasing dose. It is highly bound to albumin in plasma and widely distributed to all tissues, including synovium.

Adverse reactions. Gastrointestinal (GI) discomfort with nausea and dyspepsia is common. Increased GI blood loss occurs. Tinnitis or decreased hearing acuity, or both, are related to mild toxicity and are reversible with a decrease in dose. Central nervous system symptoms such as headache, vertigo, and irritability can occur in the elderly. Mild, reversible hepatocellular injury may be seen in acute rheumatic fever, juvenile rheumatoid arthritis, and active systemic lupus erythematosus (SLE). Platelet adhesiveness, aggregation, and adenosine diphosphate (ADP) release are inhibited by irreversible acetylation of platelet membrane protein.

Caution. Idiosyncratic reactions similar to asthma or manifested by rash occur in 0.02% of individuals. Patients with asthma and nasal polyps are at higher risk for this reaction. Cross-reactivity exists with other NSAIDs but has not been reported with sodium or magnesium salicylates. Aspirin is uricosuric at high doses (over 4 to 5 gm/24 hr), but low doses may lead to urate retention. Aspirin may displace other drugs bound to albumin, thereby potentiating the effects of oral hypoglycemics, warfarin, and other medications. Because aspirin inhibits platelet aggregation and prolongs bleeding time, it should be used with caution in patients receiving heparin or coumadin anticoagulants. Salicylate toxicity may occur during tapering of cortico steroids in patients receiving concomitant large doses of salicylates.

Supply. Aspirin, tablets 300, 325, 600, and 650 mg.

Buffered tablets, formulated with either absorbable (bicarbonate) or nonabsorbable antacids are not necessarily associated with reduced GI bleeding.

Enteric-coated tablets are often better tolerated with less dyspepsia and occult gastrointestinal blood loss but also have more variable absorption rates than either buffered or nonbuffered tablets.

Rectal suppositories are incompletely absorbed.

Time-released tablets have delayed absorption with possibly more sustained plasma levels.

Dose. 600 to 1,200 mg every 4 to 5 hours, preferably with meals. For optimal antiinflammatory effects, blood levels between 20 and 30 mg/100 ml and a total daily dose of 3 to 6 gm are usually required. Doses necessary to achieve adequate therapeutic concentrations vary with the individual patient. Maximum tolerated dose must be reached slowly, often waiting one week between dose changes. Salicylate levels are routinely available and may be useful to determine adequacy of dosage, patient compliance, and toxicity.

AZATHIOPRINE

Action. Purine antagonist. Interferes with nucleotide synthesis.

Metabolism. Well-absorbed orally and converted to the active compound 6-mercaptopurine. Urinary excretion, partial hepatic metabolism, and tissue uptake account for clearance from the blood.

Adverse reactions. Hematologic toxicity is usually mild leukopenia and thrombocytopenia; aplastic anemia is rare. Drug fever may occur. Hepatitis and pancreatitis are uncommon. Nausea, especially during initiation of therapy, is common. Stomatitis may be seen. An increased incidence of late lymphoreticular and hematopoietic malignancy is possible.

Caution. Complete blood counts and platelets counts should be obtained initially weekly and then monthly. Rapid fall in leukocyte count requires decrease in dosage or discontinuation of drug. Liver function tests should be checked periodically. Allopurinol inhibits the metabolism of azathioprine, causing high levels to accumulate; thus concomitant administration of these drugs requires marked reduction in dose of azathioprine. Contraindicated in pregnant women. Doses must be adjusted in patients with hepatic or renal impairment.

Supply. Tablets, 50 mg.

Dose. 2 to 3 mg/kg daily.

CALCITONIN

Action. Inhibits bone resorption.

Metabolism. Rapidly metabolized to smaller inactive fragments in the kidneys.

Adverse reactions. Nausea and vomiting in 10% of patients. Flushing of face and hands, peripheral paresthesias, and altered taste have been reported. Local skin reactions and urticaria. Skin testing is recommended before treatment.

Caution. Neutralizing antibodies commonly may develop with partial loss of effectiveness.

Dose. 50 to 100 Medical Research Council (MRC) units subcutaneously or intramuscularly per day. Maintenance dosage is usually 50 MRC units 3 times weekly.

Supply. Lyophilized powder, 400 MRC units per vial.

CALCIUM PREPARATIONS

Action. Increased calcium pool available for gastrointestinal absorption.

Metabolism. Renal excretion of absorbed fraction.

Adverse reactions. Nausea and gastrointestinal irritation may occur.

Caution. Hypercalcemia may occur, especially in patients receiving concomitant vitamin D. Calcium carbonate is ineffective in patients with achlorhydria.

Supply. Calcium carbonate tablets, 650 mg; calcium gluconate tablets, 450, 500, 600, 900, and 1,000 mg; calcium lactate tablets, 300 and 600 mg.

Dose. Calcium carbonate 1 to 2 gm taken with meals. Calcium gluconate 15 gm per day in divided doses. Calcium lactate 1.5 to 3 gm 3 times daily with meals.

CHLORAMBUCIL

Action. Alkylating agent. Interferes with cell function and mitotic activity by inhibition of intracellular macromolecules.

Metabolism. Adequate and reliable oral absorption. Incomplete information concerning metabolism and excretion.

Adverse reactions. Myelosuppression is usually moderate, gradual, and rapidly reversible. Gastrointestinal discomfort, dermatitis, and hepatotoxicity occasionally occur.

Caution. Frequent complete blood counts should be obtained. Delayed occurrence of acute leukemia is reported. Infertility in both sexes may occur.

Dose. 0.05 to 0.2 mg/kg per day. Total daily dose (usually 4 to 10 mg) is given as a single dose.

Supply. Tablets, 2 mg.

COLCHICINE

Action. Decreases the inflammatory response. Colchicine binds microtubular protein which interferes with granulocyte mobility. Colchicine does not influence serum uric acid levels.

Metabolism. Although complete metabolism is unknown, colchicine is deacetylated in the liver to inactive metabolites; 10% is excreted unchanged by the kidney. The drug half-life is 90 minutes; half-life is prolonged in patients with renal insufficiency.

Adverse reactions. Gastrointestinal irritation producing nausea, vomiting, and abdominal pain occurs in up to 80% of patients receiving oral colchicine for acute gout. Bone marrow depression, renal dysfunction, and hemorrhagic colitis may occur, especially with overdose or in the setting of liver or renal disease.

Caution. Intravenous colchicine should be diluted in normal saline 10 to 15 ml and administered through a free-flowing intravenous route to decrease the chance of infiltration and soft tissue necrosis.

Supply. Tablets, 0.6 mg. Intravenous ampules, 2 ml containing 1 mg colchicine.

Dose. For maintenance prophylaxis, 0.6 mg daily or BID. For acute attacks, oral colchicine, 0.6 to 1.2 mg initially, followed by 0.6 mg hourly until symptoms abate or toxicity occurs. The total cumulative dose should not exceed 7 to 8 mg. Intravenous colchicine, 1 or 2 mg initially, followed by 0.5 mg every 3 to 6 hours up to a total of 4 mg. Dosage should be reduced in the presence of renal or hepatic disease.

CORTICOSTEROIDS

Action. Glucocorticoids suppress inflammation as well as humoral and cell-mediated immune responses.

Metabolism. They are well-absorbed from the gastrointestinal tract and rapidly metabolized to inactive steroids by the liver. They are 90% protein-bound.

Adverse reactions. Cutaneous side effects include acne, hirsutism, striae, purpura, and impaired wound healing. Osteoporosis, myopathy, and asceptic necrosis of bone may occur. Gastrointestinal side effects include peptic ulceration with bleeding or perforation as well as pancreatitis. Hypertension and edema secondary to fluid retention occur. Steroid psychosis and benign intracranial hypertension are the central nervous system adverse reactions. Ocular effects include cataracts and glaucoma. Patients may suffer growth arrest, secondary amenorrhea, impotence, and suppression of hypothalamic-pituitary adrenal axis. Glucose intolerance, hyperosmolar nonketotic coma, and centripetal obesity occur. There is increased risk of infection.

Intraarticular corticosteroids may cause a crystal-induced transient synovitis. Immobilization and ice compresses will facilitate resolution; persistence of the synovitis beyond 24 hours raises the possibility of an arthrocentesis-related infectious arthritis.

Topical steroids, especially the more potent fluorinated compounds, may cause cutaneous telangiectasia, striae, epidermal and dermal atrophy, rosacea-like facial eruption, and senile-type purpura. When used with occlusive dressings, infection, folliculitis, and decreased heat exchange may occur.

Caution. Periodic determinations of blood sugar, complete blood counts, stool quaiacs, and blood pressure should be obtained. Diabetes mellitus, hypertension, pregnancy, and psychosis are relative contraindications. Patients receiving chronic steroids have a suppressed hypothalamic-pituitary adrenal (HPA) axis and require glucocorticoid supplement when undergoing surgical procedures or other physiologic stress.

Repeated administration of intraarticular injections of corticosteroid may lead to disruption of cartilage and supporting soft tissue structures. Soft tissue injections may cause similar effects.

Systemic absorption of topical steroid preparations may occur. Prolonged use, especially of the more potent compounds, may lead to suppression of the hypothalamic-pituitary adrenal axis.

Dose. Numerous schedules for administering glucocorticoids have been developed in order to limit side effects and maximize therapeutic response. Single-dose, alternate-day regimens decrease the incidence of side effects but may not suppress disease activity adequately. In such cases, daily therapy (divided or single doses) may be administered. Dosage varies widely according to the specific disease.

Intraarticular corticosteroids are useful in patients with only one or a few joints involved with inflammatory arthritis. Doses vary from several milligrams for small joints of the hand to 40 mg for large joints such as the knee.

The efficacy of topical steroids is related to both potency and percutaneous penetration. Adequate hydration of the skin, inflammation, and occlusion with plastic wraps enhance penetration. Better biologic activity is often obtained with ointment rather than cream or lotion preparations. As a general principle, therapy is started with stronger preparations and later switched to less potent strengths once control of skin manifestations is achieved.

Supply. Oral preparations (see Table G-1):

Prednisone tablets, 1, 2.5, 5, 10, 20, and 50 mg
Prednisolone tablets, 1, 2.5, and 5 mg
Methylprednisolone tablets, 2, 4, 8, 16, 24, and 32 mg
Dexamethasone tablets, 0.25, 0.5, 0.75, 1.5, and 4 mg

Table G-1. Glucocorticoid Preparations

	Equivalent Dose (mg)	Relative Antiinflammatory Potency	Relative Mineralcorticoid Potency
Hydrocortisone	20	1.0	1.0
Cortisone	25	0.8	0.8
Prednisone	5	4.0	0.8
Prednisolone	5	4.0	0.8
Methylprednisolone	4	5.0	0
Dexamethasone	0.75	30.0	0

Parenteral preparations. (see Table G-1):
Hydrocortisone vial, 100, 250, 500, and 1,000 mg
Methylprednisolone vial, 40, 125, 500, and 1,000 mg
Dexamethasone vial, 4 mg/ml in 1-, 5-, and 25-ml containers; 24 mg/ml in 5- and 10-ml containers

Intraarticular preparations:
Methylprednisolone acetate, 20 and 40 mg/ml suspension in 1-, 5-, and 10-ml containers.
Triamcinolone acetonide, 40 mg/ml suspension in 1-, 5-, and 10-ml vials; 10 mg/ml suspension in 5-ml vials
Triamcinolone hexacetonide, 20 mg/ml suspension in 1- and 5-ml vials.
Prednisolone tertiary butylacetate, 20 mg/ml suspension in 1-, 5-, and 10-ml vials.

Topical preparations. See Table G-2.

CYCLOPHOSPHAMIDE
Action. Alkylating agent. Interferes with nucleic acids and proteins by cross-linking intracellular macromolecules. Cyclophosphamide can inhibit secondary immune responses.
Metabolism. Well-absorbed from gastrointestinal tract. It requires activation by liver to produce active metabolites. Unchanged drug and metabolites are excreted in the urine.
Adverse reactions. Bone marrow depression, primarily of white cell series, and predisposition to infection, both of which may be life-threatening but reversible with discontinuation of drug. Alopecia, drug-induced infertility with amenorrhea or defec-

Table G-2. Commonly Used Topical Preparations

Very High Strength
Fluocinonide 0.05%
  Lidex cream and ointment
  Topsyn gel
Halcinonide 0.1%
  Halog cream and ointment
High Strength
Betamethasone valerate 0.1%
  Valisone cream and ointment
Betamethasone benzoate 0.025%
  Benisone
  Flurobate cream and gel
Fluocinolone acetonide 0.2%
  Synalar cream
Triamcinolone acetonide 0.1%
  Aristocort cream, ointment, and gel
  Kenalog cream, ointment, and gel
Moderate Strength
Fluocinolone acetonide 0.025%, 0.01%, Synalar cream and ointment
Flurandrenolide 0.05%, 0.025%
  Cordran cream and ointment
Triamcinolone acetonide 0.025%
  Aristocort cream, ointment, and gel
  Kenalog cream, ointment, and gel
Low Strength
Hydrocortisone 1%
  Cort-Dome cream and lotion
  Hytone cream
Other preparations with cortisone, prednisolone, and methylprednisolone acetate

tive spermatogenesis, hemorrhagic cystitis (in up to 25% of patients), fibrosing cystitis, carcinoma of the bladder, hematopoietic malignancies, anorexia, nausea, vomiting, and pulmonary fibrosis. Antidiuretic hormone–like activity may occur with large doses and result in hyponatremia.

Caution. Contraindicated in pregnant women and patients with hepatic impairment. Dosage requires adjustment in renal insufficiency. Frequent complete blood counts and platelet counts and urinalyses must be obtained. Large volume fluid intake and frequent emptying of the bladder may reduce bladder complications.

Supply. Tablets, 25 and 50 mg; vials, 100, 200, and 500 mg for intravenous injection.

Dose. 0.5 to 3.5 mg/kg per day given as single morning dose.

ETIDRONATE DISODIUM

Action. Diminishes bone resorption and new bone formation.

Metabolism. Adsorbed to developing apatite crystals during bone formation. Excreted unchanged by the kidneys.

Adverse reactions. Defective mineralization of bone with accumulation of unmineralized osteoid, and possible onset of new bone pain and pathologic fractures. Mild abdominal cramps, nausea, and diarrhea.

Caution. Patients with renal insufficiency should be treated cautiously or with another drug.

Dose. 5 mg/kg per day given as a single dose 2 hours before meals for several months. Doses above 10 mg/kg per day should be used cautiously and reserved for suppression of rapid bone turnover or for prompt reduction in elevated cardiac output.

Supply. Tablets, 200 mg.

FENOPROFEN CALCIUM

Action. Inhibits prostaglandin synthesis.

Metabolism. Fenoprofen is a arylalkanoic acid derivative. It is rapidly absorbed with peak plasma levels in 90 minutes and a half-life of 160 minutes; concomitant food ingestion decreases rate and extent of absorption. Enterohepatic circulation of the drug occurs. Ninety percent is excreted in the urine as glucuronides. Aspirin decreases the peak blood levels.

Adverse reactions. Dyspepsia and gastrointestinal bleeding occur less commonly than with aspirin. Rash, headache, sodium retention, and, rarely, interstitial nephritis and nephrotic syndrome may occur.

Caution. It reduces platelet aggregation and may increase the risk of bleeding in patients on warfarin or heparin. Fenoprofen is 90% protein-bound and may displace other protein-bound drugs with resultant drug interactions. The drug is not recommended in pregnancy. Cross-reactivity in patients with aspirin sensitivity occurs.

Supply. Tablets, 600 mg, capsules, 300 mg.

Dose. 300 to 600 mg QID. In rheumatoid arthritis, fenoprofen 2.4 gm is approximately equivalent to aspirin 3.9 gm.

FLUORIDE, SODIUM

Action. Incorporated into bone, rendering it less soluble. Stimulates new bone formation.

Metabolism. Absorbed from gastrointestinal tract and incorporated into bone.

Adverse reactions. Occasional gastrointestinal upset. Fluorosis, caused by chronic overexposure to fluoride, results in mottling of teeth and formation of thickened bones with poor mechanical quality (osteomalacia and osteosclerosis).

Caution. To prevent precipitation of CaF_2, calcium supplements and sodium fluoride are given at separate times of the day. Fluoride supplements should not be given to patients with renal insufficiency.

Supply. Tablets, 1 mg. Larger capsules available in some pharmacies.

Dose. 5 mg TID for 1 week. 15 mg TID for 1 week. 25 mg TID thereafter.

GOLD COMPOUNDS

Action. Mode of action in rheumatoid arthritis is unknown. Alters macrophage and complement functions.

Metabolism. Approximately half of the administered dose is excreted within 1 week, 30% in the urine and remainder in the stool. Gold in the circulation rapidly equilibrates with synovial fluid. It is stored by the reticuloendothelial system. It is 90% protein bound.

Adverse reactions. Forty percent of patients experience some toxicity. Eosinophilia, although common, does not necessarily predict toxicity. The most common reaction is dermatitis, which may be heralded by pruritis or eosinophilia, or both. Both dermatitis and stomatitis are reversible with discontinuation of drug and, except for the rare instances of exfoliative dermatitis, gold therapy can be reinstituted with low doses. Hematologic abnormalities occur in 1% to 2% of patients. Thrombocytopenia is most common, followed by leukopenia, agranulocytosis, and pancytopenia. Gold should not be restarted. Proteinuria may be seen in 4% of patients, but nephrotic syndrome with membranous glomerulonephritis is much less common. Proteinuria of greater than 1 gm per day requires cessation of therapy. Mild proteinuria or celluria is a signal to interrupt therapy until urinalysis is normal. Nitritoid reactions characterized by self-limited episodes of sweating, flushing, dizziness, nausea, and shortness of breath after administration of gold may occur with the thiomalate preparation. Treatment of nitritoid reactions involves switching to aurothioglucose and administering gold with the patient supine. Unusual problems, some of which may be coincidental to therapy, include enterocolitis, intrahepatic cholestasis, skin hyperpigmentation, peripheral neuropathy, pulmonary infiltrates, and deposits of gold in the cornea.

Caution. Gold is contraindicated in patients with previous gold allergy or severe toxic skin, kidney, or bone marrow reaction to gold. Relative contraindications include functional impairment of kidneys or liver. Immunosuppressives and penicillamine, agents with a potential to suppress the bone marrow, should not be given with gold. Patients should have frequent complete blood counts (including platelets) and urinalysis before each injection during the first few weeks of therapy.

Dose. Initial dose is 10 mg IM to test for idiosyncratic reactions. Thereafter, 25 mg the second week and 50 mg at subsequent weekly intervals are given. In the absence of side effects, a total dose of 1 gm may be given. If improvement has occurred, the drug is continued in 50-mg doses with an increasing time interval between injections: every 2 weeks for several months, then every 3 weeks, and finally, 50 mg monthly. Improvement is gradual but usually begins when the cumulative dose is 300 to 700 mg. Dosage for children and adolescents is 1 mg/kg up to 25 mg per injection.

Supply. Gold thioglucose, 50 mg/ml in 10-ml vials. Gold sodium thiomalate, 10, 25, 50, 100 mg/ml in 1-ml ampules; 50 mg/ml in 10-ml ampules.

HYDROXYCHLOROQUINE

Action. Mode of action is unknown. Potential actions include binding nucleic acids, stabilization of lysosomal membranes, and trapping of free radicals.

Metabolism. Well-absorbed from the gastrointestinal tract. The drug is concentrated and retained in body tissues. Excretion by the kidney is detectable months after therapy is discontinued.

Adverse reactions. Most common side effects are allergic eruptions and gastrointestinal disturbances (nausea, cramps, diarrhea). The most serious complication is ocular toxicity. Reversible corneal deposits of the drug are detectable by slit lamp examination. Retinopathy affecting macular pigmentation may be irreversible. It occurs in 0.1% to 1.5% of patients. Less common side effects include hypopigmentation of hair, neuropathy, ototoxicity, and exacerbations of psoriasis. Hematologic toxicity is rare.

Caution. Ophthalmologic examination (color testing, visual fields, fundoscopy, slit lamp exam) should be performed every four to six months. At the first sign of visual disturbance, the drug should be discontinued. Hydroxychloroquine may cause hemolytic anemia in G6PD deficient patients. The drug is contraindicated in patients with significant visual, hepatic or renal impairment, psoriasis, porphyria, and pregnancy.

Supply. Tablets, 100 and 200 mg.

IBUPROFEN

Action. An arylalkanoic acid derivative that inhibits prostaglandin synthesis.

Metabolism. It is 38% protein-bound. The half-life is 2 hours. It is primarily metabolized by the liver. No change in dosage is needed in renal failure.

Adverse reactions. Dyspepsia is common. Occult gastrointestinal bleeding may be less common than with aspirin. Occasionally headaches, rashes, and salt retention occur. Aseptic meningitis and hypersensitivity reactions in patients with lupus erythematosus have been reported.

Caution. Ibuprofen decreases platelet aggregation and prolongs bleeding time. Caution must be used with patients taking anticoagulants. Cross-reactivity in patients with aspirin sensitivity occurs. It is not recommended during pregnancy.

Supply. Tablets, 300, 400, and 600 mg.

Dose. 1,200 to 2,400 mg in 3 to 4 divided doses.

INDOMETHACIN

Action. An indole acetic acid that inhibits prostaglandin synthesis.

Metabolism. Indomethacin is 90% bound to albumin. The kidneys excrete 65%; fecal excretion of 35% suggests biliary excretion of metabolized drug. Probenecid may increase plasma levels of indomethacin by interfering with its excretion.

Adverse reactions. Gastrointestinal side effects (dyspepsia, bleeding, nausea, and vomiting) occur in 10% to 40% of patients. Central nervous system effects, occurring in 10% to 25%, include headaches, vertigo, dizziness, and psychiatric disturbances. Less common effects include sodium retention, exacerbation of hypertension, hepatitis, and bone marrow suppression.

Caution. It is not recommended for children under 14 years of age, pregnant women, or nursing mothers. It antagonizes the natriuretic and antihypertensive effects of furosemide. Indomethacin should be used cautiously in patients with coagulation defects or patients receiving anticoagulants since it does inhibit platelet aggregation. Cross-reactivity in patients with aspirin sensitivity occurs.

Supply. Capsules, 25 and 50 mg.

Dose. 25 mg TID, taken after meals. Dose can be gradually increased by 25-mg increments to 150 to 200 mg daily.

MECLOFENAMATE SODIUM

Action. Inhibits prostaglandin synthesis.

Metabolism. Meclofenamate sodium is an anthranilic acid derivative. Peak plasma levels occur in 30 to 60 minutes with a half-life of about 3 hours; concomitant antacid administration does not interfere with absorption. About two-thirds are excreted in the urine, mostly as the glucuronide conjugate, while about one-third appears in the feces.

Adverse reactions. Gastrointestinal reactions occur more frequently than with aspirin. Diarrhea may occur in up to one-third of patients; nausea in about 10%. Headache, dizziness, rash, and other reactions associated with nonsteroidal antiinflammatory agents may also occur.

Caution. Meclofenamate sodium enhances the effect of warfarin but has a smaller effect than aspirin on platelet aggregation. The drug is not recommended for use in pregnancy. Cross-reactivity in patients with aspirin sensitivity occurs.

Supply. Capsules, 50 and 100 mg.

Dose. 50 to 100 mg QID.

METHOTREXATE

Action. Folate antagonist which inhibits dihydrofolate reductase. The primary effect is inhibition of cell proliferation.

Metabolism. Readily absorbed from gastrointestinal tract in doses of less than 0.1 mg/kg body weight. Approximately 50% protein bound and susceptible to displacement by sulfonamides, salicylates, and other drugs. Rapid excretion of 50% to 90% in urine, with the rest appearing over many weeks. Urinary excretion is enhanced by an alkaline urine; impaired renal function can usually influence response to this drug.

Adverse reactions. Marrow suppression (leukopenia, thrombocytopenia, or complete aplasia) and gastrointestinal injury (ulcerative stomatitis, diarrhea, hemorrhagic enteritis, hepatic dysfunction including cirrhosis). Pulmonary infiltrates, osteoporosis, alopecia.

Caution. Use in nonmalignant disease requires emphasis on long-term side effects. The risk of hepatic cirrhosis supports intermittent administration of the drug and careful monitoring of hepatic function including liver biopsy. Renal function and complete blood count should also be monitored.

Dose. For psoriatic arthritis, 15 mg PO every 12 hours for 3 doses per week. For polymyositis, 10 to 15 mg IV weekly with gradual increase in 5-mg increments to 30 to 50 mg weekly. Dosage interval is subsequently increased to two weeks, then one month. (See also Chaps. 33 and 35.)

Supply. Tablets, 2.5 mg. Vials, 5 and 50 mg for parenteral use.

NAPROXEN

Action. An arylalkanoic derivative that inhibits prostaglandin synthesis.

Metabolism. Absorption not significantly delayed by food. Ninety-eight percent is protein bound. The half-life is 12 to 15 hours. Kidneys excrete 80% to 90% in conjugated form. Aspirin decreases peak plasma levels.

Adverse reactions. Gastrointestinal bleeding, dyspepsia, headache, dizziness, and sodium retention occur less frequently than with aspirin. Interstitial nephritis rarely occurs.

Caution. Naproxen displaces albumin-bound drugs which may lead to drug interactions. It inhibits platelet aggregation and should be used with caution in patients taking anticoagulants. Cross-reactivity in patients with aspirin sensitivity occurs.

Supply. Tablets, 250 mg and 375 mg.

Dose. 250 mg BID, which may be increased to 750 mg daily. As a result of long elimination half-life, it can be given twice daily. Naproxen 500 mg is comparable to aspirin 3.6 to 4.8 gm.

PENICILLAMINE

Action. Mode of action in rheumatoid arthritis is unknown. Penicillamine decreases circulating immune complexes, rheumatoid factor titer, and inhibits lymphocyte responsiveness to mitogens. A latent period of two to three months is often observed between initiation of therapy and clinical response.

Metabolism. Well-absorbed from gastrointestinal tract and rapidly excreted in urine. It should be administered on an empty stomach (1 to 1½ hours after a meal) to avoid interference of absorption by dietary metals.

Adverse reactions. Pruritus and skin rash represent most common side effects and can occur at any time. They can be treated by either lowering the dose or administering antihistamines. If necessary, the therapy may be interrupted until the rash resolves. Stomatitis also occurs. Alteration of taste is frequent, independent of dose, and is self-limited with resolution in 2 to 3 months despite continued drug administration. Bone marrow depression may occur precipitously at any time. If platelet count falls below 80 to 100,000, therapy must be discontinued. The most common late toxic effect is immune complex nephropathy. Proteinuria may be seen in 20% of patients. If proteinuria exceeds 1 gm per day, the dosage should be reduced. Nephrotic syndrome, hypoalbuminemia, or hematuria require discontinuation of the drug. Less common side effects include autoimmune syndromes (lupuslike syndromes, Goodpasture syndrome, myasthenia gravis, pemphigus, stenosing alveolitis, polymyositis) which necessitate prompt discontinuation of the drug.

Caution. Penicillamine administration is contraindicated in patients who are receiving gold compound, immunosuppressive drugs, or phenylbutazone. Renal insufficiency and pregnancy are further contraindications. A history of penicillin allergy does not preclude use of penicillamine. All patients should have complete blood counts with platelets and urinalysis at 2-week intervals for the first 6 months of therapy and monthly thereafter. An unreliable patient is a relative contraindication.

Supply. Capsules, 125 and 250 mg.

Dose. Initially, a single daily dose of 250 mg, which is increased in 2 to 3 months to 375 or 500 mg daily if clinical response is insufficient. Further increases to the maximum dose of 750 mg daily may be made after 2 or 3 months.

PHENYLBUTAZONE AND OXYPHENBUTAZONE

Action. Pyrazolone drugs that inhibit prostaglandin synthesis. Phenylbutazone is also a free radical scavenger and a uricosuric.

Metabolism. Phenylbutazone is 90% protein bound. The half-life is 72 hours. It is metabolized by the liver and excreted by the kidneys. Oxyphenbutazone is the major active metabolite of phenylbutazone.

Adverse reactions. Nausea and vomiting may occur in 4% of patients. Peptic ulcers may be seen in 1% to 2%. Gastrointestinal bleeding rarely occurs. Hematologic toxicity includes agranulocytosis, aplastic anemia, and thrombocytopenia. Salt and water retention often occur. Rare reactions include rashes, myocarditis, hepatitis, and sialadenitis.

Caution. Due to potential hematopoietic suppression, complete blood count and platelet count should be obtained weekly, then once every two weeks if therapy is continued beyond six weeks. Because of protein binding, phenylbutazone potentiates warfarin, tolbutamide, sulfonamides, and other protein-bound drugs. It should be used with caution with these agents. Because of fluid retention, phenylbutazone should be used with great caution in patients with congestive heart failure. It is contraindicated in children. Cross-reactivity in patients with aspirin sensitivity may occur.

Supply. Tablets, 100 mg.

Dose. 300 to 600 mg daily in 3 or 4 doses; 400 mg daily dose should not be exceeded for chronic therapy. Doses greater than 800 mg daily are not recommended. Long-term use is limited primarily to ankylosing spondylitis and related spondyloarthropathies.

PROBENECID

Action. A uricosuric agent that inhibits renal tubular reabsorption of organic acids, including uric acid. It is antagonized by low-dose salicylate (less than 3 gm/24 hr daily). Probenecid is not effective with creatinine clearances less than 40 ml/min.

Metabolism. Excreted in urine in the glucuronide form and as oxidized metabolites. Half-life is dose-dependent and ranges from 6 to 12 hours.

Adverse reactions. Gastrointestinal irritation in 10% of patients. Hypersensitivity (fever and rash) in 3%.

Caution. Maintain a large alkaline urine volume especially during the first week of therapy to prevent urate stones. Patients with a history of renal calculi should use probenecid with caution. Probenecid may alter the metabolism of other drugs by decreasing their excretion (indomethacin, ampicillin), reducing their volume of distribution (ampicillin), or delaying metabolism (heparin).

Supply. Tablet, 500 mg.

Dose. 250 mg BID for 1 week, then 500 mg BID. Maintenance colchicine should be given during the first three months of probenecid therapy and then can be stopped if the patient is asymptomatic. Probenecid is not useful in acute attacks of gout.

SALICYLATES

Action. Inhibits prostaglandin synthesis.

Metabolism. See Aspirin.

Adverse reactions. See Aspirin. Nonaspirin salicylates may cause less gastrointestinal disturbance and less gastrointestinal bleeding than aspirin. They do not inhibit platelet function.

Caution. Sodium salicylate may constitute a substantial sodium load for patients with heart failure or hypertension. Hypermagnesemic toxicity may develop with magnesium salicylate in patients with renal insufficiency. Also see Aspirin.

Supply. Sodium salicylate tablets, 300, 325, 600, and 650 mg. Choline salicylate liquid, 600 mg aspirin equivalent per 5 ml. Choline magnesium trisalicylate tablets, 500 mg. Salsalate tablets, 325 and 500 mg.

Dose. See Aspirin.

SULINDAC

Action. An indene acetic derivative of indomethacin that inhibits prostaglandin synthesis.

Metabolism. The parent sulfoxide compounds require hepatic activation to the active sulfide metabolite. Half-life of sulindac is about 8 hours, while half-life of the active sulfide metabolite is 16 to 18 hours. It is tightly protein-bound. The kidney excretes 45% to 50%, and 25% to 30% is found in feces.

Adverse reactions. Dyspepsia, nausea, gastrointestinal bleeding, tinnitis, headaches, dizziness, hepatitis, rash, and edema may occur.

Caution. Sulindac may potentiate oral hypoglycemic agents, anticoagulants, and other protein-bound drugs. It prolongs bleeding time and should be used with caution in patients receiving anticoagulants. Cross-reactivity in patients with aspirin sensitivity may occur.

Supply. Tablets, 150 and 200 mg.

Dose. Initially 150 mg tablet twice per day with meals. The dose may be increased to 200 mg BID.

SULFINPYRAZONE

Action. A uricosuric that inhibits renal tubular reabsorption of organic acids. Sulfinpyrazone is antagonized by low-dose salicylate and is ineffective in presence of renal failure.

Metabolism. Rapidly and completely absorbed with peak plasma levels in about one hour. Sulfinpyrazone is 98% protein-bound. The kidney excretes about 40% unchanged.

Adverse reactions. Gastrointestinal irritation. Hypersensitivity is rare.

Caution. Maintain a large alkaline urine output, especially during the first week of therapy to decrease risk of urate calculi formation. Sulfinpyrazone inhibits platelet aggregation and potentiates the action of protein-bound drugs such as oral hypoglycemics and oral anticoagulants. Because it has structural similarities to phenylbutazone, it should be avoided in patients with known sensitivity to phenylbutazone.

Supply. Tablets, 100 and 200 mg.

Dose. Start with 50 to 100 mg BID with meals and increase gradually over several weeks to a maintenance dose usually of 300 to 400 mg per day in 3 or 4 divided doses. Maximum recommended daily dose is 800 mg. Maintenance colchicine should be given for the first three months of therapy to prevent precipitation of an acute attack of gouty arthritis.

SUNSCREENS

Action. Absorption of ultraviolet (UV) light. Medium-wave (UVB: 280 to 320 nm) light is the major cause of sunburn and probably lupus-related skin reactions. Long-wave light (UVA: 320 to 400 nm) is the major cause of photosensitivity reactions. See Table G-3.

Metabolism. Topical use only.

Adverse reactions. Local hypersensitivity reactions to active compounds or vehicle, or both; contact dermatitis; photocontact dermatitis.

Cautions. Patients allergic to thiazides, sulfa drugs, benzocaine, procaine, analine dyes, and paraphenylene diamine may have allergic reactions to para-aminobenzoic acid (PABA), a common active ingredient.

Dose. Apply one to two hours before sun exposure and several times during exposure, especially after sweating or swimming.

TOLMETIN SODIUM

Action. Inhibitor of prostaglandin synthesis.

Metabolism. The drug half-life is 60 minutes. It is 99% excreted in urine and 99% protein-bound.

Adverse reactions. Peptic ulcers occur in 2% to 3% of patients. Gastrointestinal bleeding occurs in 1%. Other reactions include diarrhea, abdominal pain, nausea, dyspepsia, rash, sodium retention, light headedness, headache, and dizziness.

Caution. False positive tests for urinary protein are noted when sulfosalicylic acid, but not when albustix (tetrabromphenol-blue), is used. It may decrease platelet adhesiveness and prolong bleeding time. Cross-reactivity in patients with aspirin sensitivity occurs.

Supply. Tablets, 200 and 400 mg.

Dose. 400 mg TID, preferably including doses on arising and at bedtime. Doses larger than 2,000 mg daily are not recommended. Tolmetin is approved for use in children.

VITAMIN D

Action. Increases intestinal absorption of calcium and may increase mobilization of mineral from bone.

Metabolism. Hepatic and renal hydroxylation.

Adverse reactions. Vitamin D toxicity may produce elevated serum calcium and

Table G-3. Sunscreens

Strength	Product	Sun Protection Factor	Effective UV Range	Contains PABA
Very high protection	Super Shade	15	UVB, UVA	Yes
	Total Eclipse	15	UVB, UVA	Yes
	Pre-Sun 15	15	UVB, UVA	Yes
	Piz Buin 15	15	UVB, UVA	No
High protection	Original Eclipse	10	UVB	Yes
	Pabanol	8–10	UVB	Yes
	Pre-Sun 8	8	UVB	Yes
	Piz Buin 6	6	UVB, UVA	No

UVB range = 280 to 320 nm; UVA range = 320 to 400 nm.

phosphorous levels, causing drowsiness, gastrointestinal symptoms, metastatic calcifications, renal failure, and hypertension.

Caution. Monthly monitoring of serum and urinary calcium to avoid manifestations of vitamin D toxicity is recommended. If urinary calcium rises above 120 mg per day, dosage of vitamin D should be reduced.

Supply. Ergocalciferol tablets, 25,000 and 50,000 units.

Dose. 50,000 international units, 2 to 3 times weekly.

Appendix H
Normal Laboratory Values

Tests	Normal Values
Immunologic	
Latex fixation (rheumatoid factor)	<1:160 titer
Total hemolytic complement (CH_{50})	150 to 250 units/ml
Complement components:	
C1q	14 to 20 mg/dl
C2	1.6 to 3.6 mg/dl
C3	90 to 230 mg/dl
C4	15 to 35 mg/dl
C5	4.2 to 14 mg/dl
C1 esterase inhibitor	14 to 30 mg/dl
Factor B	14.8 to 31.2 mg/dl
ANA	negative (1:10 dilution)
DNA binding (Farr)	<20% binding
Cryoglobulins	<30 μg/ml
Immunoglobulin levels (radial immunodiffusion)	
IgA	106 to 668 mg/dl
IgG	635 to 1175 mg/dl
IgM	37 to 154 mg/dl
IgD (nephelometry)	0 to 6 mg /dl
IgE	<0.14 mg/dl
Antistreptolysin O titer	<125 todd units
Hematologic	
WBC	4,800 to 10,800 cells/mm^3
Hemoglobin	males: 14 to 18 gm/dl
	females: 12 to 16 gm/dl
Hematocrit	males: 45 to 52 ml/100 ml
	females: 11 to 37 ml/100 ml
Platelets	200,000 to 400,000/mm^3
Prothrombin time	11.5 seconds
Activated partial thromboplastin time	34 seconds
Sedimentation rate (Westergren)	males: 0 to 15 mm/hr
	females: 0 to 20 mm/hr
Reticulocytes	0.5% to 1.5% of RBC
Differential cell count	Neutrophils 59% to 70%
	Bands 2% to 6%
	Monocytes 2% to 8%
	Lymphocytes 25% to 40%
	Eosinophils 0% to 4%
	Basophils 0% to 2%
Biochemistry	
Acid phosphatase (Mod. Bessey Lowry)	Female: 0.03 to 0.5 μM/ml
	Male: 0.13 to 0.63 μM/ml
Albumin	3.5 to 5.0 gm/dl
Aldolase (Beisenherz)	6 mU/ml
Alkaline phosphatase (international units)	30 to 110 mU/ml

Tests	Normal Values
Amylase (Babson)	30 to 180 units/dl
Bicarbonate	20 to 30 mEq/l
Bilirubin (total)	0.12 to 1.0 mg/dl
Calcium	8.5 to 10.5 mg/dl
Chloride	95 to 105 mEq/l
Cholesterol	150 to 300 mg/dl
CPK (international units)	0 to 150 mU/ml
Fibrinogen	200 to 400 mg/dl
GGTP (substrate, gamma-glutamyl p-nitroanilide)	7 to 50 mU/ml
Glucose	70 to 105 mg/dl
Iron	60 to 160 ug/dl
Iron binding capacity	250 to 350 ug/dl
LDH (SMA 12/60)	100 to 225 mU/ml
5'NT (Schwartz)	3.2 to 11.6 mU/ml
Phosphorus (inorganic)	2.5 to 4.5 mg/dl
Potassium	3.5 to 5.0 mEq/l
Protein (total)	6.0 to 8.0 g/dl
Salicylate (therapeutic level)	15 to 25 mg/dl
SGOT (SMA 12/60)	7 to 40 mU/ml
SGPT (LKB 8600, analyzer)	1.3 to 8.2 mU/ml
Sodium	135 to 145 mEq/l
Triglyceride	74 to 172 mg/dl
Urea nitrogen	5 to 25 mg/dl
Uric acid (SMA 12/60)	2.5 to 8.5 mg/dl
Endocrine	
T4 (RIA)	4.5 to 11.5 mcg/dl
T3 (resin)	35% to 45% uptake
T3 (RIA)	60 to 160 ng/dl
Intact parathyroid hormone (PTH)	163 to 347 pg Eq/ml
C-terminal PTH	150 to 375 pg Eq/ml
*Quantitative urinary excretion**	
Calcium	50 to 400 mg/24 hr
Hydroxyproline	25 to 95 mg/24 hr
Magnesium	4 to 17 mEq/24 hr
Sodium	40 to 200 mEq/24 hr
Potassium	25 to 100 mEq/24 hr
Phosphorus (inorganic)	300 to 1100 mg/24 hr
Amylase (Babson)	1000 to 8000 units/24 hr
Protein	10 to 100 mg/24 hr
Creatinine	800 to 1800 mg/24 hr
Creatinine clearance	70 to 160 ml/min
Uric acid	
Random diet	700 to 1100 mg/24 hr
Low purine diet	<700 mg/24 hr
Cystine	None/24 hr

*In some cases, large ranges reflect variations in dietary intake.

Appendix I. ARA Criteria for Diagnosis and Classification of Rheumatic Diseases*

I. Diagnostic criteria for rheumatoid arthritis†

A. Classical rheumatoid arthritis

This diagnosis requires seven of the following criteria. In criteria 1 through 5 the joint signs or symptoms must be continuous for at least 6 weeks. (Any one of the features listed under "Exclusions" will exclude a patient from this and all other categories.)

1. **Morning stiffness.**

2. **Pain on motion** or tenderness in at least one joint (observed by a physician).

3. **Swelling** (soft tissue thickening or fluid, not bony overgrowth alone) **of at least one joint** (observed by a physician).

4. **Swelling** (observed by a physician) **of at least one other joint** (any interval free of joint symptoms between the two joint involvements may not be more than 3 months).

5. **Symmetric joint swelling** (observed by a physician) with simultaneous involvement of the same joint on both sides of the body (bilateral involvement of proximal interphalangeal, metacarpophalangeal, or metatarsophalangeal joints is acceptable without absolute symmetry). Terminal phalangeal joint involvement will not satisfy this criterion.

6. **Subcutaneous nodules** (observed by a physician) over bony prominences, on extensor surfaces or in juxtaarticular regions.

7. **Roentgenographic changes** typical of rheumatoid arthritis (which must include at least bony decalcification localized to or most marked adjacent to the involved joints and not just degenerative changes). Degenerative changes do not exclude patients from any group classified as rheumatoid arthritis.

8. **Positive agglutination test**—demonstration of the rheumatoid factor by any method that, in two laboratories, has been positive in not over 5% of normal controls—or positive streptococcal agglutination test. (The latter is now obsolete.)

9. **Poor mucin precipitate** from synovial fluid (with shreds and cloudy solution).

10. **Characteristic histologic changes in synovium** with three or more of the following: marked villous hypertrophy; proliferation of superficial synovial cells often with palisading; marked infiltration of chronic inflammatory cells (lymphocytes or plasma cells predominating) with tendency to form lymphoid nodules; deposition of compact fibrin either on surface or interstitially; foci of necrosis.

11. **Characteristic histologic changes in nodules** showing granulomatous foci with central zones of cell necrosis, surrounded by a palisade of proliferated

---

*It should be noted that these criteria were developed prior to the new classification of rheumatic diseases adopted by the ARA in 1963, in which ankylosing spondylitis, psoriatic arthritis, and arthritis associated with ulcerative colitis and regional enteritis are listed as distinct from rheumatoid arthritis (Blumberg B., et al. ARA nomenclature and classification of arthritis and rheumatism. *Arthritis Rheum.* 7:93–97, 1964).

†From M. W. Ropes, et al. Revision of diagnostic criteria for rheumatoid arthritis. *Pull. Rheum. Dis.* 9:175–176, 1958.

macrophages, and peripheral fibrosis and chronic inflammatory cell infiltration, predominantly perivascular.

B. Definite rheumatoid arthritis
This diagnosis requires five of the above criteria. In criteria 1 through 5 the joint signs or symptoms must be continuous for at least 6 weeks.

C. Probable rheumatoid arthritis
This diagnosis requires three of the above criteria. In at least one of criteria 1 through 5 the joint signs or symptoms must be continuous for at least 6 weeks.

D. Possible rheumatoid arthritis
This diagnosis requires two of the following criteria and total duration of joint symptoms must be at least 3 weeks.

1. **Morning stiffness.**

2. **Tenderness or pain on motion** (observed by a physician) with history of recurrence or persistence for three weeks.

3. History or observation of **joint swelling.**

4. **Subcutaneous nodules** (observed by a physician).

5. **Elevated sedimentation rate** or C-reactive protein.

6. **Iritis** (of dubious value as a criterion except in the case of juvenile rheumatoid arthritis).

E. Exclusions

1. **The typical rash of systemic lupus erythematosus** (with butterfly distribution, follicle plugging, and areas of atrophy).

2. **High concentration of lupus erythematosus cells** (four or more in two smears prepared from heparinized blood incubated not over 2 hours) or other clear-cut evidence of systemic lupus erythematosus.

3. **Histologic evidence of periarteritis nodosa** with segmental necrosis of arteries associated with nodular leukocytic infiltration extending perivascularly and tending to include many eosinophils.

4. **Weakness** of neck, trunk, and pharyngeal muscles or persistent muscle swelling or *dermatomyositis.*

5. **Definite scleroderma** (not limited to the fingers). (The latter is an arguable point.)

6. A clinical picture characteristic of **rheumatic fever** with migratory joint involvement and evidence of endocarditis, especially if accompanied by subcutaneous nodules or erythema marginatum or chorea. (An elevated antistreptolysin titer will not rule out the diagnosis of rheumatoid arthritis).

7. A clinical picture characteristic of **gouty arthritis** with acute attacks of swelling, redness, and pain in one or more joints, especially if relieved by colchicine.

8. **Tophi.**

9. A clinical picture characteristic of acute **infectious arthritis** of bacterial or viral origin with an acute focus of infection, or in close association with a disease of known infectious origin; chills; fever; and an acute joint involvement, usually migratory initially (especially if there are organisms in the joint fluid or response to antibiotic therapy).

10. **Tubercle bacilli** in the joints or histologic evidence of joint tuberculosis.

11. A clinical picture characteristic of **Reiter syndrome** with urethritis and conjunctivitis associated with acute joint involvement, usually migratory initially.

12. A clinical picture characteristic of the **shoulder-hand syndrome** with unilateral involvement of shoulder and hand, with diffuse swelling of the hand followed by atrophy and contractures.

13. A clinical picture characteristic of **hypertrophic osteoarthropathy** with clubbing of fingers or hypertrophic periostitis along the shafts of the long bones, or both, especially if an intrapulmonary lesion (or other appropriate underlying disorder) is present.

14. A clinical picture characteristic of **neuroarthropathy** with condensation and destruction of bones of involved joints and with associated neurologic findings.

15. **Homogentisic acid** in the urine, detectable grossly with alkalinization.

16. Histologic evidence of **sarcoid** or positive Kveim test.

17. **Multiple myeloma** as evidenced by marked increase in plasma cells in the bone marrow, or Bence-Jones protein in the urine.

18. Characteristic skin lesions of **erythema nodosum**.

19. **Leukemia** or **lymphoma** with characteristic cells in peripheral blood, bone marrow or tissues.

20. **Agammaglobulinemia.**

II. Jones criteria (revised) for guidance in the diagnosis of rheumatic fever*

A. Major manifestations†

1. **Rheumatic carditis** is almost always associated with a significant murmur. Consequently, the other manifestations listed below, when not associated with a significant murmur, should be labeled rheumatic carditis with caution.

   a. **Murmurs**

   1. In a patient without previous rheumatic fever or rheumatic heart disease, a significant apical systolic murmur, apical middiastolic murmur, or basal diastolic murmur.

   2. In a patient with previous rheumatic fever or rheumatic heart disease, a definite change in the character of any of these murmurs or the appearance of a new significant murmur.

   b. **Cardiomegaly.** Unequivocal cardiac enlargement in a patient without a history of previous rheumatic fever, or an obvious increase in cardiac size in a patient with a past history of rheumatic heart disease.

   c. **Pericarditis** is manifested by a friction rub, pericardial effusion or definite electrocardiographic evidence.

   d. **Congestive heart failure** in a child or young adult in the absence of other discernible causes.

2. **Polyarthritis** is almost always migratory and is manifested by swelling, heat, redness, and tenderness, or by pain and limitation of motion, of two or more joints. (Arthralgia alone, without other evidence of joint involvement, may occur in rheumatic fever, but is not considered a major manifestation.)

3. **Chorea.** Purposeless, involuntary, rapid movements often associated with muscle weakness are characteristic of chorea. These must be differentiated from tics, athetosis, and restlessness. Chorea is a delayed manifestation of

*From G. H. Stollerman, et al. Jones criteria (revised) for guidance in the diagnosis of rheumatic fever. *Circulation* 32:664–668, 1965.
†The presence of two major criteria, or of one major and two minor criteria, indicates a high probability of the presence of rheumatic fever. Evidence of a preceding streptococcal infection greatly strengthens the possibility of acute rheumatic fever. Its absence should make the diagnosis doubtful (except in Sydenham's chorea or long-standing carditis).

rheumatic fever, and other rheumatic manifestations may or may not be present. In the latter case, one should make the diagnosis of "rheumatic fever, chorea only."

4. **Erythema marginatum.** This evanescent, pink rash is characteristic of rheumatic fever. The erythematous areas often have pale centers and round or serpiginous margins. They vary greatly in size and occur mainly on the trunk and proximal part of the extremities, never on the face. The erythema is transient, migrates from place to place, and may be brought out by the application of heat. It is nonpruritic, not indurated, and blanches on pressure.

5. **Subcutaneous nodules.** These firm, nodules are seen or felt over the extensor surface of certain joints, particularly elbows, knees, and wrists, in the occipital region, or over the spinous processes of the thoracic and lumbar vertebrae. The skin overlying them moves freely and is not inflamed.

B. **Minor manifestations**

1. **Clinical.** These are other clinical features that occur frequently in rheumatic fever. Because they also occur in many other diseases, their diagnostic value is minor. Their usefulness consists in supporting the diagnosis of rheumatic fever when this diagnosis rests mainly on a single major manifestation.

   a. **History of previous rheumatic fever** or evidence of preexisting rheumatic heart disease increases the index of suspicion in evaluating any rheumatic complaint. The history must be well documented, or the evidence of preexisting rheumatic heart disease clear-cut.

   b. **Arthralgia** constitutes pain in one or more joints (not in the muscles and other periarticular tissues) without evidence of inflammation, tenderness to touch, or limitation of motion. The presence of arthralgia, in addition to polyarthritis, does not make the latter any more indicative of rheumatic fever, and should not be used for diagnosis when polyarthritis is a major manifestation. In the case of monoarthritis, however, arthralgia in other joints strengthens the diagnosis of rheumatic fever and can be used as a minor manifestation.

   c. **Fever** (temperature higher than 38°C rectally) is usually present early in the course of untreated rheumatic fever.

2. **Laboratory**

   a. **The acute phase reactions** offer objective but nonspecific confirmation of the presence of an inflammatory process. The erythrocyte sedimentation rate (ESR) and C-reactive protein (CRP) tests are most commonly employed. Unless the patient has received corticosteroids or salicylates, these tests are almost always abnormal in patients who present with polyarthritis or acute carditis, whereas they are often normal in patients presenting with chorea. The ESR may be markedly increased by anemia and may be decreased in congestive heart failure. The CRP is a sensitive indicator of inflammation and is negative in uncomplicated anemia. Heart failure, due to any cause, is often accompanied by a positive CRP test. Sera from normal individuals do not contain this protein, but relatively minor inflammatory stimuli may result in a positive reaction. Leukocytosis, anemia, or other nonspecific responses to inflammation may also occur in acute rheumatic fever.

   b. **Electrocardiographic changes,** mainly P-R interval prolongation, are frequent, but may occur in other inflammatory processes. Furthermore, electrocardiographic changes, whether or not associated with clinical evidence of carditis, have no bearing on the ultimate development of rheumatic heart disease. Such changes by themselves, therefore, do not constitute adequate criteria for carditis. The diagnosis of acute rheumatic fever should never be made solely on the basis of laboratory findings plus minor clinical manifestations. On the other hand, since laboratory indications of recent streptococcal infection and current inflammation occur so regularly with this disease, their unexplained absence should make the physician question the diagnosis of rheumatic fever.

C. Supporting evidence of streptococcal infection

1. **Laboratory** evidence of preceding streptococcal infection by specific antibody tests or by identification of the offending organism (positive throat culture) greatly strengthens the possibility of acute rheumatic fever. Clinical evidence of preceding streptococcal infection by a history of a recent attack of scarlet fever is the best clinical indication of antecedent streptococcal infection.

2. **Recent scarlet fever.**

III. Preliminary criteria for the classification of systemic lupus erythematosus*

The proposed criteria are based on 14 manifestations which include 21 items, as follows. For the purposes of classifying patients in clinical trials, population surveys and other such studies, a person shall be said to have systemic lupus erythematous (SLE) if any 4 or more of the following 14 manifestations are present, serially or simultaneously, during any interval of observation.

A. Manifestations

1. **Facial erythema** (butterfly rash). Diffuse erythema, flat or raised, over the malar eminence(s) or bridge of the nose, or both; may be unilateral.

2. **Discoid lupus.** Erythematous raised patches with adherent keratotic scaling and follicular plugging, atrophic scarring may occur in older lesions; may be present anywhere on the body.

3. **Raynaud phenomenon** requires a two-phase color reaction, by patient's history or physician's observation.

4. **Alopecia.** Rapid loss of large amount of the scalp hair, by patient's history or physician's observation.

5. **Photosensitivity.** Unusual skin reaction from exposure to sunlight, by patient's history or physician's observation.

6. **Oral or nasopharyngeal ulceration.**

7. **Arthritis without deformity.** One or more peripheral joints involved with any of the following in the absence of deformity: (1) pain on motion; (2) tenderness; (3) effusion or periarticular soft tissue swelling. (Peripheral joints are defined for this purpose as feet, ankles, knees, hips, shoulders, elbows, wrists, metacarpophalangeal, proximal interphalangeal, terminal interphalangeal, and temporomandibular joints.)

8. **LE cells.** Two or more classical LE cells seen on one occasion or one cell seen on two or more occasions, using an accepted published method.

9. **Chronic false-positive serologic test for syphilis.** Known to be present for at least 6 months and confirmed by *Treponema pallidum* immobilizing or Reiter's tests.

10. **Profuse proteinuria** (greater than 3.5 gm/day).

11. **Cellular casts.** May be red cell, hemoglobin, granular, tubular, or mixed.

12. One or both of the following: (1) **pleuritis,** convincing history of pleuritic pain; or rub heard by a physician; or roentgenographic evidence of both pleural thickening and fluid; (2) **pericarditis,** documented by ECG or rub.

---

*From A. S. Cohen, et al. Preliminary criteria for the classification of systemic lupus erythematosus. *Bull. Rheum. Dis.* 21:643–648, 1971.

13. One or both of the following: (1) **psychosis;** (2) **convulsions,** by patient's history or physician's observation in the absence of uremia and offending drugs.

14. One or more of the following: (1) **hemolytic anemia;** (2) **leukopenia,** white blood cell count less than 4,000/mm³ on 2 or more occasions; (3) thrombocytopenia, platelet count less than 100,000/mm³.

Current Proposed Revision of JRA Criteria*

I. General

The JRA Criteria committee has reviewed the initial criteria approved by the American Rheumatism Association in December 1971 and published in 1973. The committee determined that the criteria be revised at this time, the term *juvenile rheumatoid arthritis* be retained, and the disease should be classified into three onset subtypes (systemic, polyarticular, and pauciarticular). Confusion would result from attempts at this time to change the name to *juvenile chronic polyarthritis* and to create subclassifications. The term *Still disease,* while steeped in legitimate homage to Dr. George Frederick Still, has become a confusing term meaning different clinical patterns in different parts of the world and should not be used.

The purpose of a working classification is to allow clinicians everywhere to report experiences that can be readily categorized. A classification with appropriate subtypes allows uniform multicenter evaluation of patients with different manifestations. Clusters can then be identified with regard to prognosis or therapy.

The following classification enumerates requirements for a diagnosis of JRA and three clinical onset subtypes.

II. General criteria for JRA

Persistent arthritis of one or more joints for at least six weeks is sufficient for diagnosis if conditions listed under exclusions have been eliminated.

Arthritis is defined as swelling of a joint or limitation of motion with heat, pain, or tenderness. Pain or tenderness alone is not sufficient for the diagnosis of arthritis. Joints are counted individually with certain exceptions. The cervical spine is considered one joint. The carpal joints of each hand are counted as one joint as are tarsal joints on each foot. The metacarpophalangeal, metatarsophalangeal, proximal, distal, and interphalangeal joints will be counted individually.

III. JRA Onset subtypes

The onset subtype is determined by manifestations during the first 6 months of disease. Although manifestations more closely resembling another onset type appear later, the subtype that was present during the initial 6 months will remain the onset subtype.

A. **Systemic onset JRA.** This subtype is defined as JRA with persistent intermittent fever (daily intermittent temperature elevations to 103° F or more) with or without rheumatoid rash or other organ involvement. Typical fever and rash will be considered *probable* systemic onset JRA if not associated with arthritis. Before a definite diagnosis can be made, arthritis as defined must be present.

B. **Pauciarticular onset JRA.** This subtype is defined as JRA with arthritis in four or fewer joints. Patients with systemic onset JRA are excluded from this onset subtype.

C. **Polyarticular onset JRA.** This subtype is defined as JRA with arthritis in five or more joints. Patients with systemic JRA onset are excluded from this subtype.

D. **Other factors to be considered for purposes of continuing study.** The following factors may be important for better understanding and future classification.

*From E. J. Brewer, Jr., et al. Current proposed revision of JRA criteria. *Arthritis Rheum.* 20:195–199, 1977.

1. Rheumatoid factors
2. Antinuclear antibodies
3. Histocompatibility antigens
4. Sex
5. Age at onset
6. Iridocyclitis (chronic or acute)
7. Sacroiliitis
8. Number of affected joints
9. Distribution of affected joints
10. Family history of arthritis and related rheumatic manifestations
11. Responses to drug therapy
12. Immunologic abnormalities

IV. Definitions of certain manifestations

1. **Fever.** Any type of fever may be seen in JRA; however, a persistent intermittent fever with diurnal variation from normal to 103° F or greater is suggestive of systemic onset JRA if other diseases such as infection, malignancy, inflammatory bowel disease, and systemic lupus erythematosus are excluded.

2. **Rheumatoid rash.** Rheumatoid rash is an evanescent, pale erythematous, usually circumscribed, macular rash, with individual lesions varying in size from 2 to 10 mm. The larger lesions may have a pale center with peripheral pallor. The rash may become confluent and is found predominantly on the chest, axillae, thighs, and upper arms, and less commonly on the face and distal extremities. It occurs most frequently in patients with systemic onset disease and may occasionally precede arthritis and is occasionally pruritic.

3. **Iridocyclitis.** An anterior nongranulomatous iridocyclitis is most common in pauciarticular onset JRA patients. One or both eyes may be involved. Onset of iridocyclitis is characteristically insidious and initial physical findings may be difficult to detect. The earliest findings on slit lamp examination are cells or increased protein in the anterior chamber. Sequelae include posterior synechiae, band keratopathy, cataracts, secondary glaucoma, and phthisis bulbi. Iridocyclitis should be considered a serious complication that may lead to blindness. Frequent ophthalmologic examination should be performed to detect the lesions in the earliest stages.

4. **Cardiac involvement.** Pericarditis is not common and can be asymptomatic. It is most frequently associated with systemic onset JRA. Symptoms may include chest pain, dyspnea, and tachypnea. Signs include friction rub, tachycardia, and enlarged heart. ECG, echocardiograph, and chest x-ray may be helpful in diagnosis. Occasional patients may have myocarditis or valvular insufficiency.

5. **Rheumatoid nodules.** Rheumatoid nodules occur in a small percentage of patients with JRA. They are usually subcutaneous, vary in size up to several centimeters, and can generally be found in or about tendons of the hands, below the elbow, and around the Achilles tendon. A lesion sometimes known as a *pseudo-rheumatoid nodule* has been reported in children to have a pathological appearance indistinguishable from the adult type of rheumatoid nodules. In children these benign nodules usually appear on the anterior tibial surface or occiput.

6. **Stiffness.** Stiffness exists in the joints and muscles when they lack flexibility and ease of movement and is frequently observed after inactivity. It is ob-

served as a physical sign in young children but later also constitutes a symptom or complaint.

7. **Tenosynovitis.** Tenosynovitis may involve the sheaths of the finger extensors or flexors of the wrist as well as the posterior tibialis and peroneal tendons of the ankle. Arthritis of the adjacent joint is a frequent association.

8. **Arthritis of cervical spine.** Pain and limitation of motion of the cervical spine are frequent in systemic and polyarticular onset JRA, and less common in the pauciarticular onset JRA subtype. Clinical findings and the radiographic appearance frequently do not correlate well. Motion is usually limited in extension and lateral flexion and rotation rather than in forward flexion. Radiographic changes consist primarily of narrowing of the apophyseal joints with subsequent fusion. The C2–C3 apophyseal joint is most often involved with the other cervical vertebrae less frequently affected. Abnormalities of the vertebral bodies are much less frequent. When seen, they consist of decreased growth of the bodies and their intevertebral disks. An uncommon but potentially severe complication is subluxation of C1 on C2.

9. **Rheumatoid factors (RF).** Agglutination tests for RF are persistently positive in 5% to 20% of all JRA. Positive tests are more frequently found in older children with polyarticular onset disease. The presence of rheumatoid factor appears to correlate with a more chronic destructive arthritis.

10. **Antinuclear antibodies (ANA).** Fluorescent antibody tests for antinuclear antibodies are positive in 10% to 40% of children with polyarticular and pauciarticular onset JRA; the frequency depends somewhat upon the sensitivity of tests in individual laboratories. The majority of children with the chronic iridocyclitis of JRA have positive tests for antinuclear antibodies. Antinuclear antibodies are less commonly found in children with systemic onset JRA or with juvenile ankylosing spondylitis.

11. **Growth disturbances.** Growth disturbances occur in JRA patients as a consequence of the disease itself. Reduction of total growth can be severe. There may also be localized growth disturbances such as epiphyseal overgrowth at the knee or ankle, or undergrowth of the mandible. Resumption of growth can occur with remission. Prolonged corticosteroid therapy can also cause growth suppression.

12. **Anemia and leukocytosis.** Anemia and leukocytosis occur frequently in systemic onset JRA. Peripheral leuykocyte counts may be greatly elevated with predominance of early forms (left shift); anemia may sometimes be profound. Less pronounced leukocytosis and anemia may also be seen during periods of active disease in children with polyarticular JRA.

13. **Hepatosplenomegaly and lymphadenopathy.** Marked hepatosplenomegaly and generalized lymphadenopathy may occur in children with active systemic onset JRA. Mildly abnormal liver function tests may be associated with the disease or therapy. Less pronounced degrees of organomegaly and lymphadenopathy also occur at times with other onset types of JRA.

14. **Amyloidosis.** Amyloidosis as a complication of JRA is rarely reported in the United States. In some of the countries in Europe the incidence is said to be 4% to 6%. Amyloidosis may be a contributing factor in up to 50% of deaths in JRA patients reported in the European countries.

V. Exclusions

A. Other rheumatic diseases

1. Rheumatic fever

2. Systemic lupus erythematosus

3. Ankylosing spondylitis
4. Polymyositis and dermatomyositis
5. Vasculitis
   a. Anaphylactoid purpura (Henoch-Schönlein)
   b. Polyarteritis
   c. Serum sickness and other allergic reactions
   d. Mucocutaneous lymph node syndrome; infantile polyarteritis
   e. Other
6. Scleroderma
7. Psoriatic arthritis
8. Reiter syndrome
9. Sjögren syndrome
10. Mixed connective tissue disease
11. Behcet syndrome

B. Infectious arthritis
1. Bacterial arthritis (including tuberculosis)
2. Viral, fungal, and mycoplasmal arthritides
3. Nonbacterial arthritis associated with bacterial infections
4. Other

C. Inflammatory bowel disease

D. Neoplastic diseases including leukemia

E. Nonrheumatic conditions of bones and joints
1. Osteochrondritis
2. Toxic synovitis of the hip
3. Slipped capital femoral epiphysis
4. Trauma
   a. Battered child syndrome
   b. Fractures
   c. Joint, ligamentous, and muscular injuries
   d. Congenital indifference to pain
   e. Acute chondrolysis
5. Chondromalacia of the patella
6. Congenital anomalies and genetically determined abnormalities of musculo-skeletal system (including inborn errors of metabolism)
7. Idiopathic tenosynovitis

F. Hematologic diseases
1. Sickle cell anemia
2. Hemophilia

Table I-1. Classification of Scleroderma

1. Systemic sclerosis
   a. Classic disease with bilateral symmetrical diffuse involvement of the skin (scleroderma) affecting face, trunk, and proximal as well as distal portions of the extremities; associated with tendency toward relatively early appearance of visceral involvement
   b. With relatively limited involvement of skin, often confined to fingers and face, and tendency to long delayed appearance of visceral involvement (CREST syndrome)
   c. Overlap syndromes, including sclerodermatomyositis and mixed connective tissue disease
2. Localized (focal) forms of scleroderma
   a. Morphea (plaquelike, guttate, or generalized; subcutaneous and keloid morphea)
   b. Linear scleroderma
   c. Scleroderma *en coup de sabre*, with or without facial hemiatrophy
3. Chemical-induced sclerodermalike conditions
   a. Vinyl chloride disease
   b. Pentazocine-induced fibrosis
   c. Bleomycin-induced fibrosis
4. Eosinophilic fasciitis
5. Pseudoscleroderma
   a. Edematous (scleredema, scleromyxedema)
   b. Indurative (amyloid disease, porphyria cutanea tarda, carcinoid syndrome, phenylketonuria, acromegaly)
   c. Atrophic (progeria, Werner syndrome, lichen sclerosis et atrophicus)

Source: From Preliminary criteria for the classification of systemic sclerosis (scleroderma). *Bull. Rheum. Dis.* 31:1–6, 1981.

   G. Psychogenic arthralgia
   H. Miscellaneous
      1. Immunologic abnormalities
      2. Sarcoidosis
      3. Hypertrophic osteoarthropathy
      4. Villonodular synovitis
      5. Chronic active hepatitis
      6. Familial Mediterranean fever

Preliminary Criteria for the Classification of Systemic Sclerosis (Scleroderma)*

Systemic sclerosis (progressive systemic sclerosis, PSS, systemic scleroderma) is a disorder of the connective tissues characterized by induration and thickening of the skin (scleroderma), by abnormalities involving both the microvasculature and larger vessels (e.g., Raynaud phenomenon), and by fibrotic degenerative changes in muscles, joints, and viscera, most notably the esophagus, intestinal tract, heart, lungs, and kidneys. The disease must be differentiated from a variety of other conditions associated with similar cutaneous changes (Table I-1). Advanced systemic sclerosis with diffuse scleroderma and characteristic involvement of internal organs is unmistakable. However, the disease also

*From Preliminary criteria for the classification of systemic sclerosis (scleroderma). *Bull. Rheum. Dis.* 31:1–6, 1981.

Table I-2. Frequency of Promising Clinical Variables
Originally Considered for Criteria Analysis

Clinical Variables	Systemic Sclerosis Patients (%)			Comparison Patients (%)		
	Definite (n = 264)	Probable (n = 35)	Overlap (n = 85)	SLE (n = 172)	PM-DM (n = 120)	Raynaud Phenom- enon (n = 121)
Sclerodermatous skin changes						
Any location	98	74	75	1	3	9
Sclerodactyly*	96	74	71	1	3	9
Proximal scleroderma*	91	51	58	<1	0	0
Face or neck	79	21	41	0	0	0
Bilateral hand edema	70	76	70	24	24	28
Digital pitting scars (fingertip)*	49	43	38	9	7	15
Hand deformity or contractures	54	27	36	3	14	3
Abnormal skin pigmentation	56	29	35	21	13	8
Telangiectasia, fingers	47	26	32	8	10	8
Raynaud phenomenon	82	71	86	29	19	100

*Subsequently accepted criteria variable.
Source: From Preliminary criteria for the classification of systemic sclerosis (scleroderma). *Bull. Rheum. Dis.* 31:1–6, 1981.

exists in a form in which there is only limited skin change, often confined to the fingers and face. This latter variant is now generally known as the CREST syndrome (*C*alcinosis, *R*aynaud phenomenon, *E*sophageal dysfunction, *S*clerodactyly, and *T*elangiectasia). Also included in the spectrum of systemic sclerosis are patients in whom scleroderma and other changes typical of PSS coexist with manifestations of one or more of the other connective tissue diseases—the so-called overlap syndromes, such as mixed connective tissue disease (MCTD).

I. Design of the ARA scleroderma criteria cooperative study (SCCS)

A multicenter study was designed to gather detailed data on early-diagnosed cases of systemic sclerosis and comparison patients with certain selected rheumatic disorders. Physicians submitting cases from each of the participating centers were requested to group these into one of three categories: (1) definite, (2) probable or early stage, or (3) overlap syndrome. Comparison patients were entered from these centers with diagnoses of: (1) systemic lupus erythematosus (SLE), (2) polymyositis-dermatomyositis (PM-DM), and (3) Raynaud phenomenon, either primary or secondary (not associated with PSS or any of the comparison disorders). Patients with various forms of localized (focal) scleroderma were *excluded* from the study.

II. Results

A. Clinical features. Seven clinical variables were found to be significantly more frequent in the systemic sclerosis patients than in comparison patients (Table I-2). Interestingly, these variables all related to sclerodermatous skin changes, except for Raynaud phenomenon. Cutaneous scleroderma in any location was the most sensitive variable, but as many as 9% of the patients considered to have primary Raynaud phenomenon by center physicians also showed this change (sclerodactyly in all instances). The presence of *proximal scleroderma,* a term indicating bilateral and symmetric sclerodermatous changes in any area proximal to the metacarpophalangeal or metatarsophalangeal joints, was the most discriminating variable for systemic sclerosis, having been found in 239 (91%) of the definite systemic sclerosis cases but in only 1 (0.2%) comparison patient, a woman thought to have SLE.

B. Other findings. Digital tuft resorption and subcutaneous calcinosis, identified by clinical or roentgenographic examination (or both), were found in several-fold higher frequency among the systemic sclerosis patients than the comparison patients. Lower esophageal hypomotility detected by radiographic or manometric study was also found chiefly in the systemic sclerosis group. Colonic sacculations were confined to individuals with systemic sclerosis but occurred in relatively low frequency (17% of the definite cases). Bilateral basilar pulmonary fibrosis (determined by roentgenogram) was found in approximately one-quarter of the definite and overlap patients with systemic sclerosis and in a smaller proportion of patients with the comparison disorders.

The shin biopsy findings of dermal collagen thickening, condensation, or homogenization were the most sensitive of the laboratory features studied. These occurred in the highest frequency among the systemic sclerosis cases, but some of these changes were also found in 18% to 25% of the comparison patients studied.

C. Major criterion: proximal scleroderma. Because of its high specificity in separating systemic sclerosis from the comparison disorders, proximal scleroderma was selected as the single major criterion for systemic sclerosis. It was found in 91% of definite and in 51% of probable cases of this disease and in 58% of the cases of systemic sclerosis–overlap syndromes, as opposed to only 1 (0.2%) of 413 patients with comparison disorders (Table I-2). No other variable provided such powerful discrimination.

D. Minor criteria. Multivariate analytic techniques were applied to the remaining definite systemic sclerosis and comparison patients *without* proximal scleroderma, in order to select that combination of fewest items (minor criteria) which allowed the greatest discrimination. For simplicity, the "probable" and "overlap" systemic sclerosis patients were eliminated from these and subsequent analyses to derive criteria for early diagnosed, definite disease.

Many of the remaining "clinically promising" variables were redundant because they intercorrelated with one another or were rather nonspecific for systemic sclerosis.

Three additional variables in combination provided the most information and were selected as minor criteria: sclerodactyly, digital pitting scars of the finger tips or loss of distal finger pad substance, and bilateral basilar pulmonary fibrosis demonstrated by chest roentgenogram. An additional 17 (6%) definite and 4 (11%) probable systemic sclerosis patients satisfied at least 2 of these criteria as opposed to only 9 (2%) of the combined comparison patients (Table I-3).

E. Proposed classification criteria for definite systemic sclerosis. One major criterion or two or more minor criteria were found in 97% of the definite cases (97% sensitivity) but in only 2% of the comparison patients (98% specificity). This combination of variables constitutes the proposed preliminary classification criteria for systemic sclerosis:

1. Proximal scleroderma is the single major criterion with 91% sensitivity and greater than 99% specificity.

2. Sclerodactyly, digital pitting scars of finger tips or loss of substance of the finger pad, and bibasilar pulmonary fibrosis contribute further as minor criteria, in cases in which proximal scleroderma is absent.

3. One major or two or more minor criteria were found in 97% of patients with definite systemic sclerosis, but in only 2% of the comparison patients with SLE, PM-DM, or Raynaud phenomenon.

When the criteria were applied to patients grouped according to the original diagnoses of the participating centers (i.e., prior to any Subcommittee recommended revisions), the results were essentially identical (96% sensitivity and

Table I-3. Numbers of Patients Who Satisfied Major or Minor Criteria for Systemic Sclerosis

Criteria	Systemic Sclerosis Patients		Comparison Patients		
	Definite (n = 264)	Probable (n = 35)	SLE (n = 172)	PM-DM (n = 120)	Raynaud Phenomenon (n = 121)
Major criterion					
Proximal scleroderma	239	18	1	0	0
Minor criteria*	(25)	(17)	(171)	(120)	(121)
Sclerodactyly	19	8	1	4	11
Digital pitting scars	15	7	15	8	18
Bibasilar pulmonary fibrosis	8	1	11	22	3
2 or more minor criteria	17	4	0	3	6
Proposed criteria satisfied	256 (97%)	22 (63%)	1 (1%)	3 (3%)	6 (5%)

*Applies to the number of patients who did not satisfy the major criterion, as shown in parentheses.
Source: From Preliminary criteria for the classification of systemic sclerosis (scleroderma). *Bull. Rheum. Dis.* 31:1–6, 1981.

98% specificity). These criteria were tested with data stored in ARAMIS on over 1,300 systemic sclerosis and comparison patients and yielded 92% sensitivity and 96% specificity.

III. Discussion

A. Application of the classification criteria

The proposed classification criteria are not intended to apply to all forms of scleroderma, but only to systemic sclerosis.

Changes characteristic of scleroderma were reported in skin biopsies of a high proportion of the patients with systemic sclerosis. These included atrophy of dermal appendages, flattening of rete pegs, and thickening, condensation, and/or homogenization of dermal collagen. Some of these changes were also found, however, in approximately one-quarter of patients with the comparison disorders. More subtle histologic evaluation, including grading of the above noted abnormalities and attention to such features as the site of collagen deposition (localization and layer of the skin), small vessel alterations, and collections of lymphocytes might provide better discrimination of the sclerodermatous change. However, these measures are not as yet standardized.

When proximal scleroderma is absent, as was true in 9% of the definite cases of systemic sclerosis in this series, classification depends on a number of less discriminating minor criteria. Critical judgment must be exercised in applying the minor criteria in view of their greater variability in detection and alternate causes (e.g., the comparison disorders, frostbite, trauma, or unrelated chronic lung disease).

Raynaud phenomenon is important in the diagnosis of systemic sclerosis in the individual patient in view of its nearly uniform occurrence. However, this cold reactive state is also found in 20% to 30% of the other connective tissue diseases studied, and thus is nonspecific. Similarly, typical gastrointestinal disturbances are frequent in systemic sclerosis but may also be found in related disorders.

The presence of serum anti-RNP antibodies in very high titer was uncommon in definite and probable systemic sclerosis patients, but was found in 69% of individuals with systemic sclerosis in overlap. The latter were chiefly patients with clinical findings typical of MCTD. Recent research has revealed certain serum antibodies that appear to be highly specific for systemic sclerosis (e.g., anti-Scl 70, anti-centromere), and continuing investigation is likely to uncover the existence of still more antigen-antibody systems closely associated with this and other connective tissue disorders.

Index

Index